Veterinary Guide to Preventing Behavior
Problems in Dogs and Cats

Veterinary Guide to Preventing Behavior Problems in Dogs and Cats

Christine D. Calder, DVM, DACVB
Calder Veterinary Behavior Services
Waterboro, ME, USA

Sarah C. Wright, DVM
Catskill Veterinary Services, PLLC
Rock Hill, NY, USA

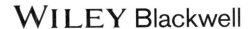
WILEY Blackwell

For general information on our other products and services or for technical support, please contact our Customer Care Department within the United States at (800) 762-2974, outside the United States at (317) 572-3993 or fax (317) 572-4002.

Wiley also publishes its books in a variety of electronic formats. Some content that appears in print may not be available in electronic formats. For more information about Wiley products, visit our web site at www.wiley.com.

Library of Congress Cataloging-in-Publication Data
Names: Calder, Christine, author. | Wright, Sarah C., author.
Title: Veterinary guide to preventing behavior problems in dogs and cats /
    Christine D. Calder, Sarah C. Wright.
Description: Hoboken, New Jersey : Wiley-Blackwell, [2025] | Includes
    bibliographical references and index.
Identifiers: LCCN 2024023164 (print) | LCCN 2024023165 (ebook) | ISBN
    9781119811756 (paperback) | ISBN 9781119811879 (adobe pdf) | ISBN
    9781119811886 (epub)
Subjects: MESH: Dogs–psychology | Behavior, Animal | Cats–psychology |
    Human-Animal Interaction | Veterinary Medicine–methods
Classification: LCC SF433 (print) | LCC SF433 (ebook) | NLM SF 433 | DDC
    636.7/0887–dc23/eng/20240703
LC record available at https://lccn.loc.gov/2024023164
LC ebook record available at https://lccn.loc.gov/2024023165

Cover Design: Wiley
Cover Images: © Christine D. Calder, © Sarah C. Wright

Set in 9.5/12.5pt STIXTwoText by Straive, Pondicherry, India

SKY10082091_081524

Dedication

This book is dedicated to my family, whose patience and understanding made this journey possible, enduring many dinners without my presence. To Roux, my patient companion, who provided silent support through countless late nights of writing, revising, and perfecting each chapter. A special dedication goes to Sarah, my co-author, whose invaluable contributions and unwavering dedication were crucial to bringing this project to fruition. Without her, the completion of this book would remain a question. My heartfelt thanks to each of you for your sacrifices, companionship, and invaluable support throughout this endeavor.

Christine D. Calder, DVM, DACVB

To my cat, Lucy Fur, a constant companion through vet school and beyond, the best educator in animal behavior I have known. To my dear friends, Jackie and Rebeca, for their unwavering support through countless French fries and endless ice cream. To Christine, for trusting me to join her in this project and for serving as a wonderful mentor in veterinary behavior. And last but certainly not least, to my family, for fostering my love of animals and encouraging me to pursue my passions. I am forever grateful.

Sarah C. Wright, DVM

Contents

Foreword

In the early days of my veterinary career I encountered a challenge that would shape my professional journey in ways I could never have anticipated. Fresh out of veterinary school, armed with knowledge on treating medical diseases but with little understanding of the complexities of animal behavior, I faced cases that left me feeling helpless. In my first year of practice as a brand new veterinarian, there was a Shepherd named Miller. From performing his first vaccinations to his neutering I witnessed his growth, only to be faced with the harrowing decision to euthanize him at just 18 months old due to him biting his caregiver. This moment, etched in my memory, propelled me toward becoming a board-certified veterinary behaviorist.

The path was not easy. Recognizing and addressing behavior problems in pets go beyond the scope of many veterinary curriculums. Veterinarians often find themselves ill-equipped to guide pet owners through the complexities of their pets' behavioral needs, unable to offer preventative advice or understand the nuances of animal body language and species-specific behaviors.

This book is born out of a deep-seated desire to bridge that gap, to empower general practice veterinarians with the knowledge and skills needed to strengthen the human–animal bond and manage these cases in their own practice. It is a culmination of years of learning and understanding and, most importantly, a tribute to the countless pets like Miller, whose stories have been cut short by lack of education and knowledge of preventative strategies. My hope is that this guide serves as a comprehensive resource for practicing veterinarians, offering insights into the whys and hows of their patients' behaviors. By equipping practitioners with this knowledge, we can aspire to create a world where animals have a chance to remain in their homes, fostering a deeper understanding of behavior, and avoid euthanasia. Let this book be your guide to enhancing the lives of your patients and fostering the important bond they share with their caregivers.

Christine D. Calder, DVM, DACVB

Looking back, the COVID-19 pandemic was a blessing in disguise. As a direct result, I had the opportunity to become deeply involved with the Behavior Service at Cornell University's College of Veterinary Medicine. I eagerly participated in virtual journal club discussions and led telehealth cases of my own after weeks of careful observation and study with none other than Dr. Katherine Houpt, a founding member of the American College of Veterinary Behaviorists. I was also able to first connect with Christine, and I learned a vast amount from our work together. These experiences allowed me to fall in love with veterinary behavioral medicine.

I was truly lucky to have had the chance to learn so much about behavior while in school. Without those extracurriculars, my knowledge and skill set would be only a fraction of what they are today, and they are very much still growing. In reflecting, I recognize areas for expansion in veterinary education, and I want to help realize that potential. This book is one step along the path to creating more widespread veterinary behavior resources. It is my hope that this text will inspire you to welcome the field of behavioral medicine into your practice, elevating the level of care that we provide as a profession.

Sarah C. Wright, DVM

Preface

Veterinary behavioral medicine is an emerging field that is rapidly gaining traction and recognition for its importance in promoting overall animal health and wellbeing. Behavior is not only a key indicator of pain and other disease states, often being the first thing that caregivers notice, it also substantially impacts an animal's quality of life and the human–animal bond. Indeed, behavior problems are some of the most common complaints presented to veterinary hospitals.

It is therefore the practitioner's responsibility to help clients prevent problematic behaviors from developing, as well as to promptly address those that arise, counseling clients to identify appropriate resources. Veterinary professionals are well positioned to help clients distinguish between training and emotional problems and to assist in selecting a suitable trainer when indicated. Client education also includes pre-adoption appointments, guidance on both general breed and individual animal selection, and information on setting up their new companions for success in a home environment. Through this, the human–animal bond is strengthened and preserved, decreasing the likelihood of relinquishment and euthanasia secondary to behavior problems.

Despite the acceptance of the vital nature of veterinary behavioral medicine, a significant number of veterinary colleges lack a robust behavioral education program, leaving the majority of graduates feeling underprepared to handle clients' concerns. Although it is imperative for veterinarians and other veterinary staff members to be equipped to address behavior questions and concerns, the profession as a whole does not yet possess the desired ability to serve as an authority in this field. Caregivers frequently turn to the internet, social media, and self-identified trainers as sources of information; however, these sources are often uncredible and unreliable, providing outdated or inaccurate information that may not only fail to help animals but also lead to worsened welfare states through exacerbated behavior problems.

In an effort to provide clinicians with resources to increase their knowledge in this field, this text delves into the world of veterinary behavioral medicine, with a focus on preventing problem behaviors from arising. To accomplish this, special attention is given to learning theory, animal body language, and normal puppy and kitten development. Furthermore, shelter animals and their unique needs are discussed; this is particularly important given the increase in popularity of shelter and rescue adoptions as sources of pets. Subsequent chapters address the veterinary clinic environment and ways to reduce the fear, anxiety, and stress associated with medical care.

As veterinarians grow their behavioral knowledge and skill set, they are better prepared to promote positive animal welfare, support the human–animal bond, and uphold the veterinary oath. Indeed, it is the veterinarian's lifelong obligation to continually improve, and veterinary behavioral medicine is an excellent area in which to fulfill that duty.

Acknowledgements

I Thank you Wiley for your support and patience throughout the creation of this book. Started during a pandemic, this journey, spanning almost four years, was met with its fair share of challenges, author, and job changes along the way. It was the addition of Sarah as a co-author that truly jumpstarted the momentum needed to cross the finish line. Her dedication and insight have been welcomed. I am thankful for her partnership and unwavering support during this challenging project. Without Sarah, the completion of this book would have remained an uncertain goal. Her contribution has been invaluable, and for that I am eternally grateful.

Christine D. Calder, DVM, DACVB

A sincere thank you to the Wiley staff and to Christine for inviting me to collaborate in the production of this book. It has been a wonderful challenge, and I am indebted to you all for your constant patience, encouragement, and mentorship. This text would not have been possible without each and every one of you.

Sarah C. Wright, DVM

1

Animal Behavior: A Key Element in Veterinary Medicine

Understanding animal behavior is important for veterinary professionals, as it helps them recognize abnormal behaviors that may be associated with medical issues including pain, dermatological conditions, gastrointestinal disorders, metabolic diseases, and neurological problems (Camps et al. 2019; Frank 2014; Mills et al. 2020; Seibert and Landsberg 2008; Stelow 2020). Despite the prevalence of behavioral problems in animals, with 85% of dogs and 61% of cats exhibiting such problems, there is a notable gap in veterinary education regarding behavior (Dinwoodie et al. 2019; Sherman and Serpell 2008; Strickler and Shull 2014). Surveys reveal that less than 43% of veterinarians feel they received adequate training in veterinary behavior during their education (Kogan et al. 2020). This lack of preparation is reflected in the fact that the majority of veterinary graduates do not feel ready to handle behavior cases from their first day in practice (Calder et al. 2017).

The availability of specialized training in veterinary behavior is limited, with Calder et al. (2017) noting that less than 40% of veterinary schools employ a Diplomate of the American College of Veterinary Behaviorists (DACVB). Additionally, Shivly et al. (2016) found that 27% of veterinary schools neither require nor offer an elective course in animal behavior. Even among schools that include behavior in their curriculum, 40% of students receive only four days or fewer of behavioral instruction (Calder et al. 2017).

This educational deficiency has considerable implications. Kogan et al. (2020) reported that over 99% of veterinarians encounter behavioral issues in their patients, even when behavior is not the primary concern. Additionally, there is a growing demand in the veterinary job market for graduates with knowledge of animal behavior, but client compliance with referrals to behavioral specialists is often limited by factors like cost and travel distance (Greenfield et al. 2004). This highlights the need for more accessible and comprehensive behavioral education within the general veterinary curriculum.

Some veterinarians may refer cases to various ways. Kogan et al. (2020) found that the majority handle most behavior cases themselves, with about 22% preferring to refer these cases to specialists. Surprisingly, a significant number of veterinarians do not routinely ask clients about behavioral issues, with only about 25% consistently inquiring about such problems (Kogan et al. 2020). Additionally, Patronek and Dodman (1999) found that 15% of veterinarians never inquire at all. Referring cases to trainers or nonveterinary behaviorists in other practices (Siracusa et al. 2017), as observed by Siracusa et al. (2017).

The importance of understanding animal behavior is further highlighted by the fact that over 78% of dogs show signs of fear, anxiety, and stress in veterinary settings, and about 38% of cat

Veterinary Guide to Preventing Behavior Problems in Dogs and Cats, First Edition. Christine D. Calder and Sarah C. Wright.
© 2025 John Wiley & Sons, Inc. Published 2025 by John Wiley & Sons, Inc.

caregivers find the thought of taking their cat to the veterinary hospital stressful (Döring et al. 2009; Volk et al. 2011). Thus, a comprehensive understanding of behavior is essential to manage and treat animals effectively, ensuring the safety and wellbeing of both staff and animals, as well as providing positive experiences for pets and their caregivers.

Proper behavior management is not only about safety but also about creating a positive and humane experience for the animals under care. Animals that are less stressed tend to respond better to treatment, leading to smoother and faster recoveries. This not only improves their interactions with caregivers but also enhances the overall veterinary care experience.

Behavior problems are a primary cause of euthanasia and surrendering of dogs and cats to shelters (Patronek and Dodman 1999; Salman et al. 2000; Scarlett et al. 2002; Seibert and Landsberg 2008). These problems strain the human–animal bond and can significantly impact the relationship between pets and their caregivers. Moreover, behavior problems can complicate a caregiver's ability to follow medical advice, perform treatments, or administer medications at home.

Prevention of Behavior Problems

Early education is critical in preventing behavior issues in pets. It is essential for prospective pet caregivers to receive guidance that helps them select pets compatible with their lifestyle. This involves understanding the specific needs, temperaments, and care requirements of different breeds or types of pets. Educating caregivers about the importance of prenatal care helps them choose pets with suitable temperaments and prepare for their arrival, thereby reducing the likelihood of future behavioral issues.

Role of the General Practitioner

Veterinarians play a key role in identifying changes in animal behavior, which can often be indicators of underlying health problems. It is critical to learn how to differentiate between normal and abnormal behaviors, which requires consideration of the context, frequency, duration, severity, and sequence of these behaviors. A comprehensive patient evaluation is necessary for an accurate diagnosis, which may include referrals to specialists when complex behavior conditions are suspected.

In emergency scenarios involving acute behavior changes, veterinarians should provide immediate guidance. This includes triaging the situation and advising pet caregivers how to manage these situations, emphasizing the avoidance of punishment and consideration of temporary boarding solutions, if needed, to prevent harm and allow for more objective decision-making (Martin et al. 2014). For nonemergency cases, scheduling ample appointment time is important to thoroughly understand the client's concerns (Martin et al. 2014). The initial step in managing these cases involves obtaining a detailed history of the pet's behavior, including when it started, how it has progressed, and what attempts have been made to address the issue, along with the outcomes of these attempts (Martin et al. 2014).

In situations where behavior problems in pets escalate suddenly, leading to an emergency or crisis, the general practitioner should offer immediate assistance. While behavior issues usually develop over time, acute changes can occur, potentially reaching a "breaking point" for caregivers and resulting in an urgent situation. In these cases, the general practitioner's role is to provide effective triage and assist caregivers in safely navigating the situation.

The practitioner should begin by validating the client's concerns and demonstrating empathy for their experience. Advise the client to avoid known triggers for the pet's behavior and all forms of punishment, both verbal and physical. In some instances temporary boarding might be beneficial, giving the client time to manage the situation more effectively and safely. Once the immediate safety of both the pet and the caregiver is assured, the practitioner should then facilitate a referral to a qualified behavior professional for specialized care and management. This approach ensures that caregivers receive the necessary support and guidance during critical behavior-related emergencies, helping to safely resolve the situation and pave the way for long-term behavioral management.

Common Behavior Problems

Behavior problems are common complaints in veterinary medicine that often indicate an underlying medical problem. These behavior changes are sometimes the first indication to caregivers that something is wrong with their pet. In determining whether a behavior problem has an underlying medical cause, a thorough differential diagnostic list and an in-depth medical workup is needed. A primary diagnosis of a behavioral condition is typically made by exclusion, meaning all potential medical differentials should be thoroughly assessed and eliminated before considering behavioral causes.

One of the most common complaints in both dogs and cats is aggression. Animals may exhibit aggression toward other animals, both familiar and unfamiliar, as well as toward people. It is important to note that aggression can be a normal behavior and does not always indicate an underlying medical or behavioral problem. However, because aggression is a nonspecific sign and can have various causes, the differential diagnosis list is extensive. Gathering a detailed history, including specifics of each aggressive incident, is important for appropriate management and treatment.

Fear, anxiety, and stress are commonly observed in veterinary patients. They occur both at the veterinary hospital and in environments away from the clinic. These problems can hinder access to medical care and often have significant impacts on the lives of both the animal and the client. The clinical signs associated with fear, anxiety, and stress can vary greatly between patients. Effective treatment and management depend on an accurate diagnosis. A complete workup and detailed history help ensure the diagnosis is specific and precise. Videos of the animal in their home environment and when alone are often invaluable and provide many additional details that the caregivers may be unable to offer.

House-soiling is another frequent complaint. This is more often brought up as a concern in cats, but it can occur in dogs as well. Again, a detailed history is highly valuable. This will help to distinguish toileting behavior from urine marking behavior and provides insights into the caregiver's management strategies. Are they appropriately providing for the animal's needs? Perhaps there is not an underlying medical or behavioral problem but rather an environmental issue that can be solved to alter the behavior.

Changes to a behavior pattern can occur at any age but are often noted with aging. Animals facing arthritis, pain, or cognitive decline can present with altered grooming, sleeping, eating, and vocalization behaviors, among others. Bloodwork, radiographs, urinalysis, and full neurologic and orthopedic examinations can provide critical insights into the underlying health of the patient and may reveal endocrine disease, urinary tract infections, seizure disorders, gastrointestinal disease, or musculoskeletal trauma; the differential diagnosis lists for underlying causes of these behavior pattern changes are extensive. Therefore, an exhaustive diagnostic screening panel is key to providing the proper treatment.

Behavior problems can manifest as new behaviors, loss of normal behaviors, or changes in the frequency of behaviors. Treating all underlying health problems is key to addressing medical components and may result in resolution of the behavioral signs. However, some cases are wholly or partially due to psychological causes; in these instances medical treatment alone will not be an effective treatment plan.

Conclusion

Understanding the common behavior complaints caregivers may mention and how to prevent them will help to build and protect the human–animal bond, thus maintaining a good quality of life for both the patient and the client.

References

Calder, C.D., Albright, J.D., and Koch, C. (2017). Evaluating graduating veterinary students' perception of preparedness in clinical veterinary behavior for "Day-1" of practice and the factors which influence that perception: a questionnaire-based survey. *Journal of Veterinary Behavior* 20: 116–120.

Camps, T., Amat, M., and Manteca, X. (2019). A review of medical conditions and behavioral problems in dogs and cats. *Animals* 9 (12): 1133.

Dinwoodie, I.R., Dwyer, B., Zottola, V. et al. (2019). Demographics and comorbidity of behavior problems in dogs. *Journal of Veterinary Behavior* 32: 62–71.

Döring, D., Roscher, A., Scheipl, F. et al. (2009). Fear-related behaviour of dogs in veterinary practice. *Veterinary Journal* 182 (1): 38–43.

Frank, D. (2014). Recognizing behavioral signs of pain and disease: a guide for practitioners. *Veterinary Clinics of North America, Small Animal Practice* 44: 507–524.

Greenfield, C.L., Johnson, A.L., and Schaeffer, D.J. (2004). Frequency of use of various procedures, skills, and areas of knowledge among veterinarians in private small animal exclusive or predominant practice and proficiency expected of new veterinary school graduates. *Journal of the American Veterinary Medical Association* 224 (11): 1780–1787.

Kogan, L.R., Hellyer, P.W., Rishniw, M., and Schoenfeld-Tacher, R. (2020). Veterinary behavior: assessment of veterinarians' training, experience, and comfort level with cases. *Journal of Veterinary Medical Education* 47 (2): 158–169.

Martin, K.M., Martin, D., and Shaw, J.K. (2014). Small animal behavioral triage: a guide for practitioners. *Veterinary Clinics of North America, Small Animal Practice* 44: 379–399.

Mills, D.S., Demontigny-Bédard, I., Gruen, M. et al. (2020). Pain and problem behavior in cats and dogs. *Animals* 10 (2): 318.

Patronek, G.J. and Dodman, N.H. (1999). Attitudes, procedures, and delivery of behavior services by veterinarians in small animal practice. *Journal of the American Veterinary Medical Association* 215 (11): 1606–1611.

Salman, M.D., Hutchison, J., Ruch-Gallie, R. et al. (2000). Behavioral reasons for relinquishment of dogs and cats to 12 shelters. *Journal of Applied Animal Welfare Science* 3 (2): 93–106.

Scarlett, J.M., Salman, M.D., New, J.G., and Kass, P.H. (2002). The role of veterinary practitioners in reducing dog and cat relinquishments and euthanasias. *Journal of the American Veterinary Medical Association* 220 (3): 306–311.

Seibert, L.M. and Landsberg, G. (2008). Diagnosis and management of patients presenting with behavior problems. *Veterinary Clinics of North America, Small Animal Practice* 38 (5): 937–950.

Sherman, B.L. and Serpell, J.A. (2008). Training veterinary students in animal behavior to preserve the human-animal bond. *Journal of Veterinary Medical Education* 35 (4): 498–502.

Shivley, C.B., Garry, F.B., Kogan, L.R., and Grandin, T. (2016). Survey of animal welfare, animal behavior, and animal ethics courses in the curricula of AVMA Council on Education-accredited veterinary colleges and schools. *Journal of the American Veterinary Medical Association* 248 (10): 1165–1170.

Siracusa, C., Provoost, L., and Reisner, I.R. (2017). Dog- and owner-related risk factors for consideration of euthanasia or rehoming before a referral behavioral consultation and for euthanizing or rehoming the dog after the consultation. *Journal of Veterinary Behavior* 22: 46–56.

Stelow, E. (2020). Behavior as an illness indicator. *Veterinary Clinics of North America, Small Animal Practice* 50: 695–706.

Strickler, B.L. and Shull, E.A. (2014). An owner survey of toys, activities, and behavior problems in indoor cats. *Journal of Veterinary Behavior* 9 (5): 207–214.

Volk, J.O., Felsted, K.O., Thomas, J.G., and Siren, C.W. (2011). Executive summary of the Bayer veterinary care usage study. *Journal of the American Veterinary Medical Association* 238 (10): 1275–1282.

2

Normal Behaviors and Body Language Interpretation

Communication in the animal world is diverse, involving vocalizations, scents, pheromones, and, most importantly, body language. Understanding animal body language is essential, particularly for humans, as it is a primary method animals use to express their emotional states. Veterinarians need to be especially attuned to even the most subtle of body language signals in order to provide humane care to their patients, as well as to help clients understand their pets in an effort to support the human–animal bond (Figure 2.1).

Animal behavior is a sequence of events (Frank 2013). Observing this entire sequence helps determine whether an animal's behavior is normal or indicative of a problem. For instance, in the context of canine aggression, this sequence might start with an initial warning such as growling or lip-lifting, indicating the initiation phase (Figure 2.2). This is typically followed by a pause, during which the dog has communicated their discomfort and is waiting for a response from the other party. In some cases the sequence may progress to a bite, representing the action phase. If a bite does occur, it often ends with an immediate voluntary release, concluding the sequence (Frank 2013).

However, when there are omissions or alterations in this behavioral sequence, it is often considered "abnormal" or indicative of an illness. For example, a dog that growls and bites simultaneously, without any prior warning, displays an altered sequence. The absence of a clear initiation phase in this instance suggests a deviation from normal behavioral patterns, which could be indicative of an underlying medical condition (Frank 2013). This principle applies not just to dogs but to other animal species as well. This understanding is important for veterinarians and pet caregivers alike in order for them to effectively manage and respond to animal behaviors appropriately.

Normal Dog Behavior

Understanding Body Language

Overall posture, tail position, and individual facial expressions are key components of a dog's body language. These elements collectively enable dogs to express a range of emotions with varying degrees, thereby adding depth and subtlety to how they communicate their emotional states (Figure 2.3).

Assertive/Aggressive (Distance-Increasing) Signals
Dogs displaying distance-increasing body language are often dogs that feel threatened; these dogs are not "mean" or "angry," and understanding their underlying emotional state is important (Frank 2013). These dogs are attempting to display signals that will prevent the threat, be it another

Veterinary Guide to Preventing Behavior Problems in Dogs and Cats, First Edition. Christine D. Calder and Sarah C. Wright.
© 2025 John Wiley & Sons, Inc. Published 2025 by John Wiley & Sons, Inc.

Figure 2.1 Yawning is considered a displacement behavior and an indicator of anxiety and stress. *Source:* Mary Swift/Adobe Stock Photos.

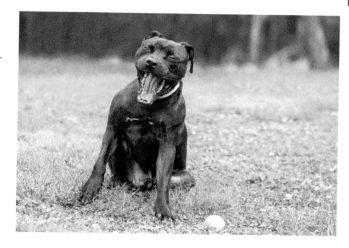

Figure 2.2 This dog is giving a warning growl. *Source:* Bonsales/Adobe Stock Photos.

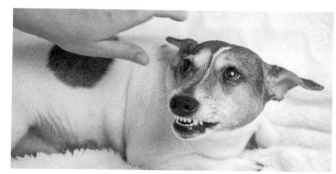

Figure 2.3 Example of whale eye (the whites of the eye are prominent). *Source:* Mary Swift/Adobe Stock Photos.

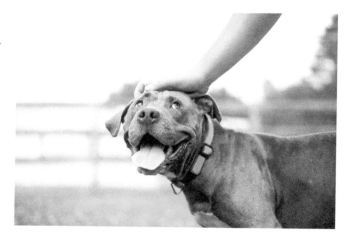

animal or a person, from continuing to approach and encourage them to back away or retreat (Figure 2.4). This type of body language typically begins subtly but increases as the signals are ignored and the threat persists. It is also important to note that dogs whose body language signs have been previously ignored or punished may start at a higher level of arousal with less subtle signs in future situations (Landsberg et al. 2013).

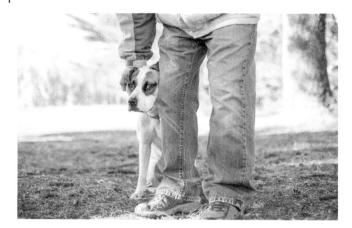

Figure 2.4 Dogs may back away or retreat when fearful or anxious. Ears may go back, mouth becomes tight, pupils dilate, and the whites of their eyes (whale eye) become prominent. *Source:* Mary Swift/Adobe Stock Photos.

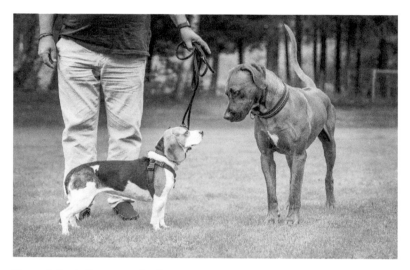

Figure 2.5 A direct stare is often the first distance-increase behavior a dog will display. *Source:* AstridAve/ Adobe Stock Photos.

One of the most subtle distance-increasing behaviors that dogs display is a direct stare (Figure 2.5) (Siniscalchi et al. 2018). This behavior can be easily overlooked by those not paying attention to mild changes in a dog's body language; awareness of these subtle signs can help prevent a situation from escalating.

Dogs whose stares have been ignored may progress in the behavioral sequence. Pulling the corners of the lips back and snarling can be the next stage. The snarl may start relatively subtly as well by involving only one side of the mouth or a very small portion of the lip (Figure 2.6). This change in facial expression may be accompanied by growling or barking. As the dog's behavior continues to escalate, they may lower their head, which can make them appear larger.

As the threat persists, the dog will shift their weight forward and stiffen their legs. They will also piloerect (raise) the hair over their tail, shoulders, and back, which indicates a state of high emotional arousal (Figure 2.7) (Siniscalchi et al. 2018). Throughout this sequence, the dog may hold their

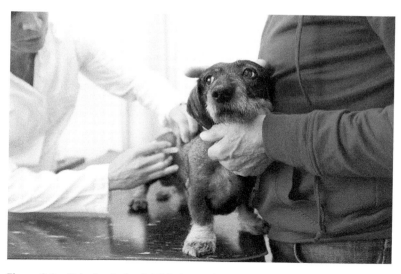

Figure 2.6 This dog is fearful. Whale eye is present, the brow is furrowed, the mouth tight. *Source:* Ivonne Wierink/Adobe Stock Photos.

Figure 2.7 Piloerection can start at the tail and indicates a state of high emotional arousal. *Source:* Wendy/Adobe Stock Photos.

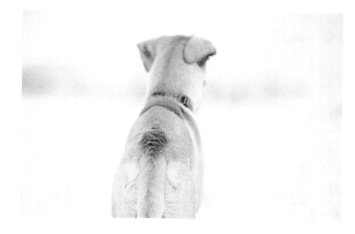

tail vertically and may move it in a slow and deliberate manner or display flagging behavior by moving their tail rapidly. Ultimately, the dog's behavior may progress to an inhibited bite (snap), which will eventually become a true bite with less inhibition if signals are still ignored (Landsberg et al. 2013).

Appeasement Signals and "Guilt"

Appeasement behaviors are displayed in an effort to diffuse tension and decrease a perceived threat. Dogs displaying appeasing signals are seeking to avoid conflict (Figure 2.8). Similar to distance-increasing signals, appeasement behaviors can range from very subtle to more overt postures. It is important to note that dogs whose appeasement behaviors have been ignored may begin to display aggressive body language.

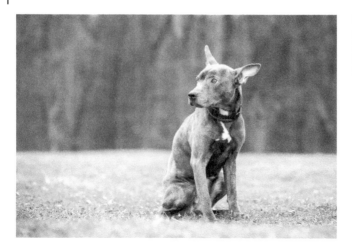

Figure 2.8 This dog is fearful, as evident by the worried look on the face, ears are back, mouth is tight, and body tense. *Source:* Mary Swift/Adobe Stock Photos.

Subtle Beginnings of Appeasement Appeasement behaviors typically start with the dog avoiding eye contact and looking away (Landsberg et al. 2013). The dog may move only their eyes or may turn their whole head and twist their neck to indicate their underlying emotional state more overtly. They may also lower their ear posture and increase the frequency of blinking (Figures 2.9 and 2.10) (Siniscalchi et al. 2018).

Progression of Appeasement Signals Dogs displaying appeasing signals may also lick their lips and yawn (Figure 2.11). They typically hold their tail low, sometimes even tucked between their back legs. The tail may wag slightly, but this behavior often ceases when the dog is touched as they enter "freeze" mode (Beaver 2009).

Extreme Fear Responses As appeasement behaviors progress, dogs may lower their body toward the ground and take up a crouched position. They may ultimately completely lay down and even roll over onto their backs, exposing their ventral abdomen (Figure 2.12) (Hargrave 2017a). Dogs may also urinate as their appeasement behaviors continue. When dogs roll over in order to express appeasement, this can be a sign of fear and conflict.

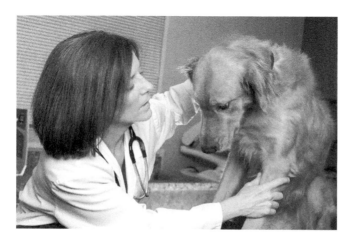

Figure 2.9 Avoiding eye contact, lowering of the head, looking away, lowered ear posture, and tight mouth are all signs of emotional discomfort or stress. This dog is uncomfortable with this interaction. *Source:* donnacoleman/Adobe Stock Photos.

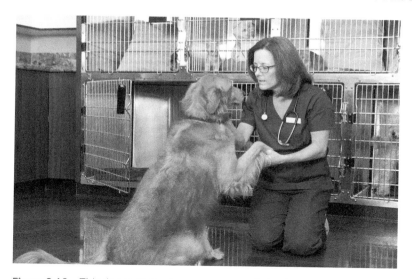

Figure 2.10 This dog is displaying appeasement behavior, ears are back, mouth is tight with a direct stare. This dog is not comfortable with this interaction. *Source:* donnacoleman/Adobe Stock Photos.

Figure 2.11 Dogs may lick their lips and nose as a sign of anxiety. *Source:* Firn/Adobe Stock Photos.

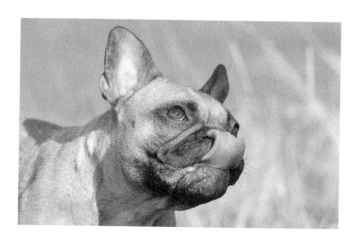

Figure 2.12 When fearful, dogs may lower their body toward the ground in a crouched position with their tail tucked between their legs. *Source:* sue/Adobe Stock Photos.

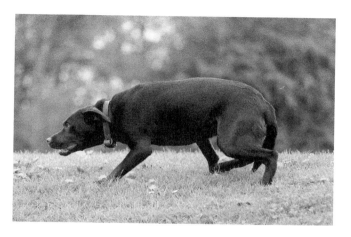

Misinterpretation as "Guilt" Many caregivers will misidentify appeasement behaviors as "guilt" (Figure 2.13) (Hecht et al. 2012; Konok et al. 2015; Pickersgill et al. 2023). However, dogs may not necessarily understand the concept of wrongdoing or why a person is upset (Martens et al. 2016). Instead, these behaviors often result from the dog sensing a potential threat from a person's body language. The dog then displays a range of appeasement behaviors, sometimes even rolling over onto their back, in an effort to avoid or diffuse any aggressive response from humans.

Conflict Behaviors

Conflict behaviors in dogs arise from a state of internal conflict, where the dog experiences opposing desires or motivations. A common example is a dog greeting a visitor: in this case the dog may want to interact with the new person but simultaneously be feeling fearful of them. These conflicting motivations can lead to significant stress and anxiety in the dog, which are evident in their body language and behavior.

Misinterpretation of Behaviors A classic example of misinterpretation is when a dog rolls onto their back. Not all instances of this behavior are solicitations for attention. It could be an invitation for a belly rub, but it could also be a sign of extreme conflict or uncertainty. In situations where the dog shows a direct stare, tight mouth, ears back, tail tucked, and stiff legs, which are indications of distance-increasing behaviors and signal discomfort, it is best to avoid an interaction. Instead, walk a few steps away and call the dog. This helps to determine their true motivational state and whether they are soliciting attention or asking for attention to stop (Figure 2.14).

Mixed Postures Due to Emotional Discomfort Conflict behaviors often manifest as a mixture of postures, reflecting a dog's emotional discomfort in a given situation. Typically, these dogs are experiencing anxiety or frustration. They may have learned that their subtle warning signs, such as avoiding eye contact, leaning away, or even growling, are routinely ignored or in some cases punished (Figure 2.15). This can lead to an escalation in behavior. For these dogs, aggressive signals can become the default behavior once they learn that they are effective in stopping uncomfortable situations. While punishment may suppress these signals, it does not address their underlying cause. Furthermore, punishment can result in the loss of early warning signs, potentially leading to an escalation in aggression with little to no warning.

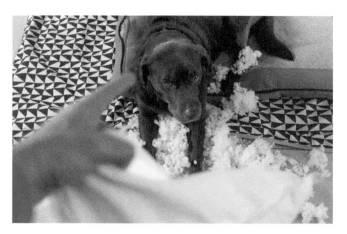

Figure 2.13 Guilt is often misunderstood. Often the body language observed is not guilt but rather fear and anxiety, such as the dog in this picture (ears back, avoiding direct eye contact, dilated pupils, closed and tight mouth). *Source:* Rawlstock/Adobe Stock Photos.

Figure 2.14 Not all dogs that roll on their back are soliciting attention. In this photo the dog has a direct stare, tight mouth, ears are back, tail is tucked, and legs are stiff, all indicating distance-increasing behaviors. *Source:* Алексей Игнатов/ Adobe Stock Photos.

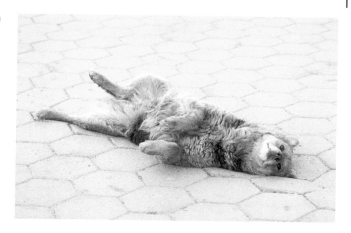

Figure 2.15 This dog is conflicted, as evidenced by him looking away with his ears back and open mouth in a pant. *Source:* Hanna/Adobe Stock Photos.

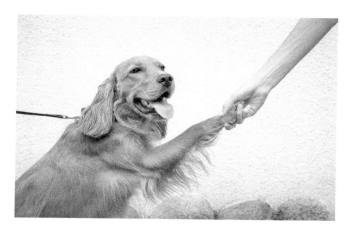

Simultaneous or Alternating Behaviors   Dogs in a state of conflict may display a combination of aggressive and appeasing behaviors at the same time. For example, a dog might tuck their tail while leaning forward, or alternate between appeasing signals like lip-licking and yawning and more aggressive behaviors such as growling. Some will display a grin (retract lips and display incisors). This alternating or simultaneous display of behaviors is indicative of the dog's internal conflict and emotional discomfort (Landsberg et al. 2013).

Display of Displacement Behaviors   Dogs experiencing conflicting emotions may also engage in displacement behaviors, which are essentially stress-relieving actions. These can include spinning in circles, shaking their heads, or other repetitive actions that do not seem to have a clear purpose in the context of the situation (Table 2.1).

Solicitous (Distance-Decreasing) Signals

Solicitous behaviors are invitations to interact and play and communicate that the dog is happy and comfortable in the environment. These dogs will have a relaxed face (Figure 2.18) and loose

Table 2.1 Signs of stress in dogs.

Appears tired or disinterested	Piloerection (raised hackles)
Barking	Raised paw (foreleg)
Biting	Rolling over
Biting/chewing on leash or caregiver's hands/clothing	Scratching at neck
Blinking	Shaking/trembling
Closing eyes	Shedding
Crouching	Showing whites of eyes (whale eye)
Ears back and/or flattened	Sitting close to caregiver
Easily startled, ears twitching as if listening	Slow deliberate movements/moving in slow motion
Excessive salivation	Snapping
Full body shake	Sniffing ground
Furrowed brow	Staring
Growling	Stiff body/muscle tension
Hypervigilant (scanning and trouble settling)	Sweaty paws
Ignoring familiar cues	Tail tucked
Involuntary urination or defecation	Tail carried high with tight wag
Lip/nose-licking	Tight mouth
Lunging	Turning body away
Lying down	Turning head away
Mounting behavior	Urine marking
Moving away, avoiding contact with hands	Walking away
Not eating/refusal of food or snatching treats	Yawning
Pawing	

Source: Adapted from Hargrave (2015).

body posture. During appropriate play, dogs may offer a play bow, lowering onto their forearms while elevating their tail, (Figures 2.16) (Beaver 2009) take turns, and use good bite inhibition (Siniscalchi et al. 2018). It is important to monitor dogs closely during play to ensure that the situation is not escalating and that all dogs are still enjoying the interaction.

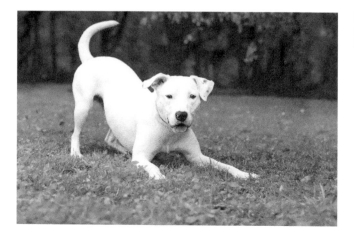

Figure 2.16 A play bow is often a distance-decreasing behavior.
Source: Mary Swift/Adobe Stock Photos.

Figure 2.17 This dog is comfortable with a "belly rub," as indicated by the almond-shaped eyes, relaxed face, and tongue position (hanging loose out of the side of the mouth). *Source:* Mary Swift/Adobe Stock Photos.

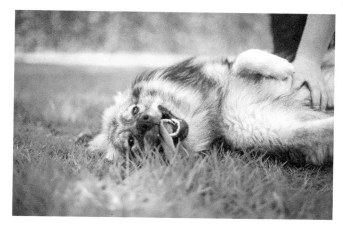

Figure 2.18 This dog is relaxed and engaged, as evidenced by the relaxed face, almond-shaped, soft eyes, and tongue out to the side. *Source:* Mary Swift/Adobe Stock Photos.

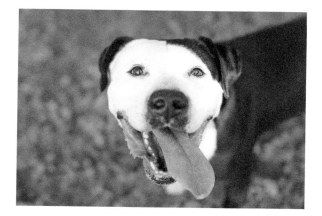

Domestication and Its Effect on Behavior

Domestication has had a substantial impact on dog behavior (Fuller and Fox 1969). In many ways, domestication has made it easier for humans and dogs to communicate with each other (Driscoll et al. 2009; Feuerstein and Terkel 2008). However, there are also several challenges that have resulted.

Domestication has brought numerous benefits to the human–dog relationship. Dogs have developed a remarkable ability to understand human social cues and can learn by observing human actions (Udell et al. 2010). Compared to wolves, dogs generally show less aggression and avoidance behavior toward people (Lazzaroni et al. 2020). Instead, they exhibit a preference for human contact and often look to humans for assistance in challenging situations (Marshall-Pescini et al. 2017). Dogs are more inclined to depend on people in dangerous scenarios and tend to form bonds with their caregivers that can easily extend to other humans. They exhibit less fear toward people and are genetically predisposed to increased sociability (Lazzaroni et al. 2020). This shift includes changes in the hypothalamic–pituitary–adrenocortical axis, which affects their stress responses. Additionally, the presence of the levator anguli oculi medialis muscle in dogs (absent in wolves) allows them to significantly raise their inner eyebrows, enhancing communication with humans (Figure 2.19) (Kaminski et al. 2019).

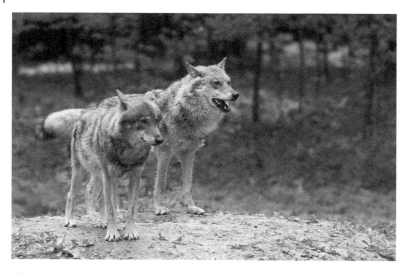

Figure 2.19 Although dogs share similar genetics to wolves, they are a different species of animal. *Source:* diartemisss/Adobe Stock Photos.

The Role of Breed in Interpretation

When considering a dog's body language, it is important to account for the dog's breed, as selective breeding has further modified physical traits (Wheat et al. 2019). For instance, brachycephalic breeds have a reduced ability to display a full range of facial expressions due to their unique physical structure. Some breeds, like the French Bulldog and Welsh Corgi, have been bred to have short tails, which limits their ability to communicate using tail position and movement. Additionally, breeds like the Spanish Water Dog and Rhodesian Ridgeback have distinctive hair coats that affect their communication abilities. These coats can impact their use of piloerection (hair standing on end) in communication and may obscure facial features. These breed-specific differences not only affect the dog's ability to perform body language signals, but they also make it more challenging for other dogs and people to accurately interpret these visual communication cues.

Social Behavior

Dogs are inherently social creatures, capable of recognizing their kind even after prolonged periods of separation (Hepper 1994). Free-roaming dogs often form social groups, though the concept of "dominance" as commonly perceived is a misconception of their social interactions. Rather than rigid hierarchies maintained by aggression, social structures among dogs are typically established through displays of appeasement and affiliative behaviors that foster group cohesion (Bradshaw et al. 2009; Bradshaw and Rooney 2016).

In any given situation, a dog's behavior is influenced by various factors, including the value they place on a resource they wish to control and their past experiences. For instance, a dog that has repeatedly experienced fear-based aggression may start to show fewer appeasement signals over time if those signals have been consistently ignored. Dogs also assess and interpret the behaviors of other dogs, making judgments about whether a situation will likely be resolved through escalation or appeasement. Interestingly, the relative sizes of the dogs involved do not appear to significantly influence these interactions (Bradshaw and Lea 1993).

Dogs also make use of a variety of vocal communications, including barks, whines, and growls. The specific acoustic profiles of each vary with the context (Yin and McCowen 2004). For example, barks are typically low-frequency sounds when directed toward a stranger but high-frequency and more musical when performed during play. As another example, a growl emitted during play has a different sound quality than a growl emitted during guarding behavior (Farago et al. 2010). Further, dogs attune to and respond to the vocalizations of other dogs in a context-dependent manner as well (Farago et al. 2010; Yin and McCowen 2004).

In fact, dogs use vocal communication as well as visual signals to initiate and maintain play. Play behaviors are usually behaviors that are also exhibited in other situations; for example, play behaviors often encompass behaviors performed while hunting or mating. However, there are major differences in the nuance and specifics between the different contexts. For example, biting during play is typically inhibited and does not lead to injury, whereas biting during a fight or hunt is often uninhibited and meant to injure.

Throughout play, dogs pay attention to the communication signals of their playmates to ensure behaviors are properly interpreted (Feuerstein and Terkel 2008).

Reproductive Behavior

Differences from Wolf Pack Structures
In contrast to wolf packs, which are family units with both paternal care and parental assistance in raising offspring, dogs, especially in feral conditions, do not form family groups. This represents a significant behavioral shift resulting from domestication and adaptation to different living environments (Pal et al. 1999). Feral dog colonies typically consist of a small group of adults, usually between five and ten individuals, along with their dependent offspring (Pal 2011). These colonies differ markedly from the structured family units observed in wolf packs, illustrating a distinct approach to social organization in dogs.

Mating Behaviors
Female domesticated dogs enter estrus annually and often mate with multiple males, most of whom are from outside their immediate social group (Pal 2011). This practice contrasts with the mating behaviors seen in wolves, where reproduction is often exclusive to the alpha pair. There are instances of seasonal monogamy in dogs, with males sometimes guarding litters for the first six to eight weeks after whelping (Pal 2005). However, unlike in wolves, the paternal role in dogs typically does not extend to long-term care of the offspring. After whelping, female dogs often separate themselves from their group for a few weeks and may display aggression toward other group members. This withdrawal is a unique aspect of canine reproductive behavior not typically observed in wolf packs.

Social Hierarchy and Reproductive Success
Unlike wolf packs, where the dominant pair usually controls reproductive rights, social hierarchies within feral dog groups do not dictate reproductive success (Bradshaw et al. 2009; Bradshaw and Rooney 2016). This highlights a significant difference in the social dynamics governing reproduction between dogs and their wolf ancestors (Table 2.2) (Pal et al. 1999).

Table 2.2 Difference in wolf vs. feral dog reproductive and social behavior.

	Wolf packs	Feral dog colonies
Structure	Family units with paternal care and paternal assistance in raising offspring	Small groups of adults (5–10 individuals) with dependent offspring, not forming family groups
Mating behaviors	Reproduction often exclusive to the alpha pair	Females enter estrus annually and mate with multiple males, usually from outside their immediate social group
Seasonal monogamy and paternal care	Strong paternal involvement in offspring care	Males may guard litters for six to eight weeks post whelping, but long-term paternal care is rare
Post-whelping behavior of females	Integrated within the pack structure	Females often isolate from the group and may exhibit aggression toward other group members
Social hierarchy and reproductive success	The alpha pair usually controls reproductive rights	Social hierarchy does not dictate reproductive success, indicating a more open reproductive system

Ingestive Behavior

Suckling

Suckling is the initial ingestive behavior in dogs, occurring within hours of birth. The process of successful nursing involves coordinated behaviors from both the mother (bitch) and her neonates (puppies). Any issues with either party can lead to inadequate milk intake, poor nutrition and growth in the puppies, and potentially fatal consequences due to failure to thrive.

Neonatal Suckling Process Neonates must locate and latch onto a nipple and then perform effective suction to nurse properly (Figure 2.20). Puppies are naturally inclined to suckle reflexively on any soft, protruding surface, which may sometimes result in attempts to nurse on inappropriate objects (James 1957). Over time, puppies generally become more proficient at nursing (Lezama-Garcia et al. 2019). Additionally, neonatal puppies exhibit rhythmic kneading movements with their forelimbs during suckling, a behavior that typically stops around 17 days of age.

The Mother's Role in Nursing The mother plays an important role in the nursing success of her litter. She must allow her puppies to nurse and is responsible for initiating nursing sessions for about the first 30 days post whelping (Lezama-Garcia et al. 2019). She stimulates her puppies by nudging and licking them, lies down to expose her mammary glands, and ensures that the puppies are latched on correctly, often licking them while they feed (Ferrell 1984). As the puppies grow older, the mother gradually becomes less tolerant of nursing, reducing the duration of nursing sessions, and she may show aggression toward puppies that attempt to nurse frequently (Fuller and Fox 1969; Markwell and Thorne 1987). The weaning process starts around 7–10 weeks of age, during which the puppies transition from nursing to eating solid food entirely (Fuller and Fox 1969; Malm and Jensen 1993).

Figure 2.20 Suckling behavior is reflexive in neonates.

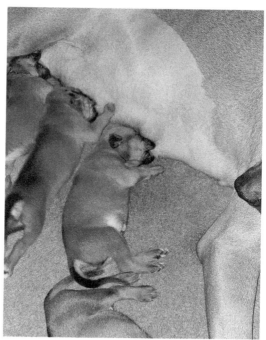

Adult Ingestive Patterns

Adult dogs often consume more calories than necessary for their maintenance (Boulcott 1967; Fuller and Fox 1969; James and McCay 1950). This tendency is partly attributed to being overfed by their caregivers. Additionally, an ancestral survival instinct drives them to eat readily available food to prepare for potential scarcity, contributing to this pattern of overeating (Bradshaw 2006; Fuller and Fox 1969). Dogs that are free fed, meaning they have continuous access to food, usually consume multiple small meals throughout the day (Boulcott 1967; Rashotte et al. 1984).

Eating Frequency and Social Housing   Dogs housed in groups eat more frequently compared to those housed individually (Houpt 1991; Houpt and Hintz 1978a). This could be due to social facilitation or competition for resources. However, many pet caregivers opt for controlled feeding schedules, offering food to their dogs at set mealtimes. This schedule of feeding can facilitate the housetraining process but may not be ideal for all dogs.

Food Preferences   While individual preferences can vary, dogs generally show a greater preference for meat over high-protein nonmeat foods (Houpt 1991; Houpt and Hintz 1978b). They also tend to favor canned food over dry kibble (Houpt 1991). This preference is influenced by their sense of smell, as dogs typically prefer warm food, which has a stronger aroma, to cold food (Houpt and Hintz 1978b).

Nonnutritional Chewing in Puppies and Dogs

Puppies and dogs regularly explore their environments with a variety of oral behaviors, including licking, chewing, tugging, and swallowing objects (Houpt 1991). Although certain breeds may be predisposed to display these mouthing behaviors, any dog can perform them. Therefore, careful observation of young puppies and redirection to appropriate chew toys are vital to ensure these types of exploratory behaviors do not become problematic.

Coprophagy

The ingestion of feces is a natural behavior in puppies. It may help to establish the normal gastrointestinal flora (Amtsberg et al. 1978). Some puppies display this behavior as part of their typical environmental exploration. Although coprophagy is normal, caregivers often perceive this behavior negatively and should be encouraged to redirect their puppy to appropriate chew toys or other activities. This behavior can be prevented by maintaining clean environments and regularly cleaning up feces in the yard. Regular deworming of all dogs in the household helps prevent the transmission of gastrointestinal parasites through coprophagy.

Plant Ingestion

Plant ingestion is a normal behavior in dogs (Beaver 2009). It is not necessarily associated with diet, gastrointestinal parasites, or behavioral problems (Sueda et al. 2005). Instead, it relates to the behavior of wolves, who often eat the viscera of herbivorous prey, which contain plant material (Beaver 2009). Because dogs are unable to properly digest cellulose, large amounts of plant material can cause gastrointestinal irritation, resulting in vomiting (Beaver 1981). Thus, some dogs learn to associate plant consumption with vomiting, and they may seek out grass or other plants when they have underlying gastrointestinal disease (Beaver 1981).

Water Consumption

Water consumption depends on a variety of factors. Body size, moisture content in food, and environmental temperature all play a role (Rashotte et al. 1984). Ultimately, body systems that regulate water balance drive water consumption. With over 70% of a dog's body made up of water, they should drink approximately one fluid ounce of water per pound of bodyweight per day, with dogs who are active or living in a hot climate drinking more.

Elimination Behavior

Neonates are born unable to eliminate on their own and therefore require stimulation from the bitch licking the perineal region to urinate and defecate. By 2–3 weeks of age puppies begin to eliminate on their own, without stimulation (Bleicher 1962). Despite this, the mother may continue to lick the perineal regions of her offspring for a few more weeks (Voith and Borchelt 1985).

As puppies age, their elimination habits change. Preferences for where they eliminate, including specific locations, substrates, and surfaces, (Voith and Borchelt 1985) and the posture they use for both urination and defecation develop (Voith and Borchelt 1985). Driven by an increase in testosterone levels as they reach sexual maturity, Male puppies typically progress from squatting to leaning forward to lifting their legs and rotating their bodies (Berg 1944; Hart 1974). Conversely, female puppies maintain a squatting position into adulthood that progressively deepens with age.

Urine marking is a normal behavior displayed by both males and females (Figure 2.21). This behavior is intended to bring attention to a certain location and provide individual identification (Voith and Borchelt 1985). Urine marking can also trigger sexual stimulation, such as when an intact male dog investigates the urine left by a female in estrus (Hart 1974).

Figure 2.21 Urine marking in a dog can be a normal behavior or a sign of anxiety. *Source:* ThamKC/Adobe Stock Photos.

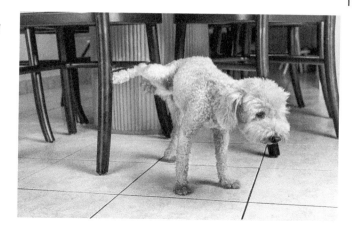

Normal Cat Behavior

Understanding Body Language

Similar to dogs, cat body language encompasses not only posture and stance but subtle changes to the face, ears, and tail (Figure 2.22). The degree of change contributes to the range of emotion that cats are able to portray through body language.

Aggressive (Distance-Increasing) Signals

Cats use a pattern of escalating behavior to communicate their desire to increase the distance from a perceived threat; often their aggressive behavior is fear based. It is important to understand the cat's underlying emotional state in order to correctly interpret their body language (Figure 2.23). In the same way that dogs may start with more overt signals when previous subtle ones have been ignored, cats may also immediately use higher arousal behaviors based on past experiences (Heath 2018).

In general, cats have a natural inclination to steer clear of direct conflict. To achieve this, they exhibit a range of signals and behaviors aimed at avoiding confrontation (Figure 2.24). Among the

Figure 2.22 Cats will maintain a sternal position, tuck in their legs, and wrap their tail when painful or stressed. *Source:* Mary Swift/ Adobe Stock Photos.

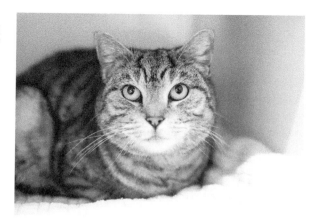

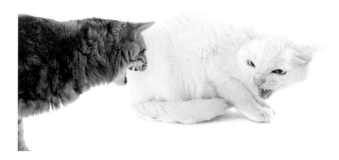

Figure 2.23 The brown tabby cat is showing more offensive behaviors (direct stare, ears forward, body leaning forward), whereas the white cat is more defensive (crouched, tail wrapped around body, ears to the side, pupils dilated). *Source:* cynoclub/Adobe Stock Photos.

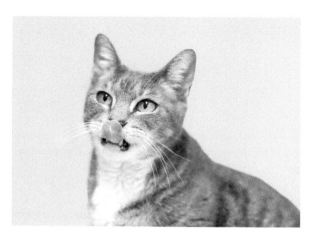

Figure 2.24 Cats will lick their lips when anxious or fearful. *Source:* Mary Swift/Adobe Stock Photos.

most subtle signs of avoidance in cats are diverting their gaze to avoid direct eye contact, turning their head away, and orienting their body in a direction away from the perceived threat (Hargrave 2017b). Additionally, cats may physically relocate to create more distance between themselves and any potential threat. The extent of space a cat requires to feel secure can vary widely, depending on both the specific situation and the individual temperament of the cat. These avoidance tactics are a key aspect of feline behavior, reflecting their preference for nonconfrontational solutions in potentially threatening scenarios.

If passive measures for increasing distance are ineffective, or if cats are unable to achieve their goal through these methods, they resort to more direct and evident signs of discomfort or agitation (Seksel 2014). There is still a range in the intensity of these behaviors, beginning with subtle changes and escalating as needed.

The subtler signs include alterations in facial expression (Holden et al. 2014). For instance, cats may turn their ears back and their pupils may dilate significantly. A direct, intense stare is another indicator of increasing discomfort. Tail position and movement also convey their emotional state; a cat may hold their tail down, either straight or with a hook at the end, and may start thrashing or slapping their tail as a sign of heightened arousal (Ellis 2022).

In states of high arousal, cats exhibit piloerection, where their fur stands on end (Figure 2.25). This is often accompanied by a defensive posture where the cat stands with an arched back and head lowered, leaning forward slightly with tensed muscles (Kolb and Nonneman 1975). These more direct signs indicate that the cat is feeling threatened and is prepared to take more assertive

Figure 2.25 Tail is down and to the side with piloerection along the spine (topline) and tail. *Source:* Kira/Adobe Stock Photos.

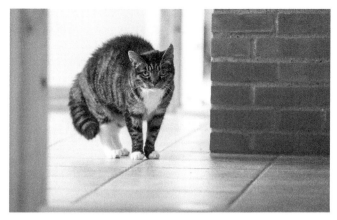

action if necessary. Understanding and responding appropriately to these signals can help prevent escalation and ensure the safety and comfort of both the cat and those around them.

When a cat's aggressive body language intensifies, it manifests in more overt and clear signals, indicating a high level of arousal and potential readiness for defensive action. For instance, vocalizations such as growling and hissing become more pronounced, and in some cases cats may even spit as a warning (Ellis 2022). These sounds are clear indicators of a cat's discomfort or threat perception.

In the most intense states of arousal, physical actions escalate. Cats may swat with their claws extended, a sign of readiness to engage in physical defense if necessary. Biting is another behavior that can occur in these heightened states, demonstrating the cat's willingness to protect themself or assert their need for space (Seksel 2014).

Additionally, if a cat's signals for increased space or avoidance are continually ignored, they may resort to displacing or actively chasing away other animals or, in some cases, people (Figure 2.26). This behavior is typically a last resort, used when all other passive and then more direct signals have failed to achieve the desired result of increased distance or reduced threat.

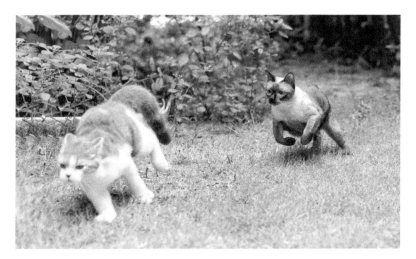

Figure 2.26 The gray tabby cat's ears are back, whiskers down, and piloerection of the tail and along the back is noted. The Siamese is displaying more offensive behavior with ears forward, direct stare, dilated pupils, whiskers out to the side, and stiff face and body. *Source:* witsawat/Adobe Stock Photos.

Appeasement Signals and "Guilt"

Due to cats' relatively solitary nature, appeasement behaviors are rather uncommon. Instead, cats typically use defensive behavior to prevent further escalation of aggressive behavior. However, these signals are still within a cat's behavioral repertoire. As with dogs, these behaviors do not indicate "guilt" but rather are displayed in order to help the cat gather information about their environment and nearby individuals in an effort to evaluate their own safety and security.

Learned Helplessness and Emotional "Shutdown" Learned helplessness or emotional shutdown in cats is a form of behavioral inhibition that serves as a survival mechanism. This behavior is a part of the "freeze" response and emotional withdrawal, which can manifest in both transient and sustained forms (Rigterink 2022). A typical transient instance is observed in hospitalized cats that may only eat at night once everyone has left for the day. In contrast, a more sustained form can occur in stressful situations, such as during a veterinary visit (Table 2.3).

Cats experiencing this emotional shutdown will often freeze in place, refuse food, and show minimal movement. They may adopt a tucked posture, with their paws drawn beneath their body and their tail wrapped around them (Figure 2.27). While this behavior might be misinterpreted as compliance or calmness, it is actually a significant indicator of compromised welfare (Heath 2018; Nicholson and O'Carroll 2021; Rigterink 2022).

Solicitous (Distance-Decreasing) Signals

While kittens actively engage in social play and seek attention for care from humans, adult cats are generally less social. Consequently, cats display distance-decreasing signals less frequently compared to other, more social animals. These behaviors in cats, indicating a desire for closeness or social interaction, can range from subtle to more overt expressions.

Subtle Solicitous Behaviors Some of the more subtle indicators of a cat's comfort with social interaction include relaxed facial features with soft eyes and round pupils that are not excessively dilated. The ears are typically forward facing and upright. Kittens may show a "play face" with their mouth half open. A common sign of a friendly approach in cats is when they hold their tail upright with a hook at the end resembling a question mark (Figure 2.28) (Nicholson and O'Carroll 2021).

Table 2.3 Signs of stress in cats.

Abdomen not exposed	Immobility
Aggression – swatting, hissing, scratching	Increased facial rubbing, scratching on surfaces
Approach to withdraw – acting conflicted	Increased resting or "feigned" sleep
Attempting to access elevated surfaces	Lack of play activity
Attempting to hide or social withdrawal	Overgrooming or decrease in grooming
Changes in behavior	Pupils fully dilated although may narrow slightly
Crouched directly on all fours, shaking, back may arch	Rapid and shallow respirations
Decrease in appetite or ravenous appetite	Redirected aggression
Ears flattened or fully flat on the back of head	Tail wrapped around body or close to body
Eyes wide and open or blinking	Vocalization – meowing, yowling, growling
Head lower than body, motionless, tense jaw	Whiskers back
House-soiling (horizontal or vertical surfaces)	
Hypervigilance, hyperactivity, easily startled	

Source: Adapted from Hargrave (2015).

Figure 2.27 This cat is in a state of emotional shutdown and withdrawal, as evidenced by the ears slightly flattened and to the side, lack of direct eye contact, stiff body, and closed mouth. *Source:* dewessa/Adobe Stock Photos.

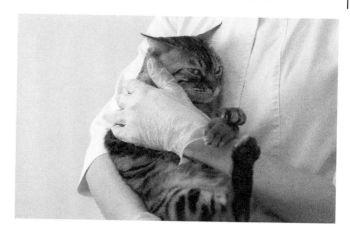

Figure 2.28 Cats will hold their tail upright with a hook (question mark) to indicate a friendly greeting. *Source:* FurryFritz/Adobe Stock Photos.

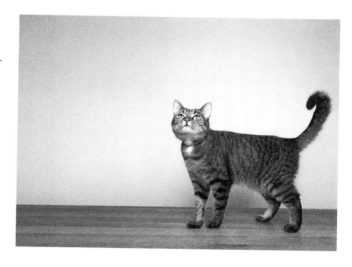

Vocalizations Indicating Friendliness Cats use a variety of sounds to express solicitous behavior. These include chattering, trilling, and purring. When seeking human interaction, cats often mew, and kittens usually initiate contact with a chirp. These vocalizations serve as a means of communication to express their desire for social interaction or attention (Nicholson and O'Carroll 2021).

Physical Gestures of Greeting and Bonding In situations of close contact, cats display friendly greetings by touching noses and engaging in sniffing behaviors. They also participate in allorubbing – rubbing their heads and bodies against each other or humans. Allorubbing serves to mix individual scents, promoting social bonding. Another bonding behavior is allogrooming, where cats groom each other. Interestingly, the cats that engage in allogrooming are often those that display aggressive behaviors in other contexts. This grooming behavior may serve as a mechanism to diffuse tension and redirect potential aggression (Figures 2.29 and 2.30) (Van den Bos 1998).

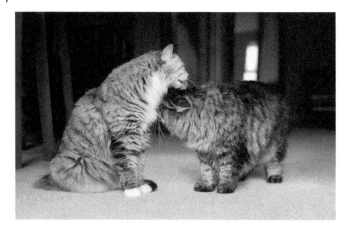

Figure 2.29 Allogrooming in cats. *Source:* Petra Richli/Adobe Stock Photos.

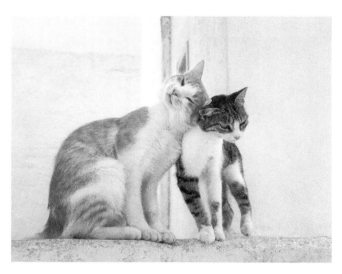

Figure 2.30 Allorubbing in cats can be a sign of a friendly greeting. *Source:* kathomenden/Adobe Stock Photos.

Domestication and Its Effect on Behavior

Cats, domesticated from their wild ancestor *Felis silvestris lybica*, experienced a domestication process that was significantly different from that of dogs (Cameron-Beaumont et al. 2002). Cats began to associate more closely with humans thousands of years after dogs, largely initiating the domestication process themselves. This occurred as humans started storing grain, which attracted rodents, thereby drawing cats into human settlements for the plentiful prey (Bradshaw et al. 2012; Vigne et al. 2004). In contrast to dogs, selective breeding pressures have been applied to cats for only about the last 200 years (Cameron-Beaumont et al. 2002; Driscoll et al. 2009; Montague et al. 2014).

Limited Change from Wild Ancestors

Given their relatively recent domestication, spanning just a few thousand years, cats have not diverged significantly from their wild ancestors (Hu et al. 2014). They are often regarded as only semi-domesticated (Montague et al. 2014). This is reflected in the minimal behavioral differences

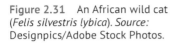

Figure 2.31 An African wild cat (*Felis silvestris lybica*). *Source:* Designpics/Adobe Stock Photos.

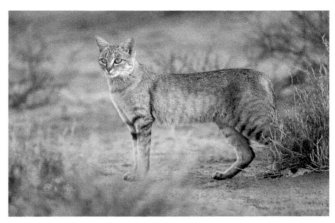

observed between domestic and wild cats (Figure 2.31). Both domestic and wild cats share a tendency to sleep for approximately 75% of the day and are crepuscular, meaning they are more active during dawn and dusk (Montague et al. 2014).

Predatory Behavior

Domestic cats retain excellent hunting skills, evident in their stalking and pouncing behaviors, which they exhibit not only when hunting prey but also when playing with toys. Cats display a full spectrum of predatory behaviors, from stalking and capturing to killing their prey. These behaviors are present from kittenhood and continue into adulthood, indicating a strong genetic predisposition and little deviation from their wild counterparts.

Temperament

Domestic cats generally exhibit less aggression and are more calm, friendly, and gentle compared to wild cats. This change in temperament is a significant aspect of domestication, making them more suitable for living in close contact with humans.

Neotenous Behaviors

Domestic cats display behaviors indicative of neoteny, which means they retain juvenile traits into adulthood. These behaviors include purring, kneading with their paws, and mewing toward their caregivers, all of which are typically associated with kitten-like behavior but continue to be expressed by adult domestic cats (Bradshaw et al. 2012).

Learning and Memory

Domestic cats have shown an increased ability to learn and to form memories. This enhanced capacity for learning and memory retention is a trait that differentiates them from their wild relatives and is likely a result of the closer interaction with humans in domestic environments.

Breed-Specific Traits and Impairments

Just as in dogs, specific breeds of domestic cats have their own unique behavioral traits and physical impairments. For example, white-coated cats with blue eyes, a phenotype not commonly found in wild cat populations, are often deaf (Figure 2.32) (Geigy et al. 2007). Siamese cats, another

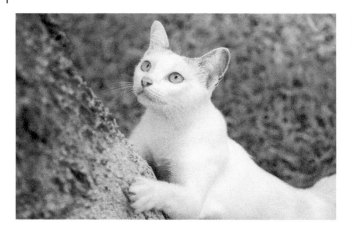

Figure 2.32 White-coated cats with blue eyes tend to be deaf. *Source:* DG PhotoStock/Adobe Stock Photos.

domestic breed, frequently experience vision impairments such as nystagmus (involuntary eye movement) and strabismus (cross-eyed appearance).

Social Behavior

Contrary to their reputation for being "aloof" and "solitary," cats do form social groups with other cats and establish bonds with humans. They sometimes even exhibit species-typical behaviors with their caregivers. The interactions within cat social colonies are structured, with cats often showing preferences for certain individuals they choose to socialize with more frequently than others.

Influence of Resources on Colony Size

The size of feral and wild cat colonies largely depends on the availability of resources in their area, which are often linked to human activities (Kerby and Macdonald 1988). Factors such as large garbage dumps, abundant grain stores leading to high rodent populations, and direct feeding by humans all contribute to this. In areas with plenty of food larger cat groups can coexist, whereas in regions with scarce resources smaller cat populations are sustained (Figure 2.33). Cats in overlapping territories tend to time-share access to resources, hunting at different times to avoid direct competition.

Multiple Social Groups in a Colony

Within a single colony there can be several social groups, although some colonies may consist of just one group. These groups are usually made up of related adult females and their offspring (Bradshaw et al. 2012). They exhibit limited tolerance for new members, often displaying aggression toward newcomers, especially when kittens are present. Some groups also include unrelated adult males, but their inclusion is less stable than that of females (Liberg and Sandell 1988).

Territorial Behavior of Male Cats

Male cats generally have larger territories than females, leading them to move between social groups more freely (Liberg and Sandell 1988). This roaming behavior is particularly pronounced during the estrus period, enhancing the males' chances of reproductive success. In low-density populations some males may control access to all females within a certain area, reducing territorial

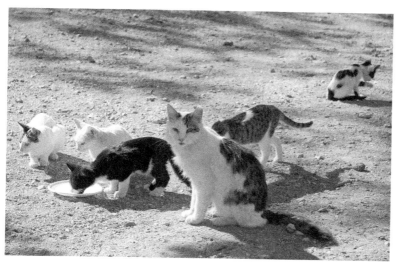

Figure 2.33 The size of a feral cat colony depends on the resources available. *Source:* ataglier/Adobe Stock Photos.

drift. In contrast, high-density areas may see significant overlap in male territories and the presence of multiple males in a group (Natoli et al. 2000; Say et al. 1999).

Solitary Nature of Male Cats

Male cats are typically more solitary than females, often engaging in fights on meeting other males. These aggressive encounters tend to decrease after repeated interactions (De Boer 1977). Affiliative behavior among male cats is usually limited to the period before they reach sexual maturity (Macdonald et al. 2000).

Reproductive Behavior

Feline behavior undergoes significant changes in response to the reproductive cycle. Although cats are generally solitary creatures, they engage in necessary social interactions during their reproductive cycle for successful mating and rearing of offspring.

Female Behavior During Estrus

When female cats enter estrus, they become more receptive to male cats. They exhibit lordosis postures, characterized by crouching and treading their hind limbs, signaling readiness for mating. Despite allowing copulation, female cats often exhibit aggressive behavior post mating, such as turning on the male to spit or scratch. This response is part of the normal mating behavior in cats. The mating process involves multiple copulatory events that are necessary to trigger ovulation in the female.

Social Behavior in Maternal Groups

Within social cat groups, female cats often den together and engage in collaborative nursing. This cooperative care extends beyond mother–daughter relationships and includes all adult females within the group. They collectively nurse and care for each other's kittens, displaying communal protective behavior. Additionally, the females in the group collectively participate in guarding and nurturing each litter (Bradshaw et al. 2012).

Ingestive Behavior

Suckling

Like puppies, kittens typically start suckling within a couple of hours after birth. The mother initiates this behavior for the first three weeks of the kitten's life. Weaning begins at around 3 weeks of age when kittens initiate nursing independently. The process usually completes by about 7 weeks, although some kittens may continue to suckle intermittently for a few weeks beyond this period.

Kitten Ingestive Patterns

Kittens dedicate a significant amount of time to learning how to hunt, with play behaviors mimicking many hunting patterns. This learning process is enhanced by prey brought back to the den by the mother, allowing kittens to practice these behaviors from around 4–5 weeks of age (Caro 1980). By the age of 5 weeks kittens develop a complete set of deciduous teeth and may begin to complete the hunting behavior pattern, including killing prey. The types of prey brought back and the mother's hunting behavior significantly influence the kittens' future prey preferences and hunting styles (Figure 2.34) (Bradshaw et al. 2012).

Adult Cat Ingestive Patterns

The eating patterns of adult cats vary depending on food availability. In an environment where food is constantly available, such as in the case of free-fed house cats, they prefer to eat multiple small meals throughout the day, slightly more during daylight hours (Mugford 1977; Overall et al. 2005). However, many cat caregivers opt for meal feeding, and cats can adjust to this schedule as well.

Hunting Behavior in Adult Cats

Adult cats that hunt for food do so solitarily and are highly skilled in this behavior. The hunting pattern involves locating prey through sight, sound, or smell, followed by a stealthy approach in a crouched position. The cat then observes the prey while concealed, flattens themself, and positions

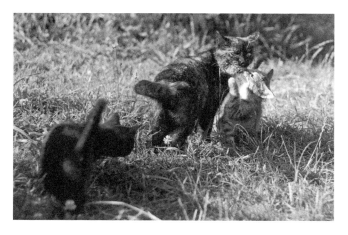

Figure 2.34 Cats learn to hunt from their mother. They also will develop food preferences based on the food their mother hunted to feed them. *Source:* Roman/Adobe Stock Photos.

their ears erect. Before capturing the prey, they shift their weight between their hind limbs and twitch their tail in preparation. The final action is a pounce or sprint toward the prey, followed by capturing it with their forepaws and delivering a bite to the nape of the neck. During this phase the cat's whiskers are positioned forward, providing additional sensory information about the prey's location.

Elimination Behavior

In the early weeks of life kittens depend on their mother (queen) for elimination. The queen stimulates urination and defecation in her kittens by licking their perineal region. As kittens grow they naturally learn to eliminate independently. During this developmental phase they instinctively seek fine-grained, sand-like substrates where they can dig to cover their urine and feces, a behavior rooted in their natural instincts for hygiene and predator avoidance (Neilson 2004).

Adult Cat Elimination Behavior

Adult cats exhibit a routine of digging in their chosen substrate before eliminating (Borchelt 1991). They typically adopt a squatting posture for both urination and defecation. However, some cats may transition from squatting to standing during elimination, which can be influenced by factors such as discomfort or pain from conditions like arthritis. The choice of location for elimination is influenced by their substrate preferences, social factors, and accessibility of the site (Borchelt 1991). For domestic cats, aspects like the size, shape, and cleanliness of the litter box influence their elimination behavior (Borchelt 1991).

Urine Marking (Spraying)

Urine marking, or spraying, is a normal behavior in cats, usually performed while standing, with urine released onto vertical surfaces (Borchelt 1991). Though it is predominantly associated with intact males and females in estrus, any cat may engage in this behavior (Bradshaw and Cameron-Beaumont 2000). Spraying serves as a form of communication, marking a cat's presence within a territory. It is typically characterized by the release of small amounts of urine, which are not covered post elimination, in contrast to regular urination behavior (Borchelt 1991; Overall et al. 2005).

Conclusion

Understanding normal canine and feline behavior is critical in order to both prevent and treat problem behaviors as well as to facilitate humane handling and promote the human–animal bond. By considering the subtleties of body language, clinicians can become more adept at recognizing subtle signs of poor health. This knowledge not only aids in diagnosis but also enables them to educate clients about their pets' emotional and physical wellbeing.

References

Amtsberg, G., Durocher, W., and Meyer, H. (1978). Influence of food composition on the intestinal flora of the dog. In: *Nutrition of the Dog and Cat* (ed. R.S. Anderson), 181–188. Oxford: Pergamon Press.
Beaver, B.V. (1981). Grass eating by carnivores. *Veterinary Clinics of North America, Small Animal Practice* 76 (7): 968.

Beaver, B.V. (2009). *Canine Behavior: Insights and Answers*. Philadelphia, PA: Saunders.

Berg, I.A. (1944). Development of behavior: the micturition pattern in the dog. *Journal of Experimental Psychology* 34 (5): 343.

Bleicher, N. (1962). Behavior of the bitch during parturition. *Journal of the American Veterinary Medical Association* 140: 1076.

Borchelt, P.L. (1991). Cat elimination behavior problems. *Veterinary Clinics of North America, Small Animal Practice* 21: 257–264.

Boulcott, S.R. (1967). Feeding behaviour of adult dogs under conditions of hospitalization. *British Veterinary Journal* 123: 498.

Bradshaw, J.W.S. (2006). The evolutionary basis for the feeding behavior of domestic dogs (*Canis familiaris*) and cats (*Felis catus*). *Journal of Nutrition* 136: 1927S–1931S.

Bradshaw, J.W. and Cameron-Beaumont, C. (2000). The signaling repertoire of the domestic cat and its undomesticated relatives. In: *The Domestic Cat: The Biology of Its Behaviour* (ed. D.C. Turner and P.P.G. Bateson), 68–93. Cambridge: Cambridge University Press.

Bradshaw, J.W. and Lea, A.M. (1993). Dyadic interactions between domestic dogs during exercise. *Anthrozoös* 5: 245–253.

Bradshaw, J.W. and Rooney, N. (2016). Dog social behavior and communication. In: *The Domestic Dog* (ed. J. Serpell), 133–159. Cambridge: Cambridge University Press.

Bradshaw, J.W., Blackwell, E.J., and Casey, R.A. (2009). Dominance in domestic dogs – useful construct or bad habit? *Journal of Veterinary Behavior* 4: 135–144.

Bradshaw, J.W.S., Casey, R.A., and Brown, S.L. (2012). *The Behaviour of the Domestic Cat*. Wallingford: CABI.

Cameron-Beaumont, C., Lowe, S.E., and Bradshaw, C.J.A. (2002). Evidence suggesting preadaptation to domestication throughout the small Felidae. *Biological Journal of the Linnean Society* 75 (3): 361–366.

Caro, T.M. (1980). Effects of the mother, object play, and adult experience on predation in cats. *Behavioral and Neural Biology* 29: 29.

De Boer, J.N. (1977). The age of olfactory cues functioning in chemocommunication among male domestic cats. *Behavioural Processes* 2: 209–225.

Driscoll, C.A., Macdonald, D.W., and O'Brien, S.J. (2009). From wild animals to domestic pets, an evolutionary view of domestication. *Proceedings of the National Academy of Sciences of the United States of America* 106 (Suppl 1): 9971–9978.

Ellis, J.J. (2022). Beyond "doing better": ordinal rating scales to monitor behavioural indicators of well-being in cats. *Animals* 12 (21): 2897.

Farago, T., Pongracz, P., Range, F. et al. (2010). "The bone is mine": affective and referential aspects of dog growls. *Animal Behaviour* 79: 917–925.

Ferrell, F. (1984). Preference for sugars and nonnutritive sweeteners in young beagles. *Neuroscience and Biobehavioral Reviews* 8 (2): 199.

Feuerstein, N.L. and Terkel, J. (2008). Interrelationships of dogs (*Canis familiaris*) and cats (*Felis catus* L.) living under the same roof. *Applied Animal Behaviour Science* 113 (1–3): 150–165.

Frank, D. (2013). Aggressive dogs: What questions do we need to ask? *Canadian Veterinary Journal* 54 (6): 554.

Fuller, J.L. and Fox, M.W. (1969). The behaviour of dogs. In: *The Behaviour of Domestic Animals* (ed. E.S. Hafez), 438–481. Philadelphia, PA: Williams & Wilkins.

Geigy, C.A., Heid, S., Steffen, F. et al. (2007). Does a pleiotropic gene explain deafness and blue irises in white cats? *Veterinary Journal* 173: 548–553.

Hargrave, C. (2015). Anxiety, fear, frustration and stress in cats and dogs – implications for the welfare of companion animals and practice finances. *Companion Animal* 20 (3): 136–141.

Hargrave, C. (2017a). Canine stress in a nutshell – why does it occur, how can it be recognised, and what can be done to alleviate it? *Veterinary Nurse* 8 (3): 140–147.

Hargrave, C. (2017b). Feline stress in a nutshell – why does it occur, how can it be recognised, and what can be done to alleviate it? *Veterinary Nurse* 8 (4): 192–199.

Hart, B.L. (1974). Normal behavior and behavioral problems associated with sexual function, urination and defecation. *Veterinary Clinics of North America* 4 (3): 589.

Heath, S. (2018). Understanding feline emotions and their role in problem behaviours. *Journal of Feline Medicine and Surgery* 20: 437–444.

Hecht, J., Miklósi, Á., and Gácsi, M. (2012). Behavioral assessment and owner perceptions of behaviors associated with guilt in dogs. *Applied Animal Behaviour Science* 139 (1–2): 134142.

Hepper, P.G. (1994). Long-term retention of kinship recognition established during infancy in the domestic dog. *Behavioural Processes* 33: 3–14.

Holden, E., Calvo, G., Collins, M. et al. (2014). Evaluation of facial expression in acute pain in cats. *Journal of Small Animal Practice* 55 (12): 615–621.

Houpt, K.A. (1991). Feeding and drinking behavior problems. *Veterinary Clinics of North America, Small Animal Practice* 21 (2): 281.

Houpt, K.A. and Hintz, H. (1978a). Obesity in dogs. *Canine Practice* 5 (2): 54.

Houpt, K.A. and Hintz, H. (1978b). Palatability and canine food preferences. *Canine Practice* 5 (6): 29.

Hu, Y., Hu, S., Wang, W. et al. (2014). Earliest evidence for commensal processes of cat domestication. *Proceedings of the National Academy of Sciences of the United States of America* 111 (1): 116–120.

James, W.T. (1957). The effect of satiation on the sucking response in puppies. *Journal of Comparative and Physiological Psychology* 50: 375.

James, W.T. and McCay, C.M. (1950). A study of food intake, activity, and digestive efficiency in different type dogs. *American Journal of Veterinary Research* 11: 412.

Kaminski, J., Waller, B.M., Diogo, R. et al. (2019). Evolution of facial muscle anatomy in dogs. *Proceedings of the National Academy of Sciences of the United States of America* 116 (29): 14677–14681.

Kerby, G. and Macdonald, D.W. (1988). Cat society and the consequences of colony size. In: *The Domestic Cat: The Biology of Its Behaviour* (ed. D.C. Turner and P. Bateson), 67–81. Cambridge: Cambridge University Press.

Kolb, B. and Nonneman, A.K. (1975). The development of social responsiveness in kittens. *Animal Behaviour* 23: 368.

Konok, V., Nagy, K., and Miklósi, Á. (2015). How do humans represent the emotions of dogs? The resemblance between the human representation of the canine and the human affective space. *Applied Animal Behaviour Science* 162: 37–46.

Landsberg, G., Hunthausen, W., and Ackerman, L. (2013). *Behavior Problems of the Dog & Cat.* Philadelphia, PA: Elsevier Health Sciences.

Lazzaroni, M., Range, F., Backes, J. et al. (2020). The effect of domestication and experience on the social interaction of dogs and wolves with a human companion. *Frontiers in Psychology* 11: 1–14.

Lezama-Garcia, K., Mariti, C., Mota-Rojas, D. et al. (2019). Maternal behaviour in domestic dogs. *International Journal of Veterinary Science and Medicine* 7 (1): 20–30.

Liberg, O. and Sandell, M. (1988). Spatial organisation and reproductive tactics in the domestic cat and other felids. In: *The Domestic Cat: The Biology of Its Behaviour* (ed. D.C. Turner and P. Bateson), 120–147. Cambridge: Cambridge University Press.

Macdonald, D.W., Yamaguchi, N., and Kerby, G. (2000). Group-living in the domestic cat: its sociobiology and epidemiology. In: *The Domestic Cat: The Biology of Its Behaviour* (ed. D.C. Turner and P. Bateson), 95–118. Cambridge: Cambridge University Press.

Malm, K. and Jensen, P. (1993). Regurgitation as a weaning strategy – a selective review on an old subject in a new light. *Applied Animal Behaviour Science* 36 (1): 47.

Markwell, P.J. and Thorne, C.J. (1987). Early behavioural development of dogs. *Journal of Small Animal Practice* 28 (11): 984.

Marshall-Pescini, S., Rao, A., Viranyi, Z., and Range, F. (2017). The role of domestication and experience in 'looking back' towards humans in an unsolvable task. *Nature Scientific Reports* 7: 46636.

Martens, P., Enders-Slegers, M.J., and Walker, J.K. (2016). The emotional lives of companion animals: Attachment and subjective claims by owners of cats and dogs. *Anthrozoös* 29 (1): 73–88.

Montague, M.J., Li, G., Gandolfi, B. et al. (2014). Comparative analysis of the domestic cat genome reveals genetic signatures underlying feline biology and domestication. *Proceedings of the National Academy of Sciences of the United States of America* 111 (48): 17230–17235.

Mugford, R.A. (1977). External influences on the feeding of carnivores. In: *The Chemical Senses and Nutrition* (ed. M.R. Kare and O. Maller), 22–50. New York: Academic Press.

Natoli, E., De Vito, E., and Pontier, D. (2000). Mate choice in the domestic cat (*F. catus*). *Aggressive Behavior* 26: 455–465.

Neilson, J. (2004). Thinking outside the box: feline elimination. *Journal of Feline Medicine and Surgery* 6: 5–11.

Nicholson, S.L. and O'Carroll, R.A. (2021). Development of an ethogram/guide for identifying feline emotions: a new approach to feline interactions and welfare assessment in practice. *Irish Veterinary Journal* 74: 8.

Overall, K.L., Rodan, I., Beaver, B.V. et al. (2005). Feline behavior guidelines from the American Association of Feline Practitioners. *Journal of the American Veterinary Medical Association* 227 (1): 70–84.

Pal, S.K. (2005). Maturation and development of social behaviour during early ontogeny in free-ranging dog puppies in West Bengal, India. *Applied Animal Behaviour Science* 126: 140–153.

Pal, S.K. (2011). Mating system of free-ranging dogs (*Canis familiaris*). *International Journal of Zoology* 2011: 314216.

Pal, S.K., Ghosh, B., and Roy, S. (1999). Inter- and intra-sexual behavior of free-ranging dogs (*Canis familiaris*) in relation to season, sex and age. *Applied Animal Behaviour Science* 59: 331–348.

Pickersgill, O., Mills, D.S., and Guo, K. (2023). Owners' beliefs regarding the emotional capabilities of their dogs and cats. *Animals* 13 (5): 820.

Rashotte, M.E., Smith, J.C., Austin, T. et al. (1984). Twenty-four-hour free-feeding patterns of dogs eating dry food. *Neuroscience and Biobehavioral Reviews* 8 (2): 205.

Rigterink, A. (2022). Fear, anxiety, stress behaviors in cats. In: *Clinical Handbook of Feline Behavior Medicine* (ed. E. Stolow), 129–141. Chichester: Wiley-Blackwell.

Say, L., Pontier, D., and Natoli, E. (1999). High variation in multiple paternity of domestic cats in relation to environmental conditions. *Proceedings of the Royal Society of London Series B* 268: 2071–2074.

Seksel, K. (2014). Fear, aggression, communication, body language and social relationships in cats. *European Journal of Companion Animal Practice* 24 (3): 20–27.

Siniscalchi, M., d'Ingeo, S., Minunno, M., and Quaranta, A. (2018). Communication in dogs. *Animals* 8 (8): 131.

Sueda, K.C., Hart, B.L., and Cliff, K.D. (2005). Plant eating in domestic dogs (*Canis familiaris*): characterization and relationship to signalment, illness, and behavior problems. In: *Current Issues and Research in Veterinary Behavioral Medicine* (ed. D. Mills, E. Levine, G. Landsberg, et al.), 230–231. West Lafayette, IN: Purdue University Press.

Udell, M.A.R., Dorey, N.R., and Wynne, C.D.L. (2010). What did domestication do to dogs? A new account of dogs' sensitivity to human actions. *Biological Reviews* 85: 327–345.

Van den Bos, R. (1998). The function of allogrooming in domestic cats (*Felis silvestris catus*): a study in a group of cats living in confinement. *Journal of Ethology* 16: 1–13.

Vigne, J.D., Guilaine, D., Debue, K. et al. (2004). Early taming of the cat in Cyprus. *Science* 304 (5668): 259.

Voith, V.L. and Borchelt, P.L. (1985). Elimination behavior and related problems in dogs. *Compendium of Continuing Education* 7 (7): 537.

Wheat, C.H., Fitzpatrick, J.L., Rowell, B., and Temrin, H. (2019). Behavioural correlations of the domestication syndrome are decoupled in modern dog breeds. *Nature Communications* 10: 2422.

Yin, S. and McCowen, B. (2004). Barking in domestic dogs: context specificity and individual identification. *Animal Behavior* 68: 343–355.

3

Basic Learning Theory and Choosing a Trainer

Learning is defined by the *Merriam-Webster Dictionary* as "knowledge or skill acquired by instruction or study" as well as "modification of a behavioral tendency by experience" (Merriam-Webster n.d.). Learning leads to a semi-permanent and long-lasting change in an animal's response. Learning can happen in a variety of ways, and it is important to consider how an animal's past experiences may affect their behavior. Further, understanding the fundamental aspects of learning theory can facilitate treatment of behavior problems through teaching animals new skills to cope with their environments, thus strengthening the human–animal bond between clients and patients.

Although teaching new skills and training specific behaviors are critical aspects of treating problem behaviors, it is equally important to understand the underlying emotional states that are contributing to the development and continuation of those behaviors. While working in conjunction with positive reinforcement-based trainers can be beneficial, not all cases should be referred to trainers. Trainers are not substitutes for medical care. Therefore, it is imperative that veterinarians understand the basics of learning theory in order to appropriately handle problem cases.

Types of Learning

Nonassociative Learning

Nonassociative learning is a change in an animal's behavior that results from repeated exposure to a single type of stimulus. It involves both habituation and sensitization.

Habituation
The gradual decrease in an animal's response to repeated exposure to a stimulus is known as habituation (Mazur 2016; McGreevy and Boakes 2011). It is important to note that habituation occurs "naturally"; that is, this change in behavior occurs regardless of whether you want it to or not. For instance, a dog might initially startle at a loud noise. Over time, if the noise has no significant consequences (neither positive nor negative), the dog may learn to ignore the noise and stop reacting.

Example of Habituation   Imagine a puppy living in a busy urban environment. Initially the puppy might be startled by the frequent sounds of sirens from emergency vehicles. However, over time, as the puppy is repeatedly exposed to this sound without any direct consequence to themselves, they

Veterinary Guide to Preventing Behavior Problems in Dogs and Cats, First Edition. Christine D. Calder and Sarah C. Wright. © 2025 John Wiley & Sons, Inc. Published 2025 by John Wiley & Sons, Inc.

begin to realize that the sirens pose no threat. Gradually, the puppy's reaction to the sirens diminishes over time. This process, where the puppy learns to ignore the sirens because they are irrelevant to daily life, is an example of habituation.

Sensitization

In contrast, sensitization involves an increase in an animal's response following repeated exposure to a stimulus (Mazur 2016; McGreevy and Boakes 2011). Unlike habituation, the stimulus in sensitization is often (but not necessarily) aversive. Sensitization can develop more quickly than habituation. It is imperative to understand that sensitization can lead to an increase in reactivity and serious behavior problems in the future.

Example of Sensitization   Consider a cat that experiences a loud, unexpected noise from a vacuum cleaner every time it is used. Instead of becoming accustomed to the noise, the cat becomes increasingly anxious and fearful each time the vacuum is turned on. Even the sight of the vacuum might start to trigger a fear response. This heightened reaction to the noise and presence of the vacuum cleaner over time is an example of sensitization. In this case, the cat's response escalates because they perceive the vacuum noise as a potential threat or discomfort, even if the vacuum has never harmed them.

Associative Learning

Associative learning involves a change in behavior that results from the association between two stimuli. There are two main types of associative learning: classical and operant conditioning.

Classical Conditioning

Classical conditioning is a type of associative learning that relies on reflexes rather than conscious effort. This learning process occurs when an unconditioned stimulus, which naturally elicits an unconditioned response, is paired with a neutral stimulus. Over time, the neutral stimulus alone begins to trigger the response, even in the absence of the unconditioned stimulus. The precise order and timing of the presentation of these stimuli are critical for classical conditioning to take place (Mazur 2016; McGreevy and Boakes 2011).

Classical conditioning can also be undone through a process called extinction. Extinction happens when the conditioned stimulus is no longer followed by the unconditioned stimulus. After enough instances where the conditioned stimulus is not reinforced, the learned behavior diminishes, and the conditioned stimulus loses its ability to predict the unconditioned response. This process should not be confused with habituation, as the mechanisms and outcomes are distinct.

A well-known example of classical conditioning is Pavlov's experiments with dogs. In these experiments, Pavlov paired the sound of a bell (neutral stimulus) with the presentation of food (unconditioned stimulus). Initially the bell had no effect on the dogs, but the food naturally caused them to salivate (unconditioned response). As Pavlov repeatedly presented the food alongside the ringing bell, the dogs began to associate the two. Eventually, the sound of the bell alone was enough to make the dogs salivate, demonstrating that the bell had become a conditioned stimulus eliciting a conditioned response.

Example of Classical Conditioning with a Puppy, a Clicker, and Food   Consider a young puppy starting their training sessions. In these sessions the trainer uses a clicker, a small device that makes a clicking sound, followed by giving the puppy a treat. At first, the clicker's sound is a neutral

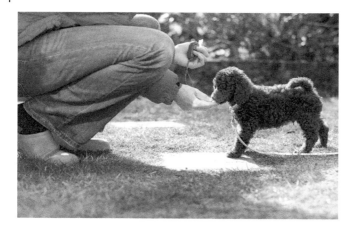

Figure 3.1 Using classical conditioning, a clicker can be conditioned to use for marking behaviors as part of positive reinforcement training. *Source:* Duncan Andison/Adobe Stock Photos.

stimulus to the puppy, meaning it does not naturally elicit any specific response, as the puppy has no prior association with this sound.

As the training continues a pattern emerges: each time the trainer clicks the clicker, a treat is promptly given to the puppy. The treat acts as an unconditioned stimulus since it naturally brings about engaging emotions from the puppy, such as expectation of food or salivation (the unconditioned response).

After repeated pairings of the clicker's sound with the treat, the puppy begins to expect the treat as soon as they hear the click. The clicker's sound has now transformed into a conditioned stimulus (Figure 3.1). It elicits a conditioned response in the puppy, which is now used to mark new and desirable behaviors.

Counterconditioning

Counterconditioning involves modifying an animal's emotional reaction to a stimulus, particularly transforming a negative emotion into a positive one (Mazur 2016; McGreevy and Boakes 2011). In other words, the goal of counterconditioning is to change an established conditioned emotional response (CER) to an alternative one. The process requires the pairing of the original conditioned stimulus, which initially elicits a negative emotional response (CER–), with a new unconditioned stimulus that triggers a strong, positive emotional response (CER+). This positive response should be incompatible with the original negative one. Over time, the association that forms between the original conditioned stimulus and the unconditioned stimulus will decrease the magnitude of the original conditioned response, and it may eventually eliminate the conditioned response entirely.

Example of Counterconditioning: A Dog Barking at the Door Consider a dog named Spot who has a habit of barking loudly every time someone knocks on the door. In this scenario, the sound of the knock is the conditioned stimulus that triggers Spot's barking (the conditioned response), which is likely a mix of alertness, fear, anticipation, and anxiety.

To modify Spot's behavior through counterconditioning, the goal is to change his reaction from barking to a calmer and quieter behavior by associating the knocking with a piece of chicken, which Spot absolutely loves and naturally responds to with excitement and anticipation.

The counterconditioning process begins by establishing a new routine. Each time someone knocks on the door, instead of responding to Spot's barking, his caregiver immediately gives him a piece of chicken. The key is to do this consistently and promptly, so Spot starts to anticipate the chicken as soon as he hears the knock.

Over time, and with consistent repetition, Spot begins to form a new association: instead of barking, he starts to sit and wait for his piece of chicken whenever he hears someone knocking. The sound of the knock, which used to trigger barking, now predicts something enjoyable, leading to a change in Spot's behavior.

Through repeated and consistent practice of this new routine, Spot's response to door knocks shifts dramatically. His initial conditioned response of barking is replaced with a more composed behavior of sitting and waiting for a treat. This change in behavior is a clear indication of successful counterconditioning, where the undesirable behavior (barking) has been transformed into a more desirable one (sitting quietly and waiting for a treat).

Fear Conditioning

Fear conditioning is a particular type of classical conditioning where an individual learns to associate a neutral stimulus with a fear-inducing stimulus, resulting in a fear response to the previously neutral stimulus. During this learning process, a neutral stimulus (e.g., a sound or visual cue) is paired with an aversive or fear-inducing stimulus (e.g., a loud noise or an electric shock). Over time, the neutral stimulus becomes a conditioned stimulus that triggers the fear response without the need for the aversive stimulus.

One example of fear conditioning involves using a shock collar to stop barking. The shock collar itself serves as the neutral stimulus. When the dog barks excessively (the undesired behavior), the caregiver activates the shock collar, delivering an electric shock to the dog as the aversive stimulus. This action is intended to deter the dog from barking.

Through repeated experiences, the dog learns to associate the presence of the shock collar with the painful electric shocks they receive when they bark excessively. Over time, the shock collar becomes a conditioned stimulus that predicts the aversive stimulus, even when it is not actively delivering a shock.

As a result of this fear conditioning, the dog may display signs of fear and anxiety when the caregiver is attempting to put the shock collar on the dog or in a particular location where the shock had previously occurred (e.g., in the yard, in the front hall, on the deck). The dog might even show signs of fear while wearing the shock collar, even when not actively in use. This fear response reflects a learned association between the presence of the collar and the aversive experiences they have endured. This is why shock collars are considered inhumane and are never recommended for training or behavior modification (Blackwell and Casey 2006; China et al. 2020; Cooper et al. 2014; Fernandes et al. 2017; Masson et al. 2018; Overall 2007; Ziv 2017).

Operant Conditioning

Operant conditioning involves a process where an animal's voluntary actions control their learning experience. This type of conditioning is centered around the concept that the consequences of an animal's behavior determine how frequently that behavior is performed in the future. In other words, the behavior itself triggers a response, which then influences the probability of the behavior's recurrence (Mazur 2016; McGreevy and Boakes 2011).

This form of conditioning can involve both positive and negative forms of punishment and reinforcement, which play a role in either increasing or decreasing the likelihood of a behavior. B.F. Skinner's experiments with mice in a box are classic examples of operant conditioning. In his experiments, a mouse placed in a box with a lever learned that pressing the lever resulted in receiving food. This positive reinforcement (receiving food) increased the likelihood of the lever-pressing behavior. Conversely, when the mice scratched the walls of the box, they were subjected to a loud noise. This positive punishment (introduction of an unpleasant stimulus) decreased the frequency of the wall-scratching behavior.

Through these experiments, Skinner demonstrated the fundamental principles of operant conditioning: behaviors that are rewarded (reinforced) are more likely to be repeated, and behaviors that result in an unpleasant outcome (punished) are less likely to occur again. This principle is a cornerstone of learning and is widely applied in various settings, including animal training. Operant conditioning is based on four contingencies, and in this context "negative" refers to the removal of a stimulus, while "positive" indicates the addition of a stimulus and not necessarily "good" or "bad."

The Four Contingencies of Operant Conditioning

See Table 3.1.

Punishment

Punishment describes methods used to decrease the frequency of a given behavior. Punishment is commonly thought to be "mean," but it does not necessarily indicate that the methodology is strongly aversive. There are specific rules for punishment to be effective, and it can have significant side effects.

Positive Punishment (P+)

This occurs when an additional element is introduced to decrease the frequency of a behavior. For instance, spraying a cat with water to prevent them from jumping on the counter is an example of positive punishment. Here, the water spray (an added factor) is meant to decrease the cat's counter-jumping behavior. (See "Effective Punishment.")

Negative Punishment (P−)

Negative punishment happens when something is taken away to decrease a behavior's frequency. For example, withdrawing attention from a dog that jumps on someone entering the home. In this case, the removal of attention (the subtracted factor) is meant to reduce the jumping behavior.

Table 3.1 The four contingencies of operant conditioning.

Contingency	Description	Example
Positive reinforcement (R+)	Adding (+) something to increase the frequency of a behavior	Giving a treat to a dog after they sit
Negative reinforcement (R−)	Removing (−) something to increase the frequency of a behavior	Releasing leash pressure when a dog is in the heel position
Positive punishment (P+)	Adding (+) something to decrease the frequency of a behavior	Spraying water on a cat to stop them while scratching furniture
Negative punishment (P−)	Removing (−) something to decrease the frequency of a behavior	Turning away (removing attention) as a dog jumps up to discourage jumping

Effective Punishment

Effective punishment in training and behavior modification should follow specific rules and guidelines to be both ethical and maximally effective. In general, punishment is never recommended for behavior modification, but here are some key guidelines that must be met for punishment to be effective:

- **Timing:** Punishment should be administered immediately after the undesirable behavior occurs. The closer the punishment is to the behavior, the more effective the association of the consequence is with the behavior.
- **Consistency:** Punishment must be applied consistently whenever the undesired behavior is displayed. Inconsistency can lead to confusion, frustration, fear, anxiety, and reduced effectiveness.
- **Appropriateness:** The learner determines what is punishment and what is reinforcement. When effective, the punishment should stop the behavior and repetition is unnecessary ("one and done"). If it does not, then the punishment was not effective. Each animal is an individual, and punishment that is too harsh can result in injuries, protective emotions, and defensive behaviors, including aggression.

When using punishment, the targeted behavior should decrease immediately. If the behavior persists after one or two instances of punishment, then reconsider the approach; further punishment will not be effective.

The goal of punishment is to decrease the frequency of a behavior by either adding or removing a stimulus. There is often confusion between what is positive punishment and negative reinforcement. While they may seem similar, the outcome is different. Positive punishment decreases behavior by adding an aversive stimulus, whereas negative reinforcement increases behavior through the removal of an unpleasant stimulus.

Reinforcement

Reinforcement is used to increase the frequency of a behavior. Reinforcement does not necessarily indicate that the method is "nice" or "kind."

Positive Reinforcement (R+)

This involves adding something to increase the frequency of a behavior. For example, giving a dog a treat after they sit is positive reinforcement.

Negative Reinforcement (R−)

Negative reinforcement occurs when removing a factor increases the frequency of a behavior. For example, easing leash pressure when a dog stops pulling on the leash is negative reinforcement. The reduction of leash tension (the removed element) encourages the dog to walk without pulling.

Escape Conditioning

Escape conditioning is a specific form of operant conditioning in which an animal learns to engage in particular behaviors to remove themselves or escape from an unpleasant situation. This type of conditioning can progress into avoidance conditioning, where the animal anticipates the unpleasant situation and proactively displays behaviors to avoid it entirely. Distinct from fear conditioning, negative reinforcement rather than positive punishment often leads to this type of behavior.

In avoidance conditioning, the animal recognizes a specific stimulus as a predictor of an unpleasant experience and alters their behavior to prevent encountering that situation. For example, as noted by Mills (1997), a dog that has a strong dislike of car rides might initially resist or struggle when being put into a car. Over time, this dog may learn to associate certain cues, such as the caregiver picking up car keys or putting on shoes, with the unpleasant experience of car rides. As a result, the dog might start to hide whenever these cues appear in an attempt to avoid the car-ride experience altogether.

Reinforcement Schedules

Reinforcement schedules are an essential concept in the field of behavior psychology, particularly in operant conditioning. These schedules determine how and when a response will be followed by a reinforcer and are used to shape and maintain behavior (Table 3.2). There are two primary types of reinforcement schedules: continuous and intermittent (or partial) (Lindsay 2013).

Table 3.2 Different reinforcement schedules for teaching and maintaining behavior.

Reinforcement schedule	Description	Response rate	Extinction resistance
Continuous reinforcement	Behavior is reinforced every single time it occurs	High	Low
Fixed interval reinforcement	Reinforcement occurs at fixed time intervals (e.g., every 15 minutes), even if behavior is displayed multiple times within that interval	Moderate	Moderate
Variable interval reinforcement	Reinforcement delivered at random time intervals (e.g., 5 minutes, 13 minutes, 2 minutes)	Moderate	Moderate
Fixed duration reinforcement	Reinforcement given after a specific amount of time of behavior display (e.g., 30 seconds)	High	Moderate
Variable duration reinforcement	Reinforcement occurs after random durations of behavior display (e.g., 10 seconds, 25 seconds)	High	Low
Fixed ratio reinforcement	Reinforcement given after a fixed number of responses (e.g., every 7 responses)	High	Moderate
Variable ratio reinforcement	Reinforcement delivered after a random number of responses (e.g., 1 response, 17 responses, 8 responses)	Very high	High

Continuous Reinforcement
In this schedule, every instance of the desired behavior is reinforced. This approach is the fastest method for teaching a new behavior but also leads to rapid extinction of the behavior if the reinforcement stops. One example is Skinner's box experiment, where every time a mouse pressed a lever, they received food. The immediate delivery of the reinforcer following the behavior is key in this schedule.

Intermittent or Partial Reinforcement
In these schedules, reinforcement is not given every time the behavior occurs. This approach is more effective for maintaining learned behaviors rather than teaching new behaviors. There are six main types of intermittent reinforcement schedules:

- **Fixed interval reinforcement:** Reinforcement is given at set time intervals (e.g., every 15 minutes), regardless of how many times the behavior is performed within that interval. This schedule results in a moderate response rate and can lead to significant pauses in response after the reinforcement is given.
- **Variable interval reinforcement:** Reinforcement is delivered at random time intervals. This leads to a moderate, steady rate of response with fewer pauses between responses compared to fixed interval schedules.
- **Fixed duration reinforcement:** Reinforcement is given after a behavior is displayed for a specific length of time. This schedule can result in high response rates but also in longer pauses after reinforcement.
- **Variable duration reinforcement:** Reinforcement occurs after the behavior is displayed for a random amount of time. This leads to high response rates with little to no pause, resulting in nearly continuous behavior.
- **Fixed ratio reinforcement:** Reinforcement is provided after a specific number of responses. This schedule typically produces a high response rate but can also lead to frequent pauses following reinforcement.
- **Variable ratio reinforcement:** Reinforcement is given after a random number of responses. This schedule generates a very high and steady rate of response and makes the behavior very resistant to extinction.

Each schedule has distinct effects on the rate and pattern of response, making them suitable for different behavioral goals and contexts. Understanding these differences helps to effectively apply operant conditioning principles in both research and practical settings.

Differential Reinforcement of Alternative Behaviors

Differential reinforcement of alternative behaviors (DRA) is a behavior modification technique in which the performance of an undesirable behavior is reduced through the reinforcement of an alternative and more desirable behavior. For successful DRA, a clear definition of the behavior is needed, including an understanding of the circumstances leading up to the behavior (antecedents), the behavior itself, and the reinforcers causing the behavior to continue (consequences). With this information, new behaviors can be learned and reinforced as alternatives and replacements for the undesired behavior in the same situation.

Antecedents

Antecedents refer to events or circumstances that precede a specific behavior. These can range from environmental cues like a vehicle arriving in the driveway or the noise of a refrigerator door opening to a direct cue like "sit." The specific antecedents associated with a given behavior will vary tremendously between each situation and individual animal. Identifying the antecedent for each behavior will require awareness of and attention to the details of the situation surrounding the animal's behavior.

Once the antecedent has been identified, it can be changed or managed in order to change the behavior that follows. In fact, environmental management is a critical component of any behavior treatment plan, since antecedent control can influence an animal's underlying emotional state (Lindsay 2013). For example, caregivers may change the time they take their dog for a walk or put up a baby gate to prevent the dog from reaching the front door (Figure 3.2). Changing the environment minimizes opportunities the animal has to practice the undesired behavior.

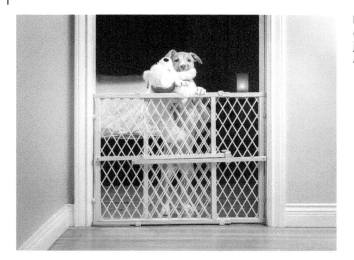

Figure 3.2 Placing a dog behind a gate can help manage and reduce jumping on visitors. Petra Richli/ Adobe Stock Photos.

Behaviors

Behaviors in the context of animal response refer to the specific actions an animal takes in response to an antecedent. It is important to be able to describe the behavior objectively. This allows for a clear understanding of the behavior, which is key to recognizing what a successful modification of that behavior would look like. Often a behavior may consist of several elements; for example, an animal might both jump and bark in response to a certain stimulus. By identifying and detailing each aspect of the behavior, it becomes possible to devise a more effective plan for reinforcing an alternative, more desirable behavior. This detailed understanding is essential for targeted behavior modification.

Consequences

Consequences refer to the outcomes or events that occur immediately following an animal's behavior. These consequences determine if an animal will repeat the behavior in the future. Reinforcing consequences, in particular, are those that increase the frequency of the behavior. These can include direct actions by the caregiver or events independent of the caregiver's presence, such as the departure of a delivery person or a bird flying away as a direct consequence of an animal barking. Both types of consequences significantly influence an animal's learning and behavior patterns.

In DRA, the strategy revolves around modifying the consequences of specific behaviors in response to an antecedent. This is achieved by providing reinforcement for alternative, more desirable behaviors, while withholding reinforcement for the original, problematic behavior. By altering the consequences in this manner, DRA effectively changes the frequency of these behaviors. As a result, the reinforced desirable behaviors become more likely to occur over time due to the positive consequences associated with them. Conversely, the undesirable behaviors, which are not reinforced, become less likely to occur. The animal learns that engaging in the alternative, reinforced behaviors leads to positive outcomes, while the original behavior, now unreinforced, becomes less appealing or rewarding. This approach leverages the principles of operant conditioning to encourage desirable behaviors and reduce the occurrence of unwanted ones by changing the behavior frequency.

Capturing, Luring, and Shaping Behavior

Capturing, luring, and shaping are three effective methods used in animal training to teach specific behaviors and associate them with cues. Each method has a distinct approach to eliciting and reinforcing the desired behavior (Lindsay 2013; Mazur 2016; McGreevy and Boakes 2011).

Capturing

One way of obtaining the desired behavior is through capturing. This method involves waiting for the animal to perform the desired behavior naturally, without a cue, luring, or prompting. When the animal offers the desired behavior, that behavior is immediately marked (using a clicker or a verbal marker like "yes") and then rewarded. This process relies on the trainer's observation skills and timing to capture the spontaneous occurrence of the behavior.

Luring

In contrast to capturing, luring actively guides the animal into performing the desired behavior. This is done by using a treat or toy to entice the animal into a specific position or action. Once the animal performs the behavior, the behavior is marked and followed by a reward. Luring involves more direct interaction and guidance from the trainer to achieve the desired behavior. Lures should be phased out as soon as the desired behavior is consistently demonstrated, and they should not be used more than two to three times to avoid dependency on the lure (Figure 3.3).

Shaping

Shaping is a more gradual method where variations of the desired behavior are incrementally reinforced. The trainer first defines the end goal of the behavior in precise terms. For example, a perfect "sit" might be defined as the dog sitting with all four feet on the ground and making eye contact. The trainer then starts by rewarding simpler versions of the behavior (e.g., the dog sitting with one foot raised) and gradually increasing the criteria. Over time, only behaviors that more closely match the predefined desired behavior (criteria) are rewarded, guiding the animal toward the final goal.

Figure 3.3 Continued luring can result in a behavior that only occurs when food is in hand and obvious. In this situation, the food becomes the cue itself rather than the reinforcement. *Source:* melounix/ Adobe Stock Photos.

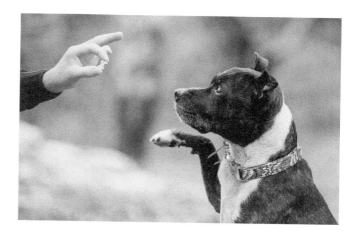

Each of these methods has its advantages and can be chosen based on the specific training context and the individual animal's learning style. They are essential tools in the trainer's toolkit for effectively teaching animals new behaviors and cues through positive reinforcement.

Pairing a Behavior with a Cue

When an animal consistently offers a specific behavior (fluency), it becomes appropriate to introduce a cue that will act as the stimulus for that behavior. Initially, this cue should be presented immediately before the behavior occurs. This stage requires careful observation of the animal to accurately predict when the animal is about to exhibit the behavior. Providing the cue at this precise moment helps in forming a clear link in the sequence of cue, behavior, and then reinforcement. As this process is repeated, the animal starts to recognize that responding to the cue with the appropriate behavior will lead to a reward. The ultimate goal is to gradually move toward a variable ratio reinforcement schedule, which helps in maintaining the behavior over the long term by making it more resistant to extinction.

Cues versus Commands

In animal training, the words *cue* and *command* are often used interchangeably, but they have different meanings and different effects on the learner.

Cues

Cues are opportunities for animals to earn rewards in response to correctly performing a desired behavior. The use of cues is a positive reinforcement approach, fostering good welfare and positive emotional responses in animals. If an animal fails to respond to a cue with the desired behavior, the typical approach is not to address or correct the lack of response directly. Instead, adjustments are made to the environment, such as reducing distractions, providing prompts, lowering the criteria, and shaping the behavior.

Commands

In contrast, commands are instructions that animals are expected to follow to avoid unpleasant consequences and corrections. This approach can lead to the animal developing and displaying protective emotions such as fear, anxiety, or frustration and may decrease their overall wellbeing. Commands are not necessary for animals to learn and perform behaviors correctly and reliably. The use of positive reinforcement using cues is a more effective and humane training method.

Stimulus Control of Behaviors

Stimulus control of behaviors is a principle where an animal consistently performs a specific behavior in response to a particular cue, even in the presence of distractions. This control is evident when the behavior reliably occurs every time the cue is presented. For instance, consider the behavior of recall in a dog, where the dog comes to the caregiver on hearing a specific cue like "come." Consistency in reinforcing the recall behavior and repetition of this stimulus–behavior pattern are key to achieving successful stimulus control. Although establishing stimulus control can be challenging and requires time and patience, the outcome is a reliably trained behavior that enhances the bond and communication between the dog and their caregiver.

The Effects of Aversive Techniques

The use of aversive techniques in animal training is a subject of significant concern, particularly regarding animal welfare standards. Despite sometimes achieving the immediate goal of eliciting desired behavior or suppressing unwanted behavior, these methods do not positively alter the animal's underlying emotional state. Research has shown that positive punishment-based training methods are not more effective than positive reinforcement-based methods (Ziv 2017).

Aversive techniques, such as positive punishment and negative reinforcement, are known to induce increased levels of fear, anxiety, and stress in animals (Blackwell et al. 2008). These elevated states of distress can lead to various adverse outcomes. Animals may exhibit escape behaviors, increased vigilance, aggression, and pose a higher risk of injury to themselves, their caregivers, or trainers (Casey et al. 2014; Chance 2003; Sidman 2000). Notably, caregivers who have used punishment-based techniques on their dogs have reported a higher incidence of behavioral problems (Hiby et al. 2004).

Furthermore, aversive methods are ineffective in teaching animals what behaviors are desired (Ziv 2017). In contrast, positive reinforcement is far more effective in teaching appropriate behaviors and changing the animal's motivation for the original behavior. Studies have demonstrated that positive reinforcement-based training methods are more effective than those based on positive punishment (Ziv 2017). Dogs trained with reward-based techniques have shown higher levels of obedience and more successful recall abilities (Blackwell et al. 2012; Hiby et al. 2004). Importantly, humane training techniques not only enhance the behavior of the animal but also strengthen the bond between humans and animals, promoting better communication and overall wellbeing.

When a Trainer Is Needed

Before referring a client to a trainer, collect a comprehensive history to better assess whether the problem behavior is primarily a training concern or stems from deeper emotional or physical health problems. While trainers can be effective in addressing certain behavioral issues, they are not equipped to resolve underlying emotional problems through training alone.

If the problem behavior is suspected to be rooted in emotional issues and the veterinarian does not feel equipped to address these themself, it is advisable to refer the client to a specialized professional, such as a board-certified veterinary behaviorist (see later and Table 3.3). These specialists have the training and experience to handle complex emotional and behavioral issues in animals, ensuring that the pet receives the most appropriate and effective care.

Trainers versus Behavior Consultants

The roles of dog trainers and behavior consultants differ significantly, with each specializing in distinct aspects of animal behavior and training.

Dog Trainers

Dog trainers primarily focus on teaching dogs specific behaviors and social skills. Their work usually involves basic training and learning of social skills, such as sit, down, and how to walk nicely on a leash. Trainers may also work on more advanced training or activities like agility, flyball, and

Table 3.3 Specialty and training organizations.

	Certification	Requirements	Methodology
American College of Veterinary Behaviorists	Diplomate of the American College of Veterinary Behaviorists (DACVB)	Licensed veterinarian, residency program, publication of case reports and research, comprehensive examination	Comprehensive behavioral, physical, and emotional animal health
Veterinarian with special interest in behavior	N/A	Licensed veterinarian, interest in behavior, continuing education courses	Behavior-focused practice, less specialized than DACVB
Veterinary technician specialist	Veterinary Technician Specialist (VTS) in Behavior	Licensed veterinary technician, specialized training, published work, practical and written examinations	Focus on management, training, and behavior modification
Veterinary technician with special interest in behavior	N/A	Licensed veterinary technician, interest in behavior, continuing education	Focus on management, training, and behavior modification
Certified Applied Animal Behaviorist (CAAB)	CAAB	Doctoral degree in animal behavior, five years of professional experience (or doctoral veterinary degree with two years in residency and three additional years of experience)	Applied behavioral analysis
Associate Certified Applied Animal Behaviorist (ACAAB)	ACAAB	Master's degree in animal behavior, two years of professional experience	Applied behavioral analysis
International Association of Animal Behavior Consultants (IAABC)	Certified Dog Behavior Consultant (CDBC) Certified Cat Behavior Consultant (CCBC) Certified Animal Behavior Consultant (CABC)	Minimum of three years and 500 hours of professional experience, 400 hours of related coursework	Least intrusive, minimally aversive (LIMA) methods
Karen Pryor Academy (KPA)	KPA Certified Training Partner (KPA CTP)	Coursework, written and hands-on components	Positive reinforcement techniques
Jean Donaldson's Academy for Dog Trainers (ADT)	Certificate in Training and Counseling (CTC)	Entirely online based, skills observed via video submissions	Positive reinforcement methods only
Victoria Stilwell Academy (VSA)	Certified Dog Trainer (VSA-CDT)	Course in positive reinforcement and basics of learning theory	Positive reinforcement techniques

Organization	Certification	Requirements	Method
Certification Council for Professional Dog Trainers (CCPDT)	Certified Behavior Consultant Canine – Knowledge Assessed (CBCC-KA)	At least 300 hours of experience, comprehensive behavior modification exam	LIMA methods
	Certified Professional Dog Trainer – Knowledge Assessed (CPDT-KA)	Knowledge assessment based	LIMA methods
	Certified Professional Dog Trainer – Knowledge and Skills Assessed (CPDT-KSA)	Knowledge and skills assessment based	LIMA methods
Control Unleashed	Certified Control Unleashed Instructor (CCUI)	Knowledge and skills assessment based	Positive reinforcement
Pet Professional Accreditation Board	Canine Training Technician (CTT-A) Professional Canine Trainer (PCT-A) Professional Canine Behavior Consultant (PCBC-A)	Online examination, video submission, PCBC-A (four written case-study reports)	Positive reinforcement

freestyle. However, their primary focus is not to address underlying behavioral disorders or emotional issues in dogs.

Behavior Consultants

In contrast, behavior consultants often take a functional approach to evaluating problem behaviors. Possessing a deeper understanding of behavioral analysis, cognition, and learning theory, behavior consultants often have advanced educational qualifications, such as a master's degree or PhD. They help caregivers understand the reasons behind their pet's behavior and how to apply behavior modification techniques to change it. While many behavior consultants are also certified trainers, this is not a requirement for their role. These consultants frequently collaborate with both certified trainers and board-certified veterinary behaviorists.

Board-Certified Veterinary Behaviorist

A board-certified veterinary behaviorist is a veterinarian with specialized training and expertise in animal behavior. These professionals are recognized as Diplomates by the American College of Veterinary Behaviorists (DACVB). Achieving this prestigious certification involves a rigorous and comprehensive process:

- **Residency program:** Candidates must complete a residency program in veterinary behavior under the mentorship of an existing DACVB. This intensive program involves hands-on experience and in-depth training in various aspects of animal behavior.
- **Publication of case reports and research:** As part of their training, these veterinarians are required to publish a case report. They also need to conduct and publish research in the field of animal behavior, with the results appearing in peer-reviewed scientific journals, contributing to the broader scientific understanding of animal behavior.
- **Rigorous examination:** Following the completion of their residency and research requirements, candidates must pass a two-day comprehensive examination. This challenging test assesses their knowledge and understanding of the behavior of all species of animals, ensuring they meet the high standards set by the American College of Veterinary Behaviorists.

Board-certified veterinary behaviorists are equipped to handle a wide range of behavioral issues across different animal species. Their training enables them to evaluate not only the behavioral aspects but also the physical and emotional health of animals. This comprehensive approach allows them to diagnose and treat complex behavioral problems effectively, often involving a combination of behavior modification techniques, environmental changes, and sometimes medical interventions. Their expertise is invaluable in cases where an animal's behavior is particularly challenging or when it may be linked to underlying medical conditions.

Veterinarian with Special Interest in Behavior

A veterinarian with a special interest in behavior is a veterinarian who, while not being a board-certified behaviorist, has chosen to focus on animal behavior in their practice. These professionals differ from board-certified veterinary behaviorists in several key aspects:

- **Level of specialization:** Unlike board-certified veterinary behaviorists who have undergone a rigorous residency program and obtained certification from the American College of Veterinary Behaviorists (DACVB), these veterinarians have not completed such an extensive specialization.

- **Continuing education:** Veterinarians with a special interest in behavior often enhance their knowledge by participating in continuing education courses related to animal behavior. These courses provide them with additional insights and techniques for managing and understanding animal behavior, though they do not equate to the comprehensive training required for board certification.
- **Behavior-focused practice:** Many of these veterinarians may choose to run a practice that primarily or exclusively focuses on behavior-related issues. This focus allows them to apply their acquired knowledge and skills in behavioral management and treatment.
- **Expertise and scope:** While these veterinarians are knowledgeable and skilled in addressing behavioral issues, their level of expertise does not match that of a DACVB. Their scope of practice in terms of treating complex behavioral cases may be more limited compared to board-certified veterinary behaviorists.

It is important for pet caregivers to understand the difference in expertise between a veterinarian with a special interest in behavior and a board-certified veterinary behaviorist, especially when seeking help for complex or challenging behavioral issues in their pets.

Specialty Veterinary Technician (Behavior)

Veterinary technicians who specialize in behavior represent a dedicated group within the veterinary field, focusing specifically on animal behavior. Like veterinarians who specialize in this area, these technicians undergo a rigorous process to gain their expertise, but there are also nonspecialist technicians who have a keen interest in behavior:

- **Veterinary technician specialist (VTS):** These professionals have completed a demanding training process that includes hands-on experience in the field of animal behavior. Their training often involves publishing work, and they must pass practical and written examinations. This level of specialization equips them with a deep understanding of animal behavior management and modification.
- **Veterinary technician with an interest in behavior:** Similar to veterinarians who have a special interest in behavior but are not board certified, there are also veterinary technicians who, while not specialized, have a strong interest in animal behavior. They may have pursued additional training or continuing education courses in this area.

Role in Veterinary Practice

Both specialized and nonspecialized technicians in animal behavior play an important role in veterinary practices. They assist veterinarians and veterinary behaviorists by overseeing treatment plans and coaching clients. Their expertise is particularly valuable in implementing behavior modification plans and providing guidance on management and training strategies for pets.

Limitations of Their Role

In the realm of animal training and behavior modification, there is no single, universal certifying authority, leading to a wide range of trainers and behavior consultants with varying levels of expertise and training methodologies. This lack of standardized regulation across different certifications means that professionals in this field come with diverse backgrounds and skills. Various certifications are available, each indicating a certain level of training and competence. However, these certifications do not necessarily guarantee that a professional is the ideal fit for every client's or animal's specific needs.

Certifications

When choosing a trainer or behavior consultant, confirm that their methods align with positive reinforcement principles and that they possess relevant experience with the behavioral issues being addressed. Organizations like the Certification Council for Professional Dog Trainers (CCPDT) and the International Association of Animal Behavior Consultants (IAABC) offer credentials such as Certified Behavior Consultant Canine – Knowledge Assessed (CBCC-KA) and Certified Dog Behavior Consultant (CDBC). These certifying bodies emphasize least intrusive, minimally aversive (LIMA) training techniques.

Additionally, well-known training programs such as the Karen Pryor Academy (KPA), Jean Donaldson's Academy for Dog Trainers (ADT), and the Victoria Stilwell Academy (VSA) provide comprehensive courses in positive reinforcement and behavior science. Graduates from these programs, who earn credentials like KPA Certified Training Partner (KPA-CTP), ADT's Certificate in Training and Counseling (CTC), and VSA Certified Dog Trainer (VSA-CDT), are all trained in humane, positive reinforcement-based methods.

Despite the ethical standards and requirements set by these certifying organizations, it remains important to conduct thorough research and screening to select a professional whose approach and expertise align with the client's specific needs and the animal's behavioral challenges. This careful selection ensures that the trainer or consultant can effectively address the unique situations and requirements presented by each case.

How to Choose a Trainer

When guiding clients in choosing a trainer for their pets, emphasize the importance of selecting someone who promotes the human–animal bond and prioritizes animal welfare. Encourage clients to seek trainers who use positive reinforcement methods, utilizing treats as rewards to motivate desired behaviors instead of viewing them as "bribes." Ask trainers about their approach when an animal performs a behavior correctly or makes a mistake in order to more fully understand their methods. Request to observe a class in order to watch the trainers interacting with both clients and animals. Everyone – including the animal – should feel comfortable with the interactions at all times, and the most subtle cues indicating discomfort should be recognized and addressed.

Trainers who use aversive methods should not be recommended, as these techniques result in increased fear, anxiety, and stress, leading to potential miscommunication and increased risk of injury (Deldalle and Gaunet 2014; Ziv 2017). This includes trainers labeled as "balanced" who use both positive and negative reinforcement and punishment, as well as those advertising using terms like "alpha" or "dominant." Trainers who use an aversive collar of any kind (which may be termed electric collar, shock collar, stim collar, e-collar, prong collar, choke collar, or bark collar) should not be recommended (Blackwell and Casey 2006; China et al. 2020; Cooper et al. 2014; Fernandes et al. 2017; Herron et al. 2009; Masson et al. 2018; Overall 2007; Ziv 2017). These types of collars can result in an increase in fear, anxiety, frustration, and stress, even if the trainer is experienced with their use (Cooper et al. 2014; Schilder and Borg 2004; Steiss et al. 2007). They also lead to an increase in aggression as well as a decrease in warning behaviors (Polsky 2000). In general, trainers who use aversive techniques can not only fail to help the dog but can actually create problem behaviors.

Furthermore, it is important for trainers to be honest and transparent about their capabilities. No trainer should guarantee complete success, and they should openly discuss their limitations and the types of problem behaviors they are equipped to handle. Some trainers may focus primarily on foundational skills rather than complex behavioral issues, but their work can still be valuable in establishing a basis for future behavior management efforts. Therefore, selecting a trainer should involve careful consideration of their methods, expertise, and the specific needs of the client and their pet.

Setting Clients Up for Success

When referring a client to a trainer, guide them in setting realistic expectations for the training process. The more knowledge clients have about dog training programs and classes, the more likely they are to understand the benefits and limitations of those options. This will help them to choose a trainer who better meets their needs and aligns with their goals.

Engaging in open and transparent discussions with clients about the capabilities and assistance that trainers can provide is essential. Clearly explain to clients the importance of their involvement in the training program. The success of any given training program depends not only on the dog learning the desired behaviors but also on the client's active participation (Stevens et al. 2021). The interactions and behaviors of caregivers toward their dogs significantly influence the dogs' behavior. Regular and consistent interactions can lead to marked improvements in behavior, while inconsistency can contribute to increased anxiety and fearfulness in dogs (Arhant et al. 2010). Additionally, a strong and positive connection between the dog and their caregiver is a key factor in the success of the training (Stevens et al. 2021). It is therefore imperative that caregivers learn and practice appropriate ways of interacting with their dogs to maximize the chances of a successful training outcome.

Furthermore, active client involvement in dog training can significantly enhance the human–animal bond (Clark and Boyer 1993). This is particularly true when training methods are based on positive reinforcement. A robust human–animal bond offers numerous benefits, including reducing the likelihood of the dog being relinquished to a shelter and providing health benefits for the caregiver (Mondelli et al. 2004; Siegel 2011). Encouraging caregivers to be actively engaged in their dog's training not only benefits the dog and the caregiver but also has a broader positive impact on public safety and health (Stevens et al. 2021).

Conclusion

There are many resources available to help veterinary professionals and clients alike work with animals with problem behaviors. In order to effectively help a given patient, it is important that the veterinarian be able not only to recognize their own limitations but to appropriately refer clients to others who may be able to help. Creating a list of trusted professionals in the area, such as behavior modification experts, can enhance the effectiveness of behavior treatment programs. Forming a collaborative team that includes the client, trainer, veterinarian, veterinary technician specializing in behavior, and a board-certified veterinary behaviorist is key to increasing the success of these programs.

References

Arhant, C., Bubna-Littitz, H., Bartels, A. et al. (2010). Behaviour of smaller and larger dogs: effects of training methods, inconsistency of owner behaviour and level of engagement in activities with the dog. *Applied Animal Behaviour Science* 123: 131–142.

Blackwell, E. and Casey, R. (2006). *The use of shock collars and their impact on the welfare of dogs*. Bristol: University of Bristol.

Blackwell, E.J., Twells, C., Seawright, A., and Casey, R.A. (2008). The relationship between training methods and the occurrence of behavior problems, as reported by owners, in a population of domestic dogs. *Journal of Veterinary Behavior: Clinical Applications and Research* 3: 207–217.

Blackwell, E.J., Bolster, C., Richards, G. et al. (2012). The use of electronic collars for training domestic dogs: estimated prevalence, reasons and risk factors for use, and owner perceived success as compared to other training methods. *BMC Veterinary Research* 8: 93.

Casey, R.A., Loftus, B.A., Bolster, C. et al. (2014). Human directed aggression in domestic dogs (*Canis familiaris*): occurrence in different contexts and risk factors. *Applied Animal Behaviour Science* 152: 52–63.

Chance, P. (2003). *Learning and Behavior*. Belmont, CA: Wadsworth Publishing.

China, L., Mills, D.S., and Cooper, J.J. (2020). Efficacy of dog training with and without remote electronic collars vs. a focus on positive reinforcement. *Frontiers in Veterinary. Science* 7: 547533.

Clark, G.I. and Boyer, W.N. (1993). The effects of dog obedience training and behavioural counselling upon the human-canine relationship. *Applied Animal Behaviour Science* 37: 147–159.

Cooper, J.J., Cracknell, N., Harriman, J. et al. (2014). The welfare consequences and efficacy of training pet dogs with remote electronic training collars in comparison to reward based training. *PLoS One* 9: e102722.

Deldalle, S. and Gaunet, F. (2014). Effects of 2 training methods on stress-related behaviors of the dog (*Canis familiaris*) and on the dog-owner relationship. *Journal of Veterinary Behavior: Clinical Applications and Research* 9: 58–65.

Fernandes, J.G., Olsson, I.A.S., and de Castro, A.C.V. (2017). Do aversive-based training methods actually compromise dog welfare? A literature review. *Applied Animal Behaviour Science* 196: 1–12.

Herron, M.E., Shofer, F.S., and Reisner, I.R. (2009). Survey of the use and outcome of confrontational and non-confrontational training methods in client-owned dogs showing undesired behaviors. *Applied Animal Behaviour Science* 117 (1–2): 47–54.

Hiby, E.F., Rooney, N.J., and Bradshaw, J.W.S. (2004). Dog training methods: their use, effectiveness and interaction with behaviour and welfare. *Animal Welfare* 13: 63–69.

Lindsay, S.R. (2013). *Handbook of Applied Dog Behavior and Training*. Oxford: Blackwell Publishing.

Masson, S., de la Vega, S., Gazzano, A. et al. (2018). Electronic training devices: discussion on the pros and cons of their use in dogs as a basis for the position statement of the European Society of Veterinary Clinical Ethology. *Journal of Veterinary Behavior* 25: 71–75.

Mazur, J.E. (2016). *Learning & Behavior*. 8. Abingdon: Routledge.

McGreevy, P. and Boakes, R. (2011). *Carrots and Sticks: Principles of Animal Training*. Sydney: Darlington Press.

Merriam-Webster. (n.d.). "Learning." www.merriam-webster.com/dictionary/learning (accessed March 20, 2024).

Mills, D.S. (1997). Using learning theory in animal behavior therapy practice. *Veterinary Clinics of North America, Small Animal Practice* 27 (3): 617–635.

Mondelli, F., Previde, E.P., Verga, M. et al. (2004). The bond that never developed: adoption and relinquishment of dogs in a rescue shelter. *Journal of Applied Animal Welfare Science* 7: 253–266.

Overall, K.L. (2007). Why electric shock is not behavior modification. *Journal of Veterinary Behavior: Clinical Applications and Research* 2: 1–4.

Polsky, R. (2000). Can aggression in dogs be elicited through the use of electronic pet containment systems? *Journal of Applied Animal Welfare Science* 3: 345–357.

Schilder, M.B.H. and van der Borg, J.M. (2004). Training dogs with help of the shock collar: short and long term behavioural effects. *Applied Animal Behaviour Science* 85: 319–334.

Sidman, M. (2000). Coercion and Its Fallout. US: Authors Cooperative Inc.

Siegel, J.M. (2011). Pet ownership and health. In: *The Psychology of the Human-Animal Bond* (ed. C. Blazina, G. Boyraz, and D. Shen-Miller), 167–177. New York: Springer Science.

Steiss, J.E., Schaffer, C., Ahmad, H.A., and Voith, V.L. (2007). Evaluation of plasma cortisol levels and behavior in dogs wearing bark control collars. *Applied Animal Behaviour Science* 106: 96–106.

Stevens, J.R., Wolff, L.M., Bosworth, M., and Morstad, J. (2021). Dog and owner characteristics predict training success. *Animal Cognition* 24: 219–230.

Ziv, G. (2017). The effects of using aversive training methods in dogs – a review. *Journal of Veterinary Behavior* 19: 50–60.

4

Meeting Basic Needs, Triage, and Management

Cats and dogs, as domesticated species, have developed distinct behavioral patterns influenced by their evolutionary history. Understanding these behaviors is essential for providing appropriate care. Often a change in behavior is the first indicator of a medical issue. Recognizing these species-specific signs is key for more accurate diagnoses and timely medical interventions. Gaining a comprehensive understanding of the specific needs of each animal is important for meeting their basic needs, playing a significant role in reducing behavioral problems and promoting optimal welfare.

Measuring Welfare

The Five Freedoms, Five Domains, and Five Provisions are central to the understanding and evaluation of animal welfare, each highlighting key aspects of an animal's wellbeing. These frameworks aid in developing criteria and scales for assessing the welfare state of animals. Watters (2021) emphasizes that inaccurately assessing an animal's welfare can result in significant negative consequences, including behavior problems.

The Five Freedoms

Originating in the 1960s in the United Kingdom, the Five Freedoms have significantly influenced animal welfare, enhancing the quality of life (QOL) for animals. Initially conceptualized as ideal states rather than standards for acceptable welfare, as noted by the UK's Farm Animal Welfare Council in 2012, these freedoms are valuable guidelines but may not fully address all aspects necessary for a comprehensive welfare assessment (Farm Animal Welfare Council 2012; Mellor 2016a,b).

The Five Domains

Building on the Five Freedoms, the Five Domains model, introduced in 1994, offers a more comprehensive framework for assessing animal welfare (Mellor et al. 2020). This model represents a significant advancement through acknowledgment of the complexity of animal welfare, which encompasses both the physical and emotional states of an animal. These are integral parts of their welfare (Mellor et al. 2020). Even if their physical needs are met, animals still may experience poor welfare if they are in a negative emotional state (Mellor 2016a,b; Mellor et al. 2020). With this recognition, the Five Domains model broadens the understanding of welfare, emphasizing the need to address both physical and emotional aspects for overall animal welfare (Mellor et al. 2020).

Limitations and the Introduction of the Five Provisions

Recognizing the limitations in the concept of "freedoms," Mellor (2016a) identified two key shortcomings. First, the focus on "freedom" from negative experiences was often misinterpreted as implying their complete elimination, whereas the realistic goal is their minimization. Second, the original framework's emphasis on avoiding negative experiences was considered insufficient given the evolving understanding that animal welfare management should not only minimize negative experiences and emotional states but also promote positive experiences and emotional states.

The Five Provisions

The Five Provisions were developed (Mellor 2016a,b) to overcome the shortcomings of the Five Freedoms. Initially aligned with the Five Freedoms, these provisions were later updated to outline welfare goals for each provision. These updates helped guide welfare management toward both minimizing negative experiences and promoting positive ones. Incorporating aspects of the European Welfare Quality assessment system and integrating elements from all domains of the Five Domains model, this updated framework provided more accessible and clear guidance for animal welfare management, applicable to a variety of species (Mellor 2016a,b).

Incorporating Positive States in Animal Welfare Frameworks

In the context of animal welfare, which encompasses the Five Freedoms, Five Domains, and Five Provisions (Table 4.1), a fundamental principle across all frameworks is that the absence of negative welfare states does not necessarily indicate the presence of positive welfare states. The Five Freedoms and Five Provisions emphasize that true animal welfare extends beyond the avoidance of harm (Mellor 2016a). These provisions provide guidance not just for reducing negative experiences but also for actively encouraging positive ones (Mellor 2016a). This approach aligns with a broader perspective of welfare that advocates the cultivation of positive states. Similarly, the Five Domains model focuses on both physical and mental wellbeing, emphasizing the importance of promoting positive emotional experiences in addition to alleviating pain or fear (Littlewood et al. 2023).

Table 4.1 The Five Freedoms, Five Domains, and Five Provisions models.

Five Freedoms	Five Domains	Five Provisions
Freedom from hunger and thirst	Nutrition	By providing ready access to fresh water and a diet to maintain full health and vigour
Freedom from discomfort	Environment	By providing an appropriate environment including shelter and a comfortable resting area
Freedom from pain, injury, and disease	Health	By prevention or rapid diagnosis and treatment
Freedom from fear and distress	Mental state	By ensuring conditions and treatment which avoid mental suffering
Freedom to express normal behavior	Behavior	By providing sufficient space, proper facilities, and company of the animal's own kind

Source: Adapted from Mellor (2016a).

Within any animal welfare framework, genuine welfare is characterized by not only the absence of discomfort but also the presence of positive wellbeing (Littlewood et al. 2023; Mellor 2016a,b, 2017). A comprehensive and humane approach to animal welfare involves addressing both the physical and emotional needs of animals. Focusing on these aspects enables early intervention and helps prevent behavioral problems, particularly those that arise from poor welfare conditions.

The Five Pillars of a Healthy Feline Environment

Organizations like the American Association of Feline Practitioners (AAFP) and the International Society of Feline Medicine (ISFM) have adapted the Five Freedoms specifically for domestic cats, creating the Five Pillars (Table 4.2) (Ellis et al. 2013). These pillars move away from the concept of enrichment, traditionally seen as adding extra features to a cat's environment, to concentrate on the fundamental aspects of a healthy feline environment. If any of these pillars are not adequately

Table 4.2 The Five Pillars of a healthy feline environment.

Pillar	Questions to ask
1) Provide a safe place	• Can you describe the environment from your cat's perspective to make sure they feel safe in their home territory? • Have you taken into account any external factors or threats, such as outdoor cats, that might impact your cat's sense of safety at home? • Are there any specific external sights, sounds, or smells that might make your indoor cat feel unsafe or threatened? • Have you noticed any unfamiliar smells, noises, or the presence of other animals or humans inside your home that could be causing stress for your cat? • What do you do to make sure your cat feels safe and comfortable at home? • Do you have spaces in your home where your cat can retreat to feel safe? Can you describe these areas?
2) Provide multiple and separate key environmental resources	• Are there separate food and water sources provided for the cats in the household? • Are the litter boxes well maintained and accessible to all the cats in the home? • Do you have resting places at various heights, including some that accommodate only one cat? • How many scratching areas are available for the cats to use? • Are the cats fed in separate rooms away from other animals or with visual barriers, and are they at least six feet apart to prevent stress during mealtime? • Are water bowls placed away from the food areas to accommodate a cat's natural preference to keep food separate from water? • Are environmental resources available in multiple locations throughout the home, allowing cats to choose based on their sense of safety and accessibility? • Have you considered adding extra litter boxes in different locations to prevent house-soiling, especially when multiple cats are present?

Table 4.2 (Continued)

Pillar	Questions to ask
3) Opportunities for play and predatory behaviors	• Do you provide opportunities for your cat to express their natural hunting instincts indoors? • Have you considered using food-dispensing and puzzle toys to encourage predatory behaviors and mental stimulation for your cat? • How often do you engage in interactive play sessions with your cat, and for how long each session? • Have you experimented with various puzzle feeders and toy styles to discover what your cat enjoys the most, and are you open to adapting these as your cat's preferences change? • Are you aware that incorporating play and predatory behaviors into your cat's routine can improve their physical fitness and provide essential mental engagement?
4) Provide positive, consistent, and predictable human–cat social interactions	• Do you provide positive, consistent, and predictable human–cat social interactions for your cat? • Are you aware that cats often form social bonds with humans but prefer to interact on their own terms? • Do you respect your cat's preferences when it comes to physical interactions, understanding that they may not always welcome such engagement? • Are you knowledgeable about the proper ways to interact with cats in a respectful and gentle manner? • Do you avoid inappropriate physical interactions with your cat, such as vigorous petting, touching unwanted body parts, holding your cat against their will, or using hands for play? • Have you considered that inappropriate interactions can lead to anxiety and defensive behaviors in cats, such as biting or scratching?
5) Provide an environment that respects a cat's sense of smell	• Do you provide an environment that respects your cat's sense of smell? • Are you aware that cats have a far more acute sense of smell than humans? • Have you considered that fragrances commonly found in households, such as perfumes, scented candles, cleaning agents, air fresheners, and even scented cat litter, can potentially compromise your cat's sense of safety? • Do you understand that these strong scents can be irritating to your cat's delicate olfactory senses?

Source: Adapted from Ellis et al. (2013).

addressed, it can lead to deficiencies, potentially causing negative behavioral outcomes in cats driven by emotions such as fear, anxiety, and frustration (Ellis et al. 2013).

The Interplay of Physical Health and Behavior in Animal Welfare

Assessing animal welfare requires a multifaceted approach that includes behavioral observations, health assessments, and evaluation of the living environment. Often changes in behavior are the initial indicators of underlying medical conditions; therefore any recent or sudden changes in behavior need to be investigated and addressed. Routine veterinary care should include comprehensive physical examinations and diagnostics such as a complete blood count, serum biochemistry, and urinalysis. Being proactive and intervening early for medical conditions can significantly improve the success rates of treatment and intervention.

Choice, Control, and Agency in Animal Welfare

Agency in animal welfare means granting animals the ability to make choices about their environment and have control over those choices (Littlewood et al. 2023), involving cognitive and physical engagement. When animals have options, their stress is reduced and their overall wellbeing improves. Recognizing and understanding an animal's choice can sometimes be challenging. However, animals often make decisions that lead to positive outcomes; therefore, relying on observations of their choices provides insight into their preferences (Littlewood et al. 2023). Not all animals will choose to participate or "opt in" every time. Therefore, choosing to "opt out" provides just as much valuable information as when they choose to opt in (Littlewood et al. 2023).

One example of this is cooperative care training, which involves teaching animals how to participate in their own veterinary care and husbandry procedures. When animals are given the opportunity to consent, defensive behaviors and protective emotions are less likely to occur (Jones 2023). For instance, in dogs, a chin-rest behavior can signal consent for an examination or venipuncture. Just as placing their chin on an object or lap is a clear "green light" to continue, lifting their chin is a clear signal to say "stop." However, some may argue that this could be coercion for food. Therefore, to ensure true consent and not coercion, animals should have alternative choices in their environment that are equally enticing, such as a mat in a different area or free access to a special food-dispensing or puzzle toy (Horowitz 2021). This way, it becomes easier to determine when an animal is providing genuine consent rather than merely offering a highly reinforced, trained behavior in anticipation of food.

Quality of Life Assessments

The concept of QOL in animals is primarily determined by their mental state and influenced by the frequency of pleasant emotional states. It is another way to measure the welfare status of an animal, with more frequent positive states indicating a better QOL. QOL can be affected by factors such as illness and physical health. For example, discomfort or distress caused by a disease has a negative impact on QOL. However, if there is no impact on comfort or pleasure, then QOL remains unaffected (McMillan 2000).

Accurately measuring QOL can be challenging in animals, as they hide pain well and cannot directly communicate their thoughts and feelings. Therefore, their QOL is evaluated through subjective and objective measures, such as validated scales and behavior observation (Taylor and Mills 2007). The goal of these measurements is to improve QOL (Yeates and Main 2009), evaluate the effectiveness of treatment plans, assist pet caregivers in making decisions such as euthanasia (Belshaw et al. 2015), determine appropriate pain management, and identify the need for more intensive treatment and intervention.

The general steps involved in a QOL assessment are as follows:

1) **Important factors:** Start by recognizing factors influencing the animal's overall physical and emotional health, such as general well-being, movement, weight, pain management, and

behavior. Since every animal is unique, consider the caregiver's viewpoint and the animal's specific circumstances and underlying health conditions when assessing QOL.

2) **Emotional state:** Watch how the animal behaves and responds to their surroundings. These states are assessed on a spectrum from comfort to discomfort (McMillan 2000). Comfort means a calm and relaxed mental state with minimal unpleasant sensations (Kolcaba and Kolcaba 1991), while discomfort can come from things like hunger, pain, fear, or frustration. However, discomfort does not always mean the animal is suffering; suffering implies a more severe or prolonged state of discomfort (DeGrazia 1996).

3) **Basic needs:** Unmet needs significantly affect an animal's health and safety. Therefore, meeting an animal's basic physiologic needs, such as adequate nutrition, free access to water, shelter, and a safe environment, is essential for their QOL. Assessments should verify if these needs are met and address any deficiencies impacting the animal's health and comfort (Dresser 1988; Hunt 1997; Hurnik 1988; Littlewood et al. 2023; Mellor 2016b, 2017; Mellor and Beausoleil 2015; Odendaal 1994).

4) **Physical health:** Health problems, whether ongoing or sudden, can make an animal uncomfortable and restrict their ability to engage in usual activities (McMillan 2000; Morse et al. 1994), significantly impacting their QOL. Therefore, it is important to thoroughly assess an animal's health to identify and address any underlying conditions that may be affecting their daily life.

5) **Agency and choices:** When an animal feels they lack control or choices, they may experience learned helplessness or emotional shutdown due to the inability to change their current situation. This lack of choices and control can lead to protective emotions and a lower QOL (Friedman et al. 2021; Littlewood et al. 2023; McMillan 2000; Seligman 1975). Assessing the living environment and daily routine helps identify opportunities for the animal to make their own choices, such as hiding, interacting with others, or engaging in normal behaviors (Littlewood et al. 2023).

6) **Social relationships:** Dogs are a social species, while cats are selectively social. Opportunities for social interaction with other animals or humans can enhance wellbeing, while isolation or inadequate opportunities for social relationships can lead to stress and protective emotions, thereby decreasing QOL (Baqueiro-Espinosa et al. 2023; Corsetti et al. 2023; Lamon et al. 2021; McMillan 2000; Mellor et al. 2020; Voith and Borchelt 1985).

7) **Health parameters:** Use validated tools and measurements to evaluate an animal's physical wellbeing, including mobility, pain levels, behavior, weight, and eating habits (Belshaw and Yeates 2018; Belshaw et al. 2015; Cobb et al. 2021; Fulmer et al. 2022; Reid et al. 2013; Roberts et al. 2021). This assessment helps understand how these factors affect the animal's QOL, which can differ depending on individual needs. For instance, a diabetic dog requires specific monitoring such as blood sugar levels and insulin dosages, while for a healthy dog the focus is more on preventative care and weight management.

8) **Comprehensive assessment:** After identifying relevant factors, conduct a thorough evaluation. This involves observing and documenting the animal's behavior and physical condition. For example, veterinarians may track an animal's movements, sleep patterns, appetite, and reactions to their surroundings, people, or other animals.

9) **Prioritize:** Evaluate each factor based on its significance and its effect on the animal's overall wellbeing and comfort. This may involve a balancing act, as what might be minor in one case could be critical in another. It might mean addressing urgent issues like severe pain before less urgent concerns.

10) **Decisions and recommendations:** Improving an animal's QOL entails addressing both their immediate and long-term needs. Depending on the assessment and the significance of

each factor, treatment plans may need adjustments. This could involve implementing new pain management strategies or making difficult decisions such as euthanasia. Other options might include changing the environment, diet, or behavior. Collaboration among veterinarians, pet caregivers, and other animal care professionals ensures decisions are made in the animal's best interest (Yeates et al. 2011).

There is an example of a QOL assessment in Table 4.3. Tiger is an indoor-only, male, neutered cat who was adopted from the shelter and is approximately seven years of age, with a body

Table 4.3 Example of a quality-of-life assessment.

Assessment category	Details for Tiger
Important factors	Life satisfaction: comfortable, limited outdoor access Mobility: reduced, overweight Weight management: critical, due to obesity Pain control: potential future issue Behavioral health: good, monitor for changes
Emotional state	Comfort: content in sunny spots, relaxed Discomfort: difficulty grooming due to weight
Basic needs	Nutrition: needs controlled diet plan Hydration: adequate Shelter: safe, comfortable, indoor environment Safety: protected but limited exercise options
Physical health	Chronic health issues: obesity, potential for diabetes, potential for osteoarthritis Activity limitation: struggles with agility due to weight
Agency and choices	Environmental control: limited due to indoor living Routine: stable but lacks variety
Social relationships	Interaction with humans: affectionate, enjoys company Interaction with other animals: limited, potential enrichment
Health parameters	Mobility: limited due to weight Pain levels: not an issue currently Behavioral signs: content but less active Physiologic measurements: overweight
Comprehensive assessment	Movement: reduced agility and stamina Appetite: overeating, needs diet regulation Responsiveness: good to humans, less overall activity Behavioral observations: more sleep, less playfulness
Prioritize	Immediate plan: weight management Less urgent concerns: social interactions, environmental changes
Decisions/ recommendations	Immediate plan: weight management program Pain management: monitor for future needs Environmental modifications: indoor enrichment Dietary changes: reduced-caloric diet Social enrichment: increase play and interaction Monitor health: regular vet exams, consult nutritionist

condition score (BCS) of 7/9. He is the only cat in the home and loves to spend his day sleeping in the big picture window in the sun.

Overall, Tiger appears to have a good QOL. However improvements are needed such as weight loss to reduce the potential for endocrine and orthopedic conditions, as well as to facilitate grooming and good hygiene. He may also benefit from increased social interactions. Next let us explore how introducing a new kitten into the household to increase these social interactions and physical activity could change his assessment and plan (Table 4.4).

Table 4.4 Impact of kitten introduction.

Assessment category	Details for Tiger with kitten addition
Important factors	Life satisfaction: may increase with feline companionship Mobility: encouragement to move and play more Weight management: more physical activity anticipated Pain control: monitor if increased activity affects any pain points Behavioral health: monitor for adjustment period and signs of stress or engagement
Emotional state	Comfort: observe Tiger's reaction to the kitten, ensure a low stress introduction Discomfort: watch for any signs of anxiety or agitation due to the new companion
Basic needs	Nutrition: separate feeding areas to prevent food competition Hydration: additional water sources Shelter: ensure both have comfortable, private resting areas Safety: supervise interactions initially to ensure safety
Physical health	Chronic health issues: monitor if increased activity with the kitten affects his health Activity limitation: observe if Tiger becomes more active with kitten's presence
Agency and choice	Environmental control: introduce kitten gradually to Tiger's environment Routine: establish a new routine including individual playtime for each
Social relationships	Interaction with humans: continue current level of human interaction Interaction with other animals: facilitate positive interactions between Tiger and kitten, monitor closely
Health parameters	Mobility: expect increase in mobility due to play Pain levels: monitor for changes Behavioral signs: look for changes indicating stress or happiness Physiologic measurements: monitor weight with increased activity
Comprehensive assessment	Movement: assess improvement in mobility with play Appetite: ensure both cats have adequate nutrition, monitor food intake Responsiveness: observe Tiger's reaction to the kitten Behavioral observations: note changes in sleep, play, and grooming habits
Prioritize	Immediate attention: monitor introduction phase and Tiger's reaction to kitten Less urgent concerns: gradual adjustment of routines and environment for both cats
Decisions/ recommendations	Immediate actions: careful, supervised introduction of kitten Environmental modifications: create spaces for both cats, including hiding spots and perches Dietary changes: maintain Tiger's diet, adjust as needed for activity Behavioral therapies: encourage joint play sessions Collaboration: monitor interactions and body language between the cats, consult veterinarian or board-certified veterinary behaviorist if needed

In summary, the addition of a kitten could help to improve Tiger's QOL assessment through increased activity and weight loss. However, it will be important to make sure both the kitten's and Tiger's individual needs are met and to monitor body language and interactions between the cats to ensure the emotional health of both cats remains protected.

Pain and Grimace Scales

Another welfare assessment is to monitor pain and overall discomfort. Various QOL scales are available, with the best choice often being a validated scale, such as those proposed by Schneider (2010) or Niessen (2010) (Belshaw et al. 2015). A scale that is representative of the individual animal's challenges should be used since generic scales may not account for significant individual differences that impact QOL (Belshaw et al. 2015).

Pain plays a significant role in behavioral changes; therefore, regardless of the scale chosen, pain assessments are often paired with QOL assessments to provide important information about an animal's comfort level and overall welfare state. Pain assessments can also be performed independently from QOL assessments.

Assessing Pain

Assessing pain in animals is complex. Unlike humans, animals cannot verbalize their pain, and many species instinctively conceal their pain. Additionally, the manifestations of pain can vary significantly between species and even among individuals within a species, often presenting as subtle signs that are challenging to recognize (Belshaw and Yeates 2018; Bloor 2017; Caddiell et al. 2023; Gruen et al. 2014, 2020, 2022; Lush and Ijichi 2018). The tendency to anthropomorphize, attributing human characteristics to animals, can further complicate the recognition and treatment of pain in animals (Hernandez-Avalos et al. 2019; Nuffield Council on Bioethics 2005).

Using a Pain Scale

Although only a limited number of pain scales have been validated for use in veterinary medicine, this does not diminish their importance. These pain scales help objectively assess a patient's comfort level, allowing veterinary professionals to determine whether intervention is needed and if the treatment plan is successful. They provide a set of reliable, sensitive, and valid criteria, facilitating consistent assessments by multiple individuals, rather than relying on subjective personal judgments (Addison and Clements 2017; Enomoto et al. 2020; Monteiro et al. 2022).

Observational Bias

Observer bias can significantly influence the accuracy of pain assessments. Consequently, these assessments are often considered best estimates of the animal's actual pain experience (Bloor 2017). Despite this limitation, subjective assessments remain valuable, as objective measures like heart rate do not always correlate with pain levels (Brondani et al. 2011).

Grimace Scales

Grimace scales are a practical method for pain assessment, especially beneficial for horses, rabbits, rats, and cats. However, there is currently no validated grimace scale for dogs. Pain may manifest as subtle changes in facial expressions, providing insights into an animal's emotional state (Evangelista et al. 2019; Mota-Rojas et al. 2021) better than vocalizations or movement (Gruen et al. 2014, 2020). Such detailed observations of facial expressions contribute to a better understanding of an animal's underlying emotions, leading to a more accurate evaluation of their overall welfare (Descovich 2017; Evangelista et al. 2019).

Enrichment

Enrichment is important for the mental and physical health of cats and dogs, and it can be broadly categorized into two main areas: environmental and social enrichment.

Environmental Enrichment

Environmental enrichment aligns with the principles of "freedom from discomfort" and "freedom to express normal behavior." This type of enrichment focuses on creating a stimulating physical space and offering various opportunities to encourage natural behaviors and provide mental stimulation. For dogs, environmental enrichment can include a variety of walks, puzzle feeders, and toys. Similarly beneficial options for cats include high perches, scratching posts, and safe outdoor access or window views, catering to needs to feel safe, scratch, and observe.

Social Enrichment

Social enrichment falls under the "mental state" domain in the Five Domains model of welfare measurement. Being social animals, some dogs enjoy playing and interacting with other dogs. For these inherently social dogs, daily social enrichment should include regular positive interactions with both other dogs and humans. Cats, on the other hand, are more selectively social. For those cats that enjoy interactions, engagement with other cats or humans can be beneficial. However, the preferences of dogs and cats who are less social should be respected, and they should not be forced to interact with other animals.

Appealing to the Five Senses

Dogs and cats view and interpret their world primarily through their senses, and their sensory input is different from that of humans. Understanding and addressing the sensory needs of dogs and cats, as part of a comprehensive enrichment plan, fulfill their basic needs and encourage exploration of their environment. Sensory enrichment is also used as part of a management and behavior modification treatment plan (Table 4.5).

Food-Dispensing and Puzzle Toys

Interactive feeding toys play a significant role in the mental stimulation of dogs and cats, mimicking their natural foraging behaviors (Table 4.6).

Games

Games provide mental stimulation and physical exercise for pets. They can also be fun and engaging, facilitating the human–animal bond (Table 4.7).

Table 4.5 The five senses and enrichment.

Sense	For dogs	For cats
Visual	Toys mimicking movement (e.g., flirt poles) for tracking and chasing instincts	Moving toys for predatory instincts, paired with food reward once play session is over and toy has been "caught"
Sound	Calming music or noise machines to reduce stress, especially in crates, safe rooms, and kennels	Soft, soothing sounds, or quiet environments for stress reduction
Smell	Scent trails or hidden treats to encourage natural foraging behaviors	Catnip (if not too arousing) or pheromone diffusers to create calming or stimulating environments
Touch	Varied textures in bedding and toys, plus regular grooming for tactile stimulation	Grooming tools (brushes, combs) and bedding with different textures for tactile needs
Taste	Variety of flavors and food textures tailored to individual preferences Food-dispensing and puzzle toys prestuffed and frozen	Diverse flavors and textures in food, considering dietary preferences and needs Variety of food-dispensing and puzzle toys

Table 4.6 Benefits of food dispensing and puzzle toys.

Dogs	Cats
Puzzle toys that dispense food during manipulation engage their problem-solving skills.	Toys that release treats when batted or rolled cater to their natural hunting instincts.
These toys can vary in complexity, providing a range of challenges that can help exercise dogs' brains and encourage exploration.	Encourage cats to use their feet and claws in a manner similar to catching prey, providing both physical exercise and mental stimulation.

Table 4.7 Games as enrichment opportunities.

Dogs	Cats
Games such as fetch, tug-of-war, and hide-and-seek can be beneficial for some dogs. Monitor for arousal.	Interactive toys that mimic prey, such as feather wands, are preferred.
These games not only engage their natural instincts but also help in building relationships between dogs and their caregivers.	These toys capture cats' attention and stimulate their natural predatory behaviors. Such games provide a fun way for cats to exercise both physically and mentally.

Management Tools

To improve safety and as part of the management plan, a variety of tools are used both in the veterinary hospital and at home. These tools not only increase safety but also help to modify behavior. Some commonly used tools are listed in Table 4.8.

Table 4.8   Tools for management and behavior modification.

Equipment type	Purpose	Details	Suitable for
Harnesses and leashes	Safe and comfortable control	Front clip harness 4–6 ft lead for regular walks Long line for sniff walks and recall training	Dogs that pull on leash or are reactive Cats needing outdoor time as part of their enrichment plan
Gates and crates	Creating safe spaces	Used to secure a safe haven Provide security Manage pet access to certain areas where undesirable behavior may occur	All pets, especially useful in multipet households or for pets needing separation
Calming caps and anxiety wraps	Reducing anxiety and stress	May help pets feel safer and more secure during veterinary visits, car rides, or thunderstorms	Pets prone to anxiety or stress, especially in new or challenging environments
Ear protection	Dampen noises	Various products are available to use for noise-sensitive dogs and cats	Dogs and cats
Basket muzzle	Safety to reduce bites	Basket muzzles of various materials, sizes, and shapes Can be custom made Should fit properly (can eat, drink, and pant while wearing it)	Dogs Not appropriate for cats
Non-slip portable mat (bathmat, yoga mat) or platform	Stationing and relaxation exercises	Used for relaxation exercises but also for stationing as treatment station for husbandry and veterinary procedures Useful to manage counter surfing and other nuisance behaviors Provides a predictable location for leashing up and harness placement	Dogs and cats

Behavioral Triage in Practice

Veterinary professionals often encounter challenges when addressing the emotional and behavioral needs of their patients. Veterinary hospitals are busy, and appointment time blocks are typically short to maximize efficiency; however, these short time slots may not allow sufficient time to address simple behavioral questions or complex problems. This is especially true when the concerning behavior is not the original reason for the scheduled appointment.

Even when the behavior is the primary reason for the visit, caregivers may be hesitant to make changes or may question the behavioral advice given. They may also have unrealistic or mismatched expectations. Integrating standard behavior first aid or management recommendations can meet the immediate needs of pets and their caregivers as well as function as a potential standalone component within a broader behavioral treatment plan, improving QOL for both the caregiver and their pet.

Understanding Normal Behavior

When addressing behavioral concerns, veterinarians and their team members should have a basic understanding of normal behavior for both their canine and feline patients. This knowledge provides insight into animals' basic needs, which can then be used to educate and support caregivers whose pets may exhibit undesirable behaviors.

In dogs and cats a range of behaviors, including barking, jumping, digging, begging for food, counter surfing, chewing, scratching furniture, increased vocalizations, waking caregivers for food, jumping on counters, engaging in hunting behavior, and urine marking, are often perceived as undesirable and problematic by caregivers. However, these behaviors are inherent and considered normal for the species. While they pose challenges, effective management and a deeper understanding of their underlying causes are needed to address and potentially modify them.

Behavioral in General Practice

Behavioral problems are a significant factor leading to the euthanasia of dogs and cats, highlighting the importance of veterinary practices as primary sources of information and guidance on behavioral care (O'Neill et al. 2013; Salman et al. 2000; Scarlett et al. 2002; Siracusa et al. 2017). Given the prevalence of behavior issues, particularly among adolescent dogs and cats who statistically face higher surrender or rehoming rates, all team members should be well informed and capable of providing reliable advice or referrals.

When it comes to referral, the number of behavioral cases reported and referred is often higher for dogs than for cats. This discrepancy might stem from the more noticeable behaviors exhibited by dogs, such as vocalizing, damaging property, or displaying aggression in public settings. In contrast, cats' stress behaviors are often subtler and typically occur at home, making them less apparent. Caregivers may not seek guidance unless faced with aggression between cats or issues of house-soiling, indicating a need for veterinary teams to help caregivers recognize and understand their pets' abnormal behaviors.

Caregivers frequently explore solutions for undesirable behaviors from a variety of sources before seeking professional help. However, not all sources are credible. Because of this, the guidance provided by the veterinary team must be evidence based, accurate, and consistent. Team members should know how to differentiate between normal and abnormal behaviors and feel comfortable discussing these behaviors and potential solutions with caregivers, even if the caregiver does not recognize that a problem exists.

Challenges and Responsibilities in Providing Behavioral Services

Providing comprehensive behavioral services can pose challenges due to varying interests, competencies, and time constraints among team members. However, every veterinary practice should offer some form of management strategy for clients. Often welfare deficiencies and medical conditions can be identified when team members recognize behaviors that clients may find unusual or problematic (Camps et al. 2019). Therefore, all team members who interact with clients and animals should possess a fundamental understanding of the basic body language and species-specific normal behaviors and welfare needs of their patients.

In cases where the clients' questions exceed a team member's level of expertise, referral to a different team member or another qualified professional should be made. This ensures that clients consistently receive the necessary support and guidance regarding their pets' emotional welfare and behavior in a timely manner and from a reliable source.

The Role of Client Service Representatives

In a veterinary practice setting, the client service representative (CSR) often serves as the first point of contact for behavior cases, since they receive the hospital's phone calls and observe the patients and caregivers as they enter the hospital. Because of this, CSRs should receive the same level of education as other team members involved in direct patient care.

CSRs (receptionists) have a key role in the early identification of behavioral problems in both dogs and cats. Positioned in the waiting area, they are uniquely equipped to observe pets and identify signs of distress or anxiety. They should be well informed about the behavioral resources the hospital offers to support caregivers, both during the wait and throughout the visit. CSRs can also provide caregivers with a checklist to help them assess their pet's behavior. Recognizing undesirable and abnormal behaviors represents the initial step in client education. This recognition offers CSRs the opportunity to encourage caregivers to discuss any behavioral concerns with the veterinary team and to ensure these observations are documented in the pet's medical record.

Observations and Documentation

Team members should also be trained to identify patterns in patients' medical records that could signal a behavioral problem. Signs to watch for include regular purchases of pheromones, frequent buys of odor eliminators, caregivers' casual comments about their pet's behavior post visit, the presence of multiple pets in the household potentially leading to chronic stress, and visible bite or scratch marks on caregivers' arms, hands, legs, and faces. These signs can be indicative of a more serious issue at home and should prompt a discussion with the veterinary team.

Utilizing the Waiting Room for Education

The time clients spend in the waiting room is an ideal opportunity for education. Whether they are waiting to be seen, picking up their pet, or waiting while their pet undergoes diagnostics, these moments offer clients a chance to explore resources and information sheets provided by the practice. Tools such as posters and books can assist caregivers in visualizing and recognizing their pets' body language and stress indicators not only within the veterinary hospital but also at home. By filling the waiting area with behavior-focused books, brochures, and articles, the practice can spark interest in common behaviors observed in dogs and cats, stimulating conversations that may not have otherwise occurred.

Special Attention to Feline Welfare

Visits to the veterinary hospital are often particularly stressful for cats. Team members can significantly improve the cat's experience by employing simple actions, such as using pheromone-infused towels and blankets to cover cat carriers. Additionally, advising caregivers on how to position carriers away from dogs and providing carrier training and travel tips can make the journey more comfortable.

The stress experienced by many cat caregivers during these visits can also contribute to delays in seeking care. Incorporating questions about behavior into routine consultations allows veterinary practices to demonstrate their commitment to feline behavioral welfare and empathize with both the cat and their caregiver. Such an approach meets the immediate needs of the cat and reassures caregivers that the practice is prepared to discuss and address these important topics.

Physical Examination as the First Step

A complete physical examination is the initial and most important step in diagnosing and treating behavioral problems. This examination helps to determine whether the observed behavior stems from physical discomfort, sensory deficits, underlying disease (e.g., metabolic, dermatologic, gastrointestinal, neurologic), or something else. During this examination veterinarians should take the opportunity to gather a more comprehensive behavioral history, including the initial onset and progression of the concerning behavior. Medical conditions must be excluded as potential causes before a behavioral diagnosis can be made (Camps et al. 2019; Frank 2014; Mills et al. 2020).

Behavioral Consultations

When a behavior identified during a physical examination requires further investigation, it is advisable to schedule an in-depth, longer appointment. This approach allows the veterinary team to thoroughly research the behavior in advance, enabling more effective communication and realistic discussions about the pet's behavior, including potential diagnostic and treatment plans. In these extended consultations the veterinarian can determine the most suitable course of action or intervention for the patient's behavior, based on their level of comfort. Options might range from providing detailed in-house behavioral advice and suggesting management strategies with plans for follow-up to referring the case to a board-certified veterinary behaviorist or another professional with more expertise in the area.

Considering Affordability and Accessibility

When deciding on a treatment or intervention plan that is effective and feasible for the caregiver to implement, always discuss with the caregiver and consider their ability to afford and access the proposed options and have a backup plan. These considerations include the costs associated with extra visits, specialized behavioral therapy, or referrals. However, the primary focus of any plan should be on management and safety. The goal is to minimize potential harm to the family, the public, the patient, and other animals in the home, as well as to prevent the progression of the behavior.

Early Detection and Prevention

Regular veterinary health assessments conducted between annual visits can facilitate the early detection of both health and behavioral issues. These visits provide an opportunity for veterinarians and their team members to identify developing health conditions and behavioral changes. It is particularly important to monitor young pets for early signs of behavioral changes, as well as to identify new or progressing behavioral changes in older pets. Being proactive with prevention and early intervention helps to stop the progression of these behaviors, which are likely to become more problematic and more difficult to change the longer they go unaddressed.

Meeting Basic Needs

Discussing the basic needs of pets and their role in preventing behavioral issues early in the process can be especially advantageous. Educating all caregivers to recognize behavioral signs that may indicate pain in their pets is crucial, as pets often do not always show obvious pain indicators. Understanding and interpreting subtler signs of pain can help break the cycle of acute or chronic pain in both dogs and cats.

A cat's home environment needs to meet their unique behavioral needs. Therefore, veterinary staff should routinely inquire about the home environment and suggest adjustments when necessary. For dogs, asking caregivers about trainers, training methods, enrichment activities, and physical exercise is essential to ensure the dogs' basic needs are satisfied, providing an opportunity for early intervention.

Behavioral First Aid

Dogs

Behavioral first aid for dogs focuses on quickly assessing behaviors and managing them to reduce risks to the dog, the family, other household pets, strangers, and other animals, while also stopping the progression of the behavior. This approach involves modifying environments to minimize the potential for harm and emphasizes preventing the escalation of behavioral issues, often referred to as "stopping the bleeding." Making sure the pet feels safe should be a priority. When an animal feels safe they are less likely to growl, bite, snarl, snap, and scratch. While these management strategies may appear to be common sense, they are frequently overlooked, particularly in stressful situations. Therefore, it is always valuable to mention practical management solutions that are easy to implement (Table 4.9).

Table 4.9 Some strategies for managing common behaviors for dogs.

Behavioral issue	Strategy
Separation-related behaviors	Arrange for someone to pet sit.
	Enroll the dog in daycare, provided the dog enjoys interacting with other dogs, people, and the daycare environment.
	Arrange for the dog to spend the day with family members or friends.
	Take the dog to work.
Barking at, jumping on, or being fearful of visitors	Establish a safe haven or space for the dog.
	Use a gate at the entrance so the dog does not have access to visitors.
	Place the dog outside in a secure and enriched location.
Resource guarding	Place the dog in a safe space during feeding time behind a closed door or gate.
	Do not attempt to remove items from the dog or take away the food dish when there is food in it.
	Practice teaching the dog to trade up for items and food of higher value.

(Continued)

Table 4.9   (Continued)

Behavioral issue	Strategy
Aggression toward family members	Identify and avoid interactions that trigger the behavior.
	Avoid reaching for, hugging, or kissing the dog.
	Avoid all forms of punishment, including scolding the dog, telling the dog no, or physically punishing the dog.
	Avoid use of aversives.
Barking, growling, and lunging when on leash	Walk during off-times.
	Avoid triggers for the behavior (other dogs, people, bikes, skateboards, etc.).
	Find quiet, secure spaces to exercise your dog (www.sniffspot.com).
Fear and aggression at the veterinary hospital	Previsit medication +/− sedation for all visits.
	Basket muzzle training.

Creating a Management Plan

- **Understand the problem:** The first step involves identifying whether a behavior is normal or abnormal. Client education includes explaining that many behaviors perceived as problematic (e.g., digging, jumping up, licking, barking) are actually normal, species-specific behaviors. Solutions should aim to manage and redirect these behaviors effectively.
- **Identify and avoid potential triggers:** A complete behavioral history is needed to identify potential triggers for the behavior. Understanding the motivation behind behaviors and assessing whether medication could be beneficial are key factors. Understanding the frequency, predictability, and intensity of triggers can also help decide which medications are appropriate. Management and avoidance strategies need to be in place to keep the dog feeling safe and to stop the progression of the behavior. Any exposure to people, animals, or situations that may elicit unwanted behavior needs to be avoided.
- **Client education:** Educating clients and communicating effectively foster empathy and prevent the misinterpretation of situations as threatening, which may indicate the dog's inability to cope. It is advisable to avoid exposing the dog to environments that could trigger aggressive behaviors. Clear objective descriptions of the behavior are needed, and the use of labels should be avoided. Caregivers need to understand that the pet is not being "bad" or trying to "dominate."
- **Avoid punishment:** Instruct caregivers to stop all forms of punishment, whether physical or verbal. This means refraining from using stern voices, pointing fingers, making physical contact, and the use of aversive tools like spray bottles, electric collars, prong collars, shock collars, or choke collars. Instead, caregivers should remain neutral or move away from the dog.
- **Reward desirable behaviors:** Reward desirable behaviors using food, toys, and play. In conditioning relaxation and reinforcing calm, resting behaviors, avoid using a clicker and opt for lower-value rewards to keep excitement levels minimal.
- **Consistency among family members:** All family members need to maintain consistent interactions with the dog and have realistic expectations about their behavior. Often long-term management will be necessary, even alongside training and behavior modification efforts.
- **Establish a safe haven:** Create a designated area like a room, crate, or exercise pen, equipped with soft and comfortable bedding, soft lighting, and preferably no windows. Enhance this space by playing classical music or audiobooks through a Bluetooth speaker. Regularly encourage the dog to spend time in this area to get accustomed to it, preparing them for moments when this safe space is needed.
- **Foundational behaviors:** Caregivers should be guided to teach foundational behaviors using positive reinforcement. These behaviors include eye contact, targeting, responding to being called, and

relaxation, among others. To maintain consistency, these behaviors should be practiced and reinforced throughout the day, in various environments, and around distractions. This approach effectively teaches and reinforces alternative behaviors that can subsequently replace undesirable ones.

- **Environmental enrichment:** Puzzle and food-dispensing toys, along with foraging activities, offer opportunities for alternative sensory input in a safe environment. They promote problemsolving skills, exploration, independence, and engaging emotions.

Reviewing Past Strategies

When discussing a pet's behavior with their caregiver, gaining an understanding of the strategies they have previously used to attempt behavior changes provides valuable insight. Encourage them to offer detailed observations and avoid using labels. Such objective information can help identify necessary changes and adjustments. For example, simply adjusting the timing and location of where rewards are placed during reinforcement might be the only adjustment needed. Discussing the use of corrections presents an educational opportunity to clarify why certain beliefs, such as correcting "bad behavior" might not be beneficial. Being specific about the techniques and methods used in these training strategies impacts recommendations and adjustments that are made.

Exercise

Exercise plays an important role in physical and mental health, yet it should not be the sole approach for addressing behavioral issues. The goal of exercise is to have short, frequent walks. "Sniff walks," where the dog leads the way and is allowed to sniff and explore at their own pace on a long line, offer numerous benefits compared to longer, endurance-focused walks or activities. The welfare of the dog should always be the priority during walks. If a dog finds walks to be stressful, these should either be discontinued or modified. Alternative activities, such as playing games in the yard, sniff walks on a long line, or walking in areas with low population and traffic during off-peak times, can be suitable replacements.

Managing Frustration

Frustration in dogs can arise from inconsistencies in rewards or using intermittent punishment (Hargrave 2015, 2017; Jakovcevic et al. 2013; McPeake et al. 2019, 2021). Placing a physical barrier between the dog and the target of their frustration can sometimes make the behavior worse. Instead, engaging the dog in a different activity, particularly one involving food, in another area of the home is more effective. To prevent frustration from building, initiate these diversions well before the dog encounters the trigger and is at a safe distance from it. Dogs that show frustration often manifest this behavior in various interactions. Treatment should focus on providing consistent and predictable rewards, along with positive reinforcement training (Table 4.10). This approach fosters clear communication, which reduces conflict and uncertainty in situations where frustration occurs.

Cats

Cats have specific environmental needs that can lead to stress when unmet. This stress manifests in a range of behavioral issues, from urine marking to aggression. Addressing these behavioral problems effectively in cats often requires managing their environment. Encouraging caregivers to draw a map of the cat's environment, detailing areas for resting, feeding, and elimination, can be very helpful. Capturing the cat's environment on video can offer valuable insights into the motivations behind their behavior and help identify unmet environmental needs. Often simple environmental adjustments can help cats cope better with stressors that are difficult to change, such as living with other pets (Table 4.11) (Ellis et al. 2013).

Table 4.10 Emergency strategies for safety in dogs.

Purpose	Strategy
Avoid all triggers	Prevent exposure to targets or triggering environments.
	Teach family members how to identify body language indicating emotional arousal and protective emotions.
Reducing escalation of aggression	Avoid positive punishment in all forms.
	If signs of protective emotions are observed, remove the dog from the environment or, if unsafe, the person should move away from the dog.
Euthanasia decision	Maintain a list of local facilities equipped to board dogs with challenging behaviors.
	Spending time away from the dog can provide immediate relief from stress and safety.
	It also helps to provide objectivity when making decisions.
Dog–dog aggression	Basket muzzle training and complete separation (if fighting is occurring between household dogs).
	The dog should learn to love their muzzle and they should wear it in areas where they may encounter other dogs.
	Education for caregivers on how to observe body language helps provide opportunities to remove the dog from situations when uncomfortable.
Aggression toward a family member	Condition the dog to wear a muzzle and separate the dog from the family member who is being targeted.
	Use secure barriers.
	Avoid conflict, direct confrontation, and interactions (do not force the relationship).
Preventing dog bites in the home	Identify and avoid known triggers.
	Keep the dog feeling safe.
	Separate the dog when appropriate.
	Muzzle training.
	Food lures can be used for safe movement of the dog, avoiding direct confrontation or force.
Aggression between familiar dogs (within the home)	Both dogs need to be muzzle trained.
	Separate dogs into different areas, avoiding reintroduction without professional help.
Aggression toward other dogs (outside the home)	Avoid crowded and busy environments and times for walks.
	Exercise the dog in less crowded spaces like parking lots.
	Condition the dog to wear a muzzle and do not greet other dogs on a short-tight leash.
	Do not allow the dog off the leash.
	Consider exercising and playing games in the backyard instead.
Destructive behavior	Place the dog in a safe environment away from potential triggers.
	Use an exercise pen or crate only if the dog is comfortable with confinement.
	A pet sitter, day boarding, or daycare may be needed (if the dog is comfortable around other dogs, people, and the daycare environment).
Reduce anxiety or fear	Never force a dog to approach triggers (fearful stimuli) or enter environments that cause anxiety or fear (e.g., meeting new people, going to a store, or walking on a busy street), which can escalate emotional arousal and defensive aggression.

Table 4.11   Enhancing the emotional wellbeing of cats.

Aspect of cat care	Suggestions for enhancement	Comment
Multimodal enrichment opportunities	Adequate resources, resting areas, vertical spaces, hiding areas, separate feeding and watering stations, puzzle toys.	Meeting a cat's basic needs is the first step in treating all behavior problems in cats.
Scratching options	Offer a variety of scratch posts made of different materials, in different locations. Often the best locations are the ones in prominent locations around the house. Choose areas where the cat is most likely to scratch.	Cats have individual preferences. Position scratch posts in well-traveled areas and spots where cats are likely to scratch (e.g., next to wear they sleep). Use a variety of different materials (rope, cardboard, burlap).
Litter boxes	Distribute litter boxes in convenient locations (for the cat) throughout the house. There should be one on each floor. The size of the litter box is the most important factor – it should be big enough for the cat to turn around and not touch the sides.	Follow the rule of one box per cat plus one extra, all in separate rooms. This is also beneficial for single cats, particularly in busy households. Avoid the use of a liner. Place away from noisy appliances.
Toys	Use toys that are small, furry, or feathery and rotate them frequently.	Toys that flitter and float tend to attract the most interest. Fast and erratic movements, similar to those of fishing-rod toys, are popular among cats. Always end play sessions with a treat find to conclude the seeking cycle and reduce frustration.
Games	Playing games like fetch using balls, small toys, or scrunched-up paper can be fun for some cats.	Use tunnels or stairs to enhance the fun and stimulate more complex play behavior. Avoid direct use of hands and feet.
Positive reinforcement training	Start training at any age using food rewards. A clicker can be beneficial.	Provides social and mental enrichment, improves communication, and builds a positive relationship between caregiver and cat.
Pheromones	Cheek or mammary gland pheromones.	Pheromones can be deposited using a towel on new items or on items around the house where urine marking and scratching is likely to occur. Mammary gland pheromones may help to reduce social conflict among cats.

Emotional States and Environmental Stress

Educating caregivers about cats' emotional states and how to interpret their body language allows for early detection and intervention in potential behavioral problems. A cat's lack of engagement with toys or changes in resting place can be signals of stress or discomfort, not necessarily disinterest. Cats typically show nonconfrontational body language, therefore close observation of their interactions can help identify conflicts. Such signs may include a cat causing another to leave as they enter the room or cats choosing to rest in separate areas or on different furniture pieces. Hiding or seeking high perches on countertops, cabinets, shelves, and cat trees often signal environmental stress. These behaviors may also point to conflicts with other pets or humans in the home.

Management

Just as with dogs, the primary goals in managing feline behavioral issues are to manage the environment and avoid triggers. This approach minimizes the risk of injury to both humans and animals, prevents environmental damage, and reduces the occurrence of unwanted behaviors (Table 4.12).

Table 4.12   Basic management advice for cat caregivers.

Objective	Method
General advice	Stop all forms of punishment (verbal and physical).
	Ignore then redirect unwanted behavior and reinforce desirable behavior.
Damage	Cover areas that are scratched or urine marked with protective material.
	Use barriers to prevent access to areas where damage is likely to occur.
	Window film helps to reduce visual access to other cats or environmental triggers outside the home.
	Determine the reason for the damage (e.g., not enough or appropriate scratching posts, inadequate litter box numbers or location, conflict among cats).
Nocturnal waking	Close the bedroom door to manage space and privacy.
	Feed the cat using food-dispensing or puzzle toys to encourage engagement.
	Set up a remote treat dispenser to disassociate food from the caregiver.
	Install a cat door to a catio or provide access to the outdoors.
	Ensure adequate multimodal enrichment to stimulate the cat's senses.
	Remember that cats are crepuscular, meaning they may be more active at dawn and dusk.
Bringing prey home	Limiting the cat's outdoor access is the only way to reduce or stop this behavior.
	A catio could be used instead.
Vocalizations and begging for food	Provide multiple small meals per day via puzzle feeding.
	Understand that rubbing and vocalizing may also be a greeting, not just a request for food.
	Use a remote treat dispenser.
	Positive reinforcement training to teach alternative behaviors such as touch or go to a mat.
Play-related aggression	Avoid playing using hands or body parts.
	Use toys for short bursts of play, ending with a treat to minimize frustration and end the seeking cycle.
Aggression between household cats	Separate the cats.
	Provide adequate resources and multimodal enrichment to reduce environmental stress.
	In unavoidable situations, use thick protective clothing or blankets to remove cats if an altercation occurs.
Scratching furniture and carpets	Wash scratched areas with enzymatic cleaner.
	Use a cheek pheromone spray on scratched items and preferred scratching surfaces.
	Cover previously scratched surfaces.
	Provide suitable scratching items near these areas.
House-soiling (urine marking and toileting)	Make sure there are adequate resources (litter boxes, hiding spaces, vertical spaces, resting areas, separate feeding and watering stations).
	Clean soiled areas with enzymatic cleaner.
	Block the sight of outdoor cats using window film.
	Identify triggers for urine marking.
	Identify and treat underlying medical conditions.

Table 4.13   Resource management and placement in multicat homes.

Creating a suitable environment	Comment
Resources of plenty	All resources should have two access points to avoid blocking access.
	Provide individual resources (beds, litter trays, water, food) for each cat in a secure location, avoiding forced proximity during feeding.
Vertical spaces	Vertical spaces such as shelves are prime locations for cats.
	Provide varied cat trees and raised areas in every room used by a cat, with both open observation and a closed resting area.
Safe access in the home	Use tunnels and boxes, especially in hallways, with two openings to enable escape and safety while moving around.
	Shelves should allow cats to pass each other and should vary in height and angle to avoid confrontation.
Sleeping areas	Provide individual sleeping areas like beds or mats, sized for one cat only.
	Elderly cats should have access to ramps and low steps for raised areas.
Outdoor access and visibility	Provide secure access out a door or window into a catio for safety.
	Use window film to limit visibility of other cats or environmental stimuli.

Medical Conditions and Behavior

Behavior changes often signal disease, and both behavior and medical conditions can contribute to undesirable behaviors. Therefore a complete physical examination and any necessary diagnostics should be conducted to maintain the cat's overall health. Prompt diagnosis and treatment of medical conditions, along with adequate pain control, are essential for improving welfare.

Multicat Households

Cats tend to be selectively social and nonconfrontational (Seksel 2016). In households with multiple cats, the inability to resolve social tensions through ritualized body language can lead to ongoing conflict and behavioral concerns. Veterinary team members should be comfortable educating and advising caregivers on how to properly introduce new cats into the household. Understanding cats' basic needs helps team members provide environmental management advice and recognize body language that may indicate conflict between cats (Table 4.13).

Conclusion

The implementation of behavioral first aid and management significantly enhances the emotional wellbeing and quality of life of both dogs and cats. By understanding and addressing species-specific behaviors and providing appropriate environmental enrichment, veterinarians and their teams can profoundly impact the lives of their patients. Engaging the five senses through activities, along with effective management strategies, is key to preventing and addressing behavioral problems. Adopting a comprehensive approach to wellness and animal care not only benefits pets but also strengthens the bond between them and their caregivers.

References

Addison, E.S. and Clements, D.N. (2017). Repeatability of quantitative sensory testing in healthy cats in a clinical setting with comparison to cats with osteoarthritis. *Journal of Feline Medicine and Surgery* 19 (12): 1274–1282.

Baqueiro-Espinosa, U., Lo, T.H., Hunter, R. et al. (2023). Positive human interaction improves welfare in commercial breeding dogs: evidence from attention bias and human sociability tests. *Applied Animal Behaviour Science* 262: 105904.

Belshaw, Z. and Yeates, J. (2018). Assessment of quality of life and chronic pain in dogs. *Veterinary Journal* 239: 59–64.

Belshaw, Z., Asher, L., Harvey, N.D., and Dean, R.S. (2015). Quality of life assessment in domestic dogs: an evidence-based rapid review. *Veterinary Journal* 206: 203–212.

Bloor, C. (2017). Pain scoring systems in the canine and feline patient. *Veterinary Nurse* 8 (5): 252–258.

Brondani, J.T., Luna, S.P., and Padovani, C.R. (2011). Refinement and initial validation of a multidimensional composite scale for use in assessing acute postoperative pain in cats. *American Journal of Veterinary Research* 72: 174–183.

Caddiell, R.M., Cunningham, R.M., White, P.A. et al. (2023). Pain sensitivity differs between dog breeds but not in the way veterinarians believe. *Frontiers in Pain Research* 4: 1165340.

Camps, T., Amat, M., and Manteca, X. (2019). A review of medical conditions and behavioral problems in dogs and cats. *Animals* 9 (12): 1133.

Cobb, M.L., Otto, C.M., and Fine, A.H. (2021). The animal welfare science of working dogs: current perspectives on recent advances and future directions. *Frontiers in Veterinary Science* 8: 666898.

Corsetti, S., Natoli, E., Palme, R., and Viggiano, E. (2023). Intraspecific interactions decrease stress affecting welfare in shelter dogs: a comparison of four different housing conditions. *Animals* 13 (11): 1828.

DeGrazia, D. (1996). *Taking Animals Seriously*. Cambridge: Cambridge University Press.

Descovich, K. (2017). Facial expression: an under-utilised tool for the assessment of welfare in mammals. *Alternatives to Animal Experimentation* 34: 409–429.

Dresser, R. (1988). Assessing harm and justification in animal research: federal policy opens the laboratory door. *Rutgers Law Review* 4: 723–729.

Ellis, S.L.H., Rodan, I., Carney, H.C. et al. (2013). AAFP and ISFM feline environmental needs guidelines. *Journal of Feline Medicine and Surgery* 15 (3): 219–230.

Enomoto, M., Lascelles, B.D.X., and Gruen, M.E. (2020). Development of a checklist for the detection of degenerative joint disease-associated pain in cats. *Journal of Feline Medicine and Surgery* 22 (12): 1137–1147.

Evangelista, M.C., Watanabe, R., Leung, V.S.Y. et al. (2019). Facial expressions of pain in cats: the development and validation of a Feline Grimace Scale. *Nature Scientific Reports* 9: 19128.

Farm Animal Welfare Council. (2012). *Five Freedoms*. The National Archives. https://webarchive.nationalarchives.gov.uk/ukgwa/20121007104210/http:/www.fawc.org.uk/freedoms.htm (accessed March 21, 2024).

Frank, D. (2014). Recognizing behavioral signs of pain and disease: a guide for practitioners. *Veterinary Clinics of North America. Small Animal Practice* 44 (3): 507–524.

Friedman, S.G., Stringfield, C.E., and Desmarchelier, M.R. (2021). Animal behavior and learning: support from applied behavior analysis. *Veterinary Clinics of North America. Exotic Animal Practice* 24 (1): 1–16.

Fulmer, A.E., Laven, L.J., and Hill, K.E. (2022). Quality of life measurement in dogs and cats: a scoping review of generic tools. *Animals* 12 (3): 400.

Gruen, M.E., Griffith, E., Thomson, A. et al. (2014). Detection of clinically relevant pain relief in cats with degenerative joint disease associated pain. *Journal of Veterinary Internal Medicine* 28 (2): 346–350.

Gruen, M.E., White, P., and Hare, B. (2020). Do dog breeds differ in pain sensitivity? Veterinarians and the public believe they do. *PLoS One* 15 (3): e0230315.

Gruen, M.E., Duncan, B., Lascelles, X. et al. (2022). 2022 AAHA pain management guidelines for dogs and cats. *Journal of the American Animal Hospital Association* 58 (2): 55–76.

Hargrave, C. (2015). Anxiety, fear, frustration and stress in cats and dogs—implications for the welfare of companion animals and practice finances. *Companion Animal* 20 (3): 136–141.

Hargrave, C. (2017). Ouch! Understanding and reducing patients' frustration to improve patient welfare and reduce staff injuries. *Companion Animal* 22 (9): 510–515.

Hernandez-Avalos, I., Mota-Rojas, D., Mora-Medina, P. et al. (2019). Review of different methods used for clinical recognition and assessment of pain in dogs and cats. *International Journal of Veterinary Science and Medicine* 7 (1): 43–54.

Horowitz, A. (2021). Considering the "dog" in dog–human interaction. *Frontiers in Veterinary Science* 8: 642821.

Hunt, S.M. (1997). The problem of quality of life. *Quality of Life Research* 6: 205–212.

Hurnik, J.F. (1988). Welfare of farm animals. *Applied Animal Behaviour Science* 20: 105–117.

Jakovcevic, A., Elgier, A.M., Mustaca, A.E., and Bentosela, M. (2013). Frustration behaviors in domestic dogs. *Journal of Applied Animal Welfare Science* 16 (1): 19–34.

Jones, E. (2023). Preparing fearful dogs for vaccinations with cooperative care. *Animal Behaviour and Welfare Cases* 2023: abwcases20230011.

Kolcaba, K.Y. and Kolcaba, R.J. (1991). An analysis of the concept of comfort. *Journal of Advanced Nursing* 16: 1301–1310.

Lamon, T.K., Slater, M.R., Moberly, H.K., and Budke, C.M. (2021). Welfare and quality of life assessments for shelter dogs: a scoping review. *Applied Animal Behaviour Science* 244: 105490.

Littlewood, K.E., Heslop, M.V., and Cobb, M.L. (2023). The agency domain and behavioral interactions: assessing positive animal welfare using the Five Domains Model. *Frontiers in Veterinary Science* 10: 1284869.

Lush, J. and Ijichi, C. (2018). A preliminary investigation into personality and pain in dogs. *Journal of Veterinary Behavior* 24: 62–68.

McMillan, F.D. (2000). Quality of life in animals. *Journal of the American Veterinary Medical Association* 216 (12): 1904–1910.

McPeake, K.J., Collins, L.M., Zulch, H., and Mills, D.S. (2019). The canine frustration questionnaire—development of a new psychometric tool for measuring frustration in domestic dogs (Canis familiaris). *Frontiers in Veterinary Science* 6: 152.

McPeake, K.J., Collins, L.M., Zulch, H., and Mills, D.S. (2021). Behavioural and physiological correlates of the Canine Frustration Questionnaire. *Animals* 11 (12): 3346.

Mellor, D.J. (2016a). Moving beyond the "five freedoms" by updating the "five provisions" and introducing aligned "animal welfare aims". *Animals* 6 (10): 59.

Mellor, D.J. (2016b). Updating animal welfare thinking: moving beyond the "five freedoms" towards "a life worth living". *Animals* 6 (3): 21.

Mellor, D.J. (2017). Operational details of the five domains model and its key applications to the assessment and management of animal welfare. *Animals* 7 (8): 60.

Mellor, D.J. and Beausoleil, N.J. (2015). Extending the 'five domains' model for animal welfare assessment to incorporate positive welfare states. *Animal Welfare* 24 (3): 241–253.

Mellor, D.J., Beausoleil, N.J., Littlewood, K.E. et al. (2020). The 2020 five domains model: including human–animal interactions in assessments of animal welfare. *Animals* 10 (10): 1870.

Mills, D.S., Demontigny-Bédard, I., Gruen, M. et al. (2020). Pain and problem behavior in cats and dogs. *Animals* 10 (2): 318.

Monteiro, B.P., Lascelles, B.D.X., Murrell, J. et al. (2022). 2022 WSAVA guidelines for the recognition, assessment and treatment of pain. *Journal of Small Animal Practice* 64 (4): 177–254.

Morse, J.M., Bottorff, J.L., and Hutchinson, S. (1994). The phenomenology of comfort. *Journal of Advanced Nursing* 20: 189–195.

Mota-Rojas, D., Marcet-Rius, M., Ogi, A. et al. (2021). Current advances in assessment of dog's emotions, facial expressions, and their use for clinical recognition of pain. *Animals* 11 (11): 3334.

Niessen, S., Powney, S., Guitian, J. et al. (2010). Evaluation of a quality-of-life tool for cats with diabetes mellitus. *Journal of Veterinary Internal Medicine* 24: 1098–1105.

Nuffield Council on Bioethics (2005). *The Ethics of Research Involving Animals*. Southampton: Latimer Trend.

Odendaal, J.S.J. (1994). Veterinary ethology and animal welfare. *Revue Scientifique et Technique* 13: 291–302.

O'neill, D.G., Church, D.B., McGreevy, P.D. et al. (2013). Longevity and mortality of owned dogs in England. *Veterinary Journal* 198 (3): 638–643.

Reid, J., Wiseman-Orr, M.L., Scott, E.M., and Nolan, A.M. (2013). Development, validation and reliability of a web-based questionnaire to measure health-related quality of life in dogs. *Journal of Small Animal Practice* 54 (5): 227–233.

Roberts, C., Armson, B., Bartram, D. et al. (2021). Construction of a conceptual framework for assessment of health-related quality of life in dogs with osteoarthritis. *Frontiers in Veterinary Science* 8: 741864.

Salman, M.D., Hutchison, J., Ruch-Gallie, R. et al. (2000). Behavioral reasons for relinquishment of dogs and cats to 12 shelters. *Journal of Applied Animal Welfare Science* 3 (2): 93–106.

Scarlett, J.M., Salman, M.D., New, J.G., and Kass, P.H. (2002). The role of veterinary practitioners in reducing dog and cat relinquishments and euthanasias. *Journal of the American Veterinary Medical Association* 220 (3): 306–311.

Schneider, T.R., Lyons, J.B., Tetrick, M.A., and Accortt, E.E. (2010). Multidimensional quality of life and human-animal bond measures for companion dogs. *Journal of Veterinary Behavior: Clinical Applications and Research* 5: 287–301.

Seksel, K. (2016). *Providing appropriate behavioral care. Feline Behavioral Health* (ed. I. Rodan and S. Heath), 90–100. Philadelphia, PA: Elsevier.

Seligman, M.E. (1975). *Helplessness: On Depression, Development, and Death*. New York: W. H. Freeman.

Siracusa, C., Provoost, L., and Reisner, I.R. (2017). Dog-and owner-related risk factors for consideration of euthanasia or rehoming before a referral behavioral consultation and for euthanizing or rehoming the dog after the consultation. *Journal of Veterinary Behavior* 22: 46–56.

Taylor, K.D. and Mills, D.S. (2007). Is quality of life a useful concept for companion animals? *Animal Welfare* 16: 55–65.

Voith, V.L. and Borchelt, P.L. (1985). Separation anxiety in dogs. *Compendium on Continuing Education for the Practicing Veterinarian* 7: 42–52.

Watters, J.V., Krebs, B.L., and Eschmann, C.L. (2021). Assessing animal welfare with behavior: onward with caution. *Journal of Zoological and Botanical Gardens* 2 (1): 75–87.

Yeates, J. and Main, D. (2009). Assessment of companion animal quality of life in veterinary practice and research. *Journal of Small Animal Practice* 50: 274–281.

Yeates, J.W., Mullan, S., Stone, M., and Main, D.C.J. (2011). Promoting discussions and decisions about dogs' quality-of-life. *Journal of Small Animal Practice* 52 (9): 459–463.

5

Setting Puppies Up for Success

The early life of a puppy is marked by a series of developmental stages, each playing an important role in shaping the puppy's behavior and physical maturation. These stages are categorized as neonatal, transitional, socialization, juvenile, sexual maturity, and social maturity (Scott and Fuller 1965). Understanding the events that occur during these stages and their impacts on a puppy's future behavior is important so that appropriate care and guidance can be offered to caregivers.

Furthermore, it is important to recognize that developmental rates can vary among different breeds, and environmental factors may play a role in influencing genetic expression (Morrow et al. 2015). The diet and health of the mother, or dam, are prenatal conditions that can significantly impact a puppy's development. Studies in other species have shown that offspring of mothers who experience stressful handling during pregnancy are often more sensitive to stressors (Champagne 2008). These findings highlight the need for a nurturing and stable environment throughout the developmental stages of a puppy's life, emphasizing the connection between physical, environmental, and emotional factors in their overall growth.

Developmental Periods of Behavior with Kittens for Neonatal Period through Social Maturity

Neonatal Period (0–2 Weeks)

The neonatal period, which begins with the birth of a puppy and lasts until about 13 days of age, is a critical phase in their development (Figures 5.1–5.4). During these initial two weeks puppies are dependent on their mother for survival. They are born with closed eyes and ears, which start to open toward the end of this period. At this stage a puppy's experience of the world is primarily through touch and smell, as their nervous system is still maturing (Houpt 2018; Serpell 2017).

In this phase puppies cannot regulate their own body temperature and thus heavily rely on the warmth from their mother and littermates. This warmth, along with physical contact, plays an important role in their early emotional development. The experiences puppies undergo in this period have a lasting impact on their future. Studies have indicated that puppies receiving attentive maternal care are more socially and physically engaged as adults compared to those with less attentive mothers (Foyer et al. 2016). Additionally, puppies that receive gentle human handling from as early as 3 days old are observed to be calmer and more confident at 8 weeks of age (Gazzano et al. 2008). This gentle handling not only affects their behavioral development but also contributes to faster neurodevelopment. This is evidenced by the earlier opening of their eyes and ears, as well as quicker hair growth.

Veterinary Guide to Preventing Behavior Problems in Dogs and Cats, First Edition. Christine D. Calder and Sarah C. Wright. © 2025 John Wiley & Sons, Inc. Published 2025 by John Wiley & Sons, Inc.

Figure 5.1 Newborn puppies spend most of their time eating and sleeping in the first two weeks of life. *Source:* Christine Calder (book author).

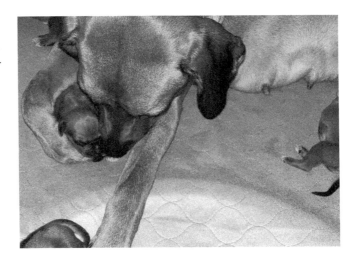

(a)

(b)

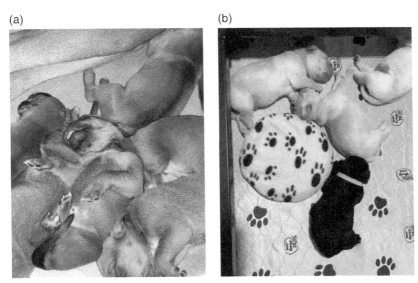

Figure 5.2 (a) During the neonatal stage puppies are completely dependent on their mother and each other for warmth. (b) An external heat source can help regulate temperature at this time. This one is warmed in the microwave to a safe temperature before placing it in with the puppies. It is important that they have an option to move away and there are various temperature gradients offered to them. *Source:* (a) Christine Calder (book author); (b) Rachel Thornton.

Figure 5.3 The mother licks to stimulate elimination and will ingest it. This is normal dog behavior. *Source:* Rachel Thornton.

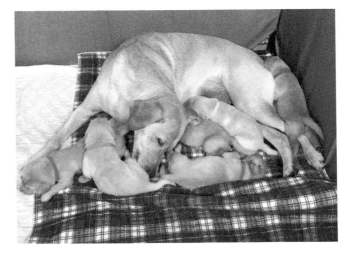

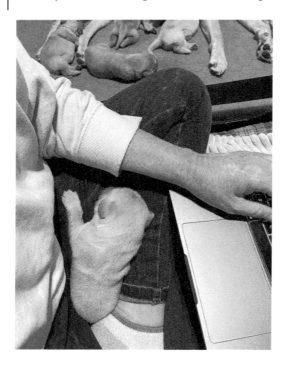

Figure 5.4 Early handling and time spent with humans have many benefits for a puppy's physical and emotional development. *Source:* Rachel Thornton.

Transitional Period (3 Weeks)

The transitional period in a puppy's development typically lasts around seven days, beginning as puppies open their eyes around day 13 and concluding when they start responding to sounds, generally by day 20 (Figure 5.5) (Houpt 2018). This stage is marked by notable advancements in visual

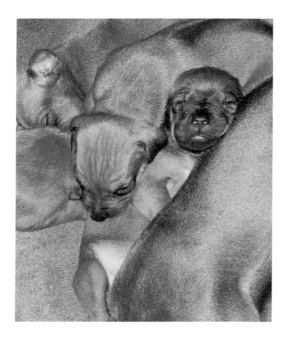

Figure 5.5 Eyes start to open at around 10–14 days. *Source:* Christine Calder (book author).

and auditory abilities, as well as improved muscle coordination. The onset of functioning eyes and ears leads to a significant change in how puppies perceive their environment.

During this period puppies acquire the skills to lap and chew food, eliminate waste independently of their mother's stimulation, and engage in physical activities like standing, walking, and tail wagging. Social communication behaviors such as growling and interactive play develop during this stage. As puppies become more mobile and explore their environment, their interactions with their mother and littermates grow in complexity. This helps them learn important canine communication skills, including bite inhibition and understanding body language cues, which are fundamental for social interactions among dogs.

As puppies increasingly move away from their nesting area, it is an appropriate time to introduce an elimination substrate (Figure 5.6). The ongoing development of their sensory organs makes it beneficial to gradually introduce various sounds and visual stimuli. Giving opportunities for puppies to explore these stimuli at their own pace and avoiding high-intensity noises helps create a nurturing environment that supports their sensory development without causing undue stress or sensitization.

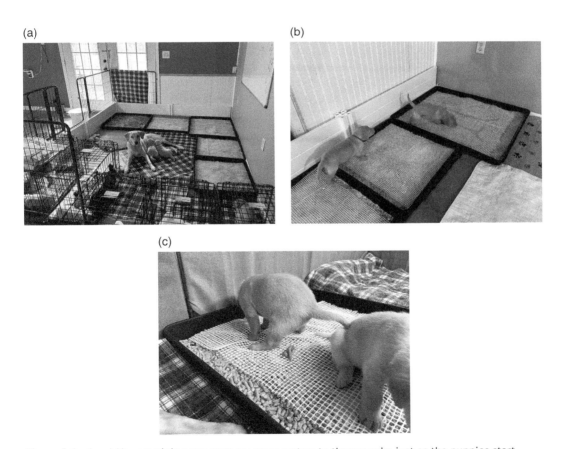

Figure 5.6 (a–c) Housetraining can start as young as two to three weeks, just as the puppies start to move around and eliminate without stimulation from their mother. Setting up elimination areas (large litter pans) can help with this and also helps to keep the whelping and play/exploration area clean. *Source:* Rachel Thornton.

Socialization Period (4–14 Weeks)

Socialization in puppies involves developing appropriate social behaviors toward their own species (conspecifics) and, more broadly, toward beings of any species while adapting to various environmental stimuli. The sensitive period, beginning at about 3 weeks and lasting until approximately 12–14 weeks of age, is critical for a puppy's development (Houpt 2018; Serpell 2017). During this time puppies are particularly open to forming preferences and are influenced significantly by external stimuli (Figure 5.7).

Quality over Quantity in Socialization

During the socialization period, puppies start to explore new objects, engage in social play, follow others, and form strong attachments. Lack of adequate socialization in this phase may lead to puppies developing fearfulness toward unfamiliar humans or situations (Scott and Fuller 1965). The focus should be on the quality of experiences, ensuring they are positive and suitable for the puppy's developmental stage, and avoiding overwhelming them with excessive stimulation (Figures 5.8 and 5.9).

Long-Term Effects of Early Separation

Weaning typically starts around 5 weeks of age and ends between 7 and 10 weeks of age and is an important time for learning social behaviors, especially with other dogs. Puppies separated from their dam and litter before 6 weeks of age tend to show more fear and undesirable behaviors as adults than those who stay with their litter until at least 8 weeks of age (Pierantoni et al. 2011; Slabbert and Rasa 1993). Sudden weaning and abrupt separation from littermates can result in long-term behavioral issues.

Juvenile Period (3–6 Months)

The juvenile period follows the end of the socialization period, which typically occurs around 14 weeks of age and extends until sexual maturity, at around 6 months of age. This stage is marked by rapid physical growth and building curiosity about the puppy's environment. During this phase puppies may exhibit behaviors that seem challenging to their caregivers, such as chewing on furniture or shoes, jumping on people, or seemingly ignoring previously learned cues. These actions are normal canine behaviors and a natural part of their exploratory and learning process.

Adolescent Period (6–12 Months)

The adolescent period in puppies, spanning from 6 to 12 months of age, marks a significant transition as they reach sexual maturity. Notably in larger and giant breeds the onset of sexual maturity may be delayed. This stage is often likened to the teenage years in humans and brings its own set of unique challenges for both puppies and their caregivers. As puppies reach sexual maturity, certain sexually dimorphic behaviors may become more pronounced. These behaviors can include urine marking, displays of aggression, roaming tendencies, and mounting.

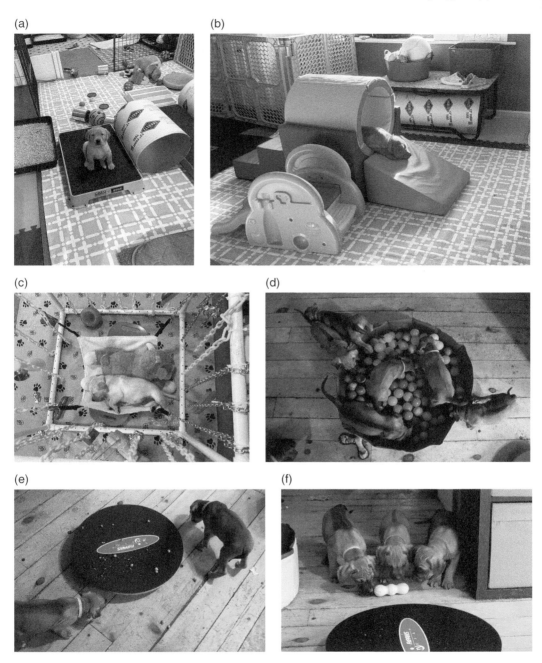

Figure 5.7 (Continued)

(g) (h)

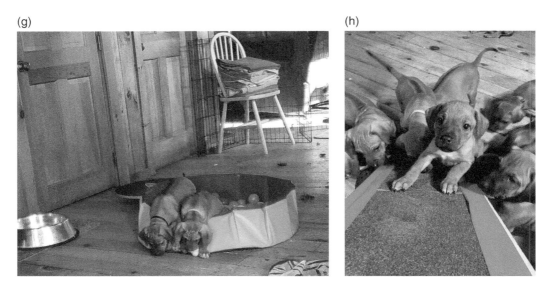

Figure 5.7 (a–h) Establishing a mentally stimulating and enriching environment while still living with the breeder helps set puppies up for success, builds confidence, and eases the transition into a new home. *Source:* (a–c) Rachel Thornton; (d–h) Christine Calder (book author).

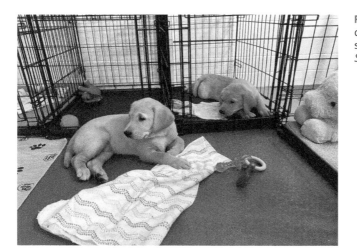

Figure 5.8 Confinement training can start with puppies while still at the breeder's house. *Source:* Rachel Thornton.

(a) (b)

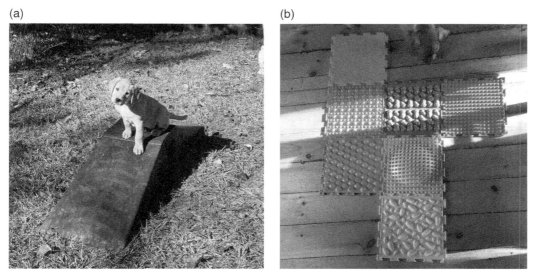

Figure 5.9 (a, b) Opportunities to explore different surfaces and environments help to build confidence and familiarity. *Source:* (a) Rachel Thornton; (b) Christine Calder (book author).

During the adolescent phase puppies may exhibit increased independence and can sometimes challenge established boundaries. Behaviors such as excessive barking, ignoring cues, or attempting to escape from the yard are not uncommon. Caregivers should be prepared for these changes in behavior during the adolescent period and continue to provide consistent training and guidance.

Social Maturity (2–3 Years)

As dogs transition out of adolescence and into social maturity, usually around 2–3 years of age, they exhibit more predictable behavior patterns. However, it is during the latter part of the adolescent period and the onset of social maturity that dogs are most frequently surrendered to shelters or rehomed due to behavioral issues. Understanding and effectively managing these behaviors are critical during this time.

Socialization: Understanding the Concept

The socialization process with a puppy should be begin as soon as possible, and continue as long as the puppy is not fearful (Figure 5.10). The caregiver's goals and future living environment should be considered in customizing a socialization program, incorporating stimuli relevant to the puppy's future environment.

Goals of Socialization

The main goal of socialization is to help puppies grow into well-adjusted adults who are comfortable and adapt to various situations and environments. This involves positive introductions to different people, environments, animals, and situations (Figure 5.11). Puppies should explore at their own pace, using treats and toys to enhance experiences. If a puppy becomes overly frightened, the session should end.

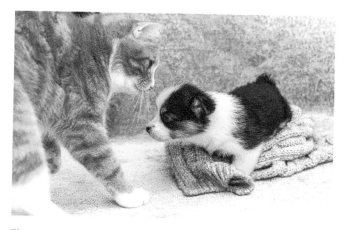

Figure 5.10 While young, interactions with other animals can help puppies learn appropriate social skills around these animals. *Source:* lusyaya/Adobe Stock Photos.

(a)

(b)

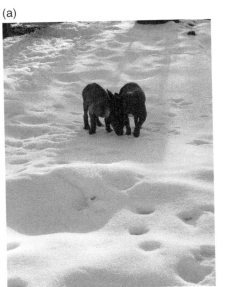

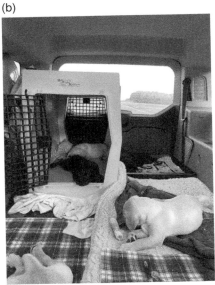

Figure 5.11 (a, b) New environments, interactions with other animals and car rides should all occur during the critical socialization period. Be sure the puppies are comfortable with these interactions and experiences. *Source:* (a) Christine Calder (book author); (b) Rachel Thornton.

Introducing Puppies to People

During the socialization process, puppies should be introduced to individuals of varying ages, genders, ethnicities, and appearances, including those wearing different types of clothing. Gentle handling by children helps puppies become comfortable around energetic young individuals.

Meeting Other Animals

Puppies should be socialized with other dogs and cats with supervision. Playdates with dogs of known vaccination status and various ages facilitate learning social cues and behaviors. This period is also ideal for introducing puppies to other animals they might encounter later in life, such as cats, chickens, horses, and goats (Figures 5.12–5.14).

Acclimating to Different Environments

Acclimating a puppy to different environments involves taking them for walks in both urban and rural settings, giving them an opportunity to experience different sights, smells, and sounds. For instance, walking on a busy city street exposes them to cars and crowds, while a hike in the countryside introduces them to wildlife and natural water bodies. Even simple changes like walking on different surfaces such as grass, gravel, or pavement can be beneficial (Figures 5.15–5.17).

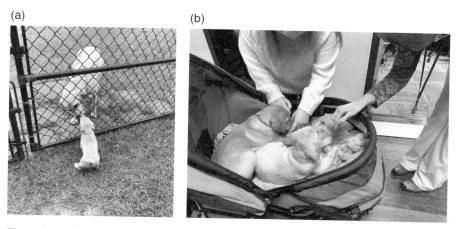

Figure 5.12 (a) Safety barriers such as fences help protect puppies yet give an opportunity to interact with other dogs. (b) Using strollers and carts gives a puppy an opportunity to be kept safe yet interact with people. *Source:* Rachel Thornton.

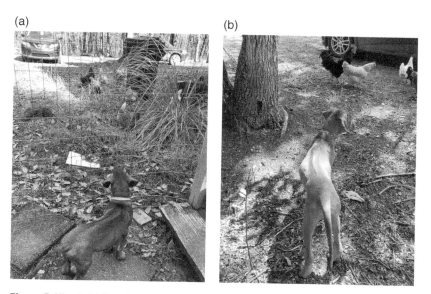

Figure 5.13 (a, b) Puppies should have opportunities to interact with other animals they may encounter or be expected to spend time around in the future. *Source:* Christine Calder (book author).

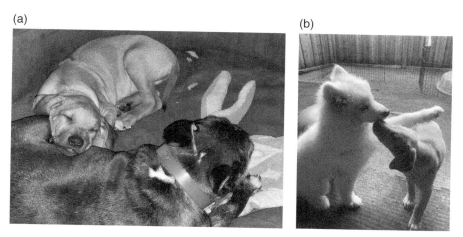

Figure 5.14 (a, b) Introduction to other puppies and adult dogs with known vaccination status gives opportunities for play and to develop critical social skills with other dogs. *Source:* (a) Christine Calder (book author); (b) Rachel Thornton.

(a)   (b)   (c)

(d)   (e)

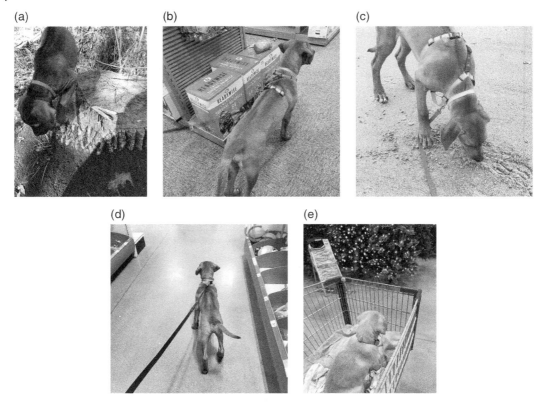

Figure 5.15 (a–e) Trips to dog friendly stores and various natural environments provide opportunities for puppies to experience new sights, sounds, smells, and people. Make sure the puppy is comfortable and interactions should not be forced. *Source:* (a–d) Christine Calder (book author); (e) Rachel Thornton.

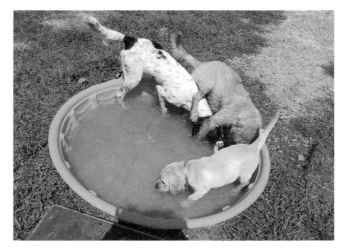

Figure 5.16 Different surfaces should be introduced including opportunities for swimming, especially if time will be spent near the water later in life. *Source:* Rachel Thornton.

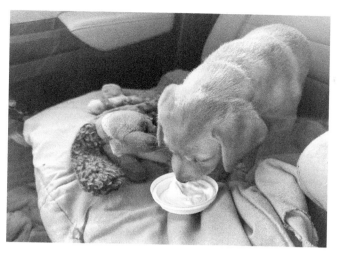

Figure 5.17   The addition of food helps to form a positive conditioned emotional response to situations such as car rides. *Source:* Rachel Thornton.

Familiarization with Various Sounds

Acclimating puppies to a variety of sounds is an important part of their socialization process. This involves exposing them to everyday household noises like the vacuum cleaner's hum, the washing machine's rhythm, and the doorbell's chime. Additionally, outdoor sounds such as traffic, sirens, and the noise from construction sites should also be introduced.

One effective method for familiarizing puppies with these sounds is to play recorded versions at a low volume initially and then gradually increase the volume. This approach, known as habituation, allows puppies to become accustomed to the sounds in a controlled, nonthreatening way. Alongside this, pairing the sounds with positive experiences such as food or playtime, known as desensitization and counterconditioning, enables puppies to form positive associations with these sounds.

By integrating habituation with desensitization and counterconditioning, puppies are encouraged to associate these sounds with enjoyable experiences. This strategy can significantly reduce the chances of puppies developing phobias or anxieties in response to these auditory stimuli later in life.

Gentle Handling

Gentle handling is an important part of behavioral development. Research shows that handling puppies from a young age can have beneficial effects (Figure 5.18). Puppies that are not handled until 7 weeks of age may be more hesitant to approach humans than those handled between 3 and 5 weeks (Freedman et al. 1961). If handling is delayed until 14 weeks these puppies often remain persistently fearful and resistant to handling (Freedman et al. 1961).

Regular, careful touching of a puppy's paws, ears, and mouth helps prepare them for routine experiences such as grooming sessions and veterinary examinations. Handling should always be a positive experience from the puppy's perspective. The puppy should always have a choice to engage

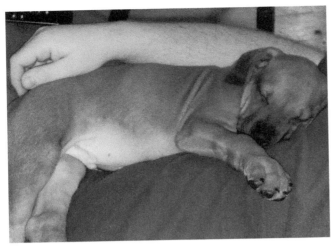

Figure 5.18 Early handling helps build trusting relationships with people. *Source:* Christine Calder (book author).

or walk away. Providing treats during the handling process can make it a more enjoyable and rewarding experience for the puppy. This approach not only familiarizes them with being handled but also helps in building trust and a sense of safety around humans (Figure 5.19).

(a)
(b)

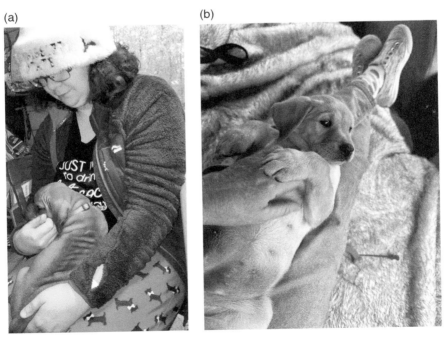

Figure 5.19 (a, b) Gentle handling helps a puppy to feel more comfortable and prepare them for the future. Puppies should always have the option to leave if they choose. *Source:* (a) Christine Calder (book author); (b) Rachel Thornton.

Safety and Vaccination

During the socialization process, to minimize disease, puppies should not be exposed to areas frequented by unvaccinated dogs. Socialization classes provide an opportunity for a safe and healthy learning environment while minimizing the risk for disease transmission (Duxbury et al. 2003; Stepita et al. 2013). All puppies should be healthy and up to date on their vaccination requirements to attend.

Adjusting the Socialization Plan

For some puppies, especially those who seem overwhelmed by mild stimuli, the socialization plan should be modified. Fear should not be ignored or underestimated in young puppies. Unlike some developmental phases, puppies are unlikely to naturally "get over" their fears without intervention (Godbout and Frank 2011). When fear in puppies is profound, persistent, and still evident at 12 weeks of age, seek the expertise of a board-certified veterinary behaviorist.

Puppy Kindergarten Classes

Puppy kindergarten classes provide a structured environment for puppies to learn basic behaviors and an opportunity to socialize with other dogs and people. These classes also provide an opportunity for caregivers to learn about dog behavior, training techniques, and ways to effectively communicate with their pets.

Setting Puppies Up for Success

Housetraining

Housetraining a puppy can be straightforward if caregivers diligently follow five key steps: supervision, frequent elimination opportunities on a schedule, cleaning up soiled areas, avoiding punishment, and rewarding the puppy as they complete voiding. To maximize housetraining success, adult supervision is a necessity. Caregivers must be continually aware of their puppy's location and activities. If direct supervision is not possible, the puppy should be confined to a safe area.

Scheduled Elimination Opportunities

Frequent trips to a designated toileting spot out the same door and to the same area, preferably on a leash, helps establish a routine. Puppies typically need to go outside after waking up, during and after vigorous play (approximately every 15 minutes), and within 15–30 minutes after eating. Avoiding free feeding helps predict this timeframe.

Alternative Elimination Area

If the puppy does not eliminate during a trip outside and it has been an hour or two since their last elimination, they should be returned to their safe space where an alternative elimination area is available, like a litter box with appropriate substrate (turf or pellets) or a puppy pad. After 10–15 minutes return to the elimination area for another opportunity to eliminate and receive reinforcement.

Rewarding Good Behavior

Each time the puppy successfully eliminates outside, they should immediately receive a special treat. Keeping a jar of treats by the door can facilitate this process and make sure treats are easy to grab on the way out the door. Avoid punishing the puppy. Punishment leads to fear and teaches the puppy it is safer to eliminate away from people, making future leash walks for elimination frustrating.

Cleaning and Monitoring

If the puppy eliminates indoors, use an enzyme-based cleaner for clean-up. Keeping a log helps identify and maintain a regular elimination schedule. Monitor the puppy for displacement behaviors such as circling, sniffing, or wandering off, which often indicate an immediate need to eliminate. If the puppy starts to squat, calmly take the puppy outside without yelling. If the puppy needs to be picked up, a towel can be placed under it to reduce messes while being carried outside.

Understanding Individual Differences

Puppies usually form a substrate preference by 8–9 weeks of age. With consistency and patience most puppies can be housetrained in a short period of time, although it could take up to a year for them to be completely reliable. The timeframe for housetraining can vary based on breed, with smaller dogs traditionally more challenging to train due to their size. They have smaller bladders, resulting in a higher frequency of elimination, and are closer to the ground, making it harder to observe behaviors indicating the need to eliminate.

Troubleshooting the Process

Puppies require frequent elimination breaks and should not be crated for extended periods. Caregivers should always provide an indoor elimination area during the housetraining process while encouraging outdoor elimination. If a puppy eliminates in a crate, they may require a larger enclosure or a medical evaluation for potential medical conditions, confinement anxiety, or other separation-related behaviors.

Confinement Training

Confinement areas can be used for both short-term and long-term confinement. They have many benefits beyond housetraining, including teaching puppies how to self-soothe and be comfortable alone. For those who work from home, providing a safe space for the puppy to relax or play while work gets done helps reduce the development of separation-related behaviors. This confinement space also serves as an opportunity to develop important social skills and acts as a peaceful retreat

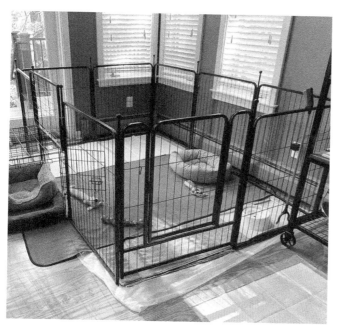

Figure 5.20 A long-term confinement space should have an elimination area, resting area, and watering station. The floor can be protected with a scrap piece of laminate flooring or washable puppy pads. *Source:* FXW/https://fxw.life/ (accessed February 5, 2024).

during busy times, such as when visitors arrive, children are playing, or during mealtimes, thereby reducing door dashing and counter surfing. Once the environment is calm or guests are settled, the puppy can be brought out for greetings and opportunities to reinforce calm and desirable behaviors.

Long-Term Confinement Areas

A long-term confinement area for a puppy is a space larger than their crate that includes an appropriate elimination area, play area, access to water, and a resting area (often the puppy's crate). The size of this pen should be tailored to the puppy's size but not so large that they might have accidents outside the designated elimination area. Such a setup aids in housetraining, prevents destructive chewing, "puppy proofs" the home from hazards, and teaches puppies that being alone is acceptable. By managing their environment, puppies can be guided to make better choices about where to eliminate, what to chew, and how to entertain themselves in the absence of their caregiver (Figure 5.20).

Placement of the Puppy Confinement Area

Choose a fully enclosed, easy-to-clean space for the puppy confinement area, free from items or furniture the puppy might chew such as a laundry room or bathroom where the door can be blocked securely. If a small room is not available then, an exercise pen around the puppy's usual crate area works well. This pen should be securely attached to the dog's crate or against a wall to prevent the puppy from knocking it over and escaping.

Using a Portable Confinement Area

If possible, having two puppy playpens is ideal. The first should be a more permanent setup attached to the puppy's crate. The second, a portable playpen, allows for flexibility, enabling movement throughout the day or for outdoor time. This portable pen should have access to water, a comfortable area to rest, and some puppy-safe toys or food puzzles. Add puppy pads if they are part of the housetraining routine.

Setting Up the Confinement Space

Setting up a playpen for a puppy involves creating a safe, comfortable, and functional space where the puppy can play, rest, eat, and relieve themselves while unsupervised. A pheromone diffuser can promote relaxation and calm behavior, but it should be placed out of the puppy's reach to prevent chewing. Providing chew and puzzle toys offers opportunities for licking, chewing, and problem-solving, which help form positive associations with being alone.

Age-appropriate exercise before confinement can help expend their energy, making them more likely to rest or engage calmly with their toys while confined. As the puppy matures, gradually increasing the size of their confinement area can ease the transition to larger spaces when they are ready.

A camera in the confinement area allows for monitoring, making it easier to observe the puppy and respond quickly if needed. There are many affordable options for cameras that record in real time with the addition of a SIM card and are accessible with a smartphone app (Table 5.1).

Table 5.1   Confinement space setup.

Crate or sleeping area	**Crate placement:** Position the puppy's regular crate on one side of the playpen, leaving the door open for easy access.
	Bedding: Use chew-proof bedding inside the crate. For power chewer puppies, an indestructible raised cot is a great option.
	Securing the bed: Tape down the dog's bed to prevent it from being pulled out and chewed. Opt for a bed that is durable and chew-proof for puppies likely to chew up their bed and the tape.
Designated elimination area	**Location**: Set up the elimination area as far away from the crate and sleeping area as possible.
	Setup: Use puppy pads or an indoor turf elimination spot. For puppies that push toys into their elimination area, consider a dog litter box with raised edges.
	Floor protection: Choose a location with durable flooring, like a laundry room or tiled kitchen, to avoid damage to more sensitive floor surfaces. Also, flooring remnants may be available at the local home improvement store that can be placed under the pen for floor protection.
Appropriate chew toys	Select toys that are safe for unsupervised play. Interactive treat toys are mentally stimulating, build confidence, and encourage exploration.
Food	**Feeding method:** Offer food in stuffed puzzle toys to engage the puppy.
	Tethering Kongs®: Tether Kongs® to the edge of the playpen to prevent them from rolling into the potty area. Thread a rope through the Kong®, tie a knot inside it before stuffing, and then tether. For avid chewer puppies, consider a different style of puzzle toy for safety.
	Interactive feeders: Explore various interactive feeders suitable for puppies to encourage active feeding.
Water	Place a spill-proof water bowl or hang up a no-drip water bottle near the sleeping area to make sure access to water is always available.

Table 5.2   Teaching a puppy to settle and be independent in their safe confinement area.

Step	Instructions
Elimination break or walks	Take the puppy out for an elimination break or walk.
Introduce the confinement area	Place the puppy in the playpen and provide a stuffed puzzle toy or another high-value chew toy.
Leave puppy alone for short periods	Allow the puppy to enjoy their treat alone for a few minutes. This step is important to help prevent separated-related behaviors and can be done while still at home or leaving for a very short period.
Low-key return	Let the puppy out of their playpen, preferably before they finish their toy. The return should be low key to teach that humans coming and going is normal and to give an opportunity to capture and reinforce calm and relaxed behaviors.
Gradually increase alone time	Repeat the previous steps, progressively increasing the time the puppy spends alone in their playpen. Begin by leaving the house for short durations such as checking the mail or taking out the trash. Gradually extend these periods to running short errands and other brief outings.

Independence Training

A basic skill for all puppies and dogs is learning how to settle and be comfortable when alone. A safe space can be used for preventative measures as well as an intervention and management strategy. When confined, if the puppy barks or whines and they are not in distress, do not ignore them but also do not immediately return to them, open the door, or speak to them. Responding to these behaviors can inadvertently teach the puppy that barking or whining is an effective strategy to get attention or to be let out of the confinement space. Instead, wait nearby (within sight) until the puppy has been quiet for at least 10–15 seconds before speaking to them and opening the door. This is the perfect opportunity to use a clicker and treats to reinforce calm and quiet behavior in this space or use a remote treat dispenser (Table 5.2).

Meeting Basic Needs

Meeting basic needs is fundamental to animal welfare. Although needs can vary by species, they typically include access to food and water, proper nutrition, healthcare, a safe and comfortable resting place, the ability to move according to temperature, appropriate exercise, and enrichment opportunities with both animals and humans (see Chapter 4). Positive reinforcement training, opportunities for choice and control over their environment, and positive human-animal interactions are essential for enhancing welfare and overall emotional health (Table 5.3).

Exercise

Exercise is a basic need for dogs, but the right amount varies based on age, breed, and health, even among dogs of the same breed. For example, an energetic, older Labrador Retriever might require more exercise than a younger, calmer one. Generally, dogs need 30–60 minutes of physical activity daily to satisfy their exercise needs, with the goal of achieving noticeable tiredness but not exhaustion.

Table 5.3 Enrichment options for dogs.

Category	Details
DIY dog enrichment ideas	Use household items like empty cereal boxes, toilet paper rolls, cardboard boxes, packing papers, and egg cartons to make homemade dog enrichment toys like food tube dog puzzles, DIY lick mats, muffin tin dog puzzles, and rolled-up treat burrito towels.
Enrichment games for your dog	Engage in activities such as a planned scavenger hunt, playing hide-and-seek, taking sniff walks, watching TV for dogs, and sitting with your dog to watch the world.
Create a dig area for your dog	Provide a designated area for digging using a kiddie pool, sandpit container, or a specific corner of the yard. Bury toys, treats, or chews for your dog to find.
Blow some bubbles	Blowing bubbles can be fun for dogs as they activate different senses. Use dog-safe bubbles with scents like peanut butter or bacon and consider a bubble blower machine.
Create a scent garden	Create a scent garden with dog-safe smells like lavender or rosemary or use dried herbs. Allow your dog to explore the new scents.
Food toppers	Increase meal enrichment with different food toppers or garnishes like wet dog food, dog-safe fruits, or vegetables.

Active breeds like Border Collies need at least 30 minutes of intense aerobic exercise almost every day. Smaller breeds, such as Beagles, often mistakenly thought to get enough exercise indoors, also require significant activity to prevent obesity.

Exercise alone is not a universal solution for abnormal behaviors like anxiety; mental stimulation is equally important. Activities like exploring new hiking trails provide opportunities for sniffing and exploring, which build confidence, improve social skills, and offer both mental and physical enrichment. In extreme weather, indoor activities that mentally engage dogs, such as teaching tricks or playing fetch, are safer options.

Positive Social Interactions and Training

Dogs are inherently social creatures, requiring positive interactions with both other dogs and humans. Over time, they have evolved to include humans in their social circles, actively seeking contact and showing distress when isolated. A lack of social interaction can hinder a dog's learning and social development, while positive interactions often lead to reduced stress and fear-related behaviors, providing long-term benefits.

Dog–Dog Social Interactions
- Dogs benefit from spending time with other dogs, as social play with other dogs enhances welfare differently than interactions with humans (Rezvani et al. 2021a).
- Group or pair housing for dogs and puppies offers essential social experiences. It is important to match dogs by age, size, and sex as well as to ensure enough space and resources are available to minimize conflict.
- Without sufficient social interaction, dogs may experience increased stress and exhibit undesirable behaviors.

- Dogs that are socially housed tend to be more active, bark less, and display fewer behavioral issues. They also show more positive behaviors, including play and sleep.
- Social play is beneficial for enrichment, the development of motor and social skills, and both short- and long-term welfare.

Introducing Puppies to Other Dogs

- During their socialization period, introducing puppies to friendly dogs is important to prevent fearful and aggressive behaviors later in life.
- Dogs can become selective about their canine companions as they mature.
- Each dog has their own comfort level with other dogs, and interactions should never be forced.

Dog–Human Interactions

- Time spent with human caretakers, including that involving touch and play, is essential for dogs (Rezvani et al. 2021b).
- Activities like petting and playing lower cortisol levels and reduce stress indicators, such as increased vocalization and panting. They result in decreased frustration and strengthen the dog–human relationship.
- Even adult dogs can quickly form attachments to human caretakers, who provide a "safe base" and help dogs feel secure around other people.
- Secure relationships with humans build confidence in dogs and reduce stress when encountering new situations.

Social interactions with both dogs and people are necessary for a dog's overall welfare. While playing with other dogs is important, it does not replace the need for quality time with human caretakers. Both types of socialization contribute to a dog's emotional wellbeing and physical health.

Foundational Behaviors

The foundation for a behaviorally sound adult dog is laid during the early stages of their development. Basic training should focus on establishing clear communication and reinforcing desirable behaviors. Socialization should involve positive experiences in a variety of environments, with different people, and with animals.

SMART x 50

The SMART x 50 method, created by Kathy Sdao (www.kathysdao.com) and highlighted in her book *Plenty in Life Is Free*, is a straightforward yet effective dog training technique. The method encompasses **S**ee, **M**ark, **A**nd **R**eward **T**raining with 50 pieces of food or treats (Table 5.4).

The essence of the SMART x 50 method is to shift focus from the dog's undesirable behaviors to recognizing and reinforcing the desired ones. By consistently rewarding desired behaviors, these behaviors are more likely to be repeated, effectively shaping the dog's behavior and building a repertoire of default behaviors. This method not only improves training skills but also encourages dog caregivers to actively look for and acknowledge their dog's desired behaviors, rather than focusing solely on correcting the undesired ones.

Table 5.4 The steps to SMART x 50.

Step	Instructions
Get treats ready	Prepare 50 low-calorie, high-value treats and store them in a bowl or container in a central location at home, out of the dog's reach. The treats should be appealing to the dog but also low in calories. These can be the dog's own food or a mixture of food and treats.
Observe behavior	Actively observe and identify instances when the dog exhibits desirable behaviors without being prompted. Examples include lying down quietly while watching TV, not barking at distractions, sitting instead of jumping, or going to their crate or bed voluntarily.
Mark and reward	On observing a desired behavior, immediately mark it with a clicker or by saying a marker word like "yes," and then give the dog a treat. This step reinforces the desired behavior, encouraging the dog to repeat it.
Repeat 50 times each day	The process of observing, marking, and rewarding should be repeated 50 times daily, which is where the name SMART x 50 comes from. Over time the number can be increased as desired.

Eye Contact

Eye contact is a fundamental aspect of communication for social animals like humans and dogs, serving different purposes depending on the context (Figure 5.21). Natural, voluntary eye contact is more meaningful and comfortable, while forced eye contact can be perceived as uncomfortable or even threatening. In human social interactions, brief eye contact followed by a slight aversion of gaze is typically a sign of peaceful intentions, whereas prolonged and forced eye contact can feel unnatural and confrontational.

In dog training, eye contact should be used as an indicator of attention and readiness for engagement rather than a forced action. Coercing a dog into maintaining eye contact does not always result in true engagement or interest. A dog's hesitation to make eye contact during training can be due to various factors, such as the intensity of the training, external distractions, or discomfort felt by the dog. Recognizing and understanding these underlying reasons improves and fine-tunes straining methods. Effective and compassionate dog training involves interpreting a dog's reactions and adapting the approach to meet their individual needs.

In daily life, constant direct eye contact is not essential. It is more important to understand and address a dog's distractions, fears, and anxieties than to insist on maintaining eye contact. Effective positive reinforcement training cultivates voluntary focus and attention through enjoyable, engaging activities without the need for force.

Come When Called (Recall)

Training a dog to respond to a recall cue effectively revolves around the principle that returning to their caregiver should be a consistently rewarding experience. The approach involves using treats as rewards and making the training process engaging to keep the dog's interest and to develop an instinctive response to the recall cue.

It is never too early to begin recall training for dogs. The training process begins with using high-value rewards and gradually increasing the distance based on the dog's reliability to return for a reward. Punishment should never be used, even if the dog does not return immediately. Instead,

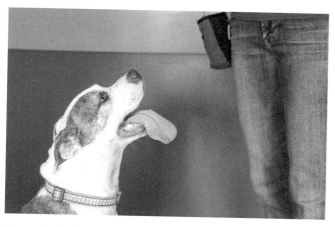

Figure 5.21 Eye contact is an important foundational behavior that should be reinforced for every dog. *Source:* Jennifer/Adobe Stock Photos.

try turning away, walking in the opposite direction, or getting down on the ground as if you are in distress or finding something interesting in the grass to encourage the dog to return quickly.

A fun recall game to play involves intently looking at the grass and counting "1-2-3" as you place food in the grass. This can entice the dog to come investigate. Once the dog arrives, move to a different location and repeat the process to maintain their interest.

Incorporating various games into recall training adds diversity and keeps the dog engaged. Here are a few more examples:

- **Name game:** This involves saying the dog's name and rewarding them when they respond, helping them associate their name with positive experiences.
- **Catch me game:** In this game the dog receives a treat each time they approach the caregiver, making it ideal for both indoor and outdoor training.
- **Chase me game:** The caregiver tosses a treat, moves away, and then rewards the dog when they catch up, simultaneously calling their name as they approach.
- **Round Robin:** Family members, spaced apart, take turns calling the dog, rewarding them with treats on arrival. This game not only reinforces recall but also involves multiple caregivers, enhancing the dog's response to different people.
- **Whiplash Turn and Give Me A Break:** From Control Unleashed® Pattern Games (www.cleanrun.com), both of these encourage the dog to turn back toward their caregiver for engagement and check-ins, which are the basic foundational behaviors for recall.

The training process should be enjoyable, turning recall into a game that creates positive memories and strengthens the bond between the dog and their caregivers. This behavior is especially beneficial for puppies or newly adopted dogs to learn. Incorporating favorite activities like tug or fetch as rewards further enriches the training experience, making it more engaging and rewarding for the dog.

Loose Leash Walking

Teaching a dog to walk calmly on a leash and using appropriate walking equipment helps make outings more engaging and safe. A front clip harness paired with a long line helps reduce leash tension, which might otherwise encourage the dog to pull. A waist leash offers the added benefit of freeing up hands and providing better stability if pulling occurs. Aversive tools such as prong collars, choke collars, and electronic or shock collars are never appropriate for walking a dog on or off leash.

When teaching a dog to walk nicely on a leash, begin training without a leash in a non-distracting environment, such as inside the house or in a fenced yard. As the dog becomes proficient at loose leash walking, gradually introduce more distractions. Techniques such as hand targeting and Control Unleashed Pattern Games, like the 1-2-3 Game, offer predictable and structured activities that foster engagement and provide opportunities for reinforcing check-ins. Using positive reinforcement makes loose leash training a rewarding experience for both the dog and the handler.

Targeting

Teaching a dog nose targeting is a fundamental skill with numerous applications in dog training and behavior modification (Figure 5.22 and Table 5.5). It effectively sharpens a caregiver's clicker mechanics, allowing them to physically feel the behavior to be marked and reinforced. The dog is taught to touch and follow a target, typically the caregiver's hand, with their nose. This technique not only maintains the dog's attention but also provides direction and motivation to follow the caregiver's lead.

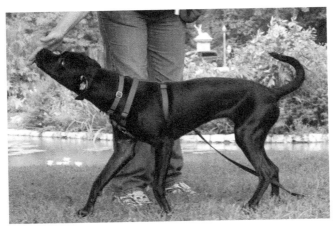

Figure 5.22 Example of nose targeting in a dog. *Source:* Bumble Wolf Gifts / Naomi Barnes / https://bumblewolf.com/blogs/dog-tips-tricks (accessed February 5, 2024).

Mat Training and Relaxation on a Mat

Mat training is a form of targeting and a fundamental aspect of dog training that focuses on teaching dogs to settle and relax on a specific mat or blanket (Table 5.6). This training promotes relaxed behavior in various environments, from busy cafés to quiet homes. By learning to associate the mat with relaxation and rewards, dogs develop the ability to regulate their emotional arousal and remain relaxed in situations that might otherwise induce fear and cause anxiety, frustration, or overexcitement. Mat training improves a dog's ability to cope in different settings and equips them with a practical skill that is useful in everyday life, particularly in circumstances where fear and anxiety might be prevalent (Figure 5.23).

Nipping

Nipping is a normal behavior for puppies, especially as they go through their teething phase, typically between 3 and 7 months old. This period can be marked by an increase in nipping due to the discomfort of growing new teeth. Different reasons can trigger a puppy's nipping behavior such as the desire to play, overstimulation, tiredness, seeking attention, or teething discomfort (Figure 5.28). Understanding these motivations helps caregivers tailor their responses and training methods (Table 5.7).

(a)   (b)

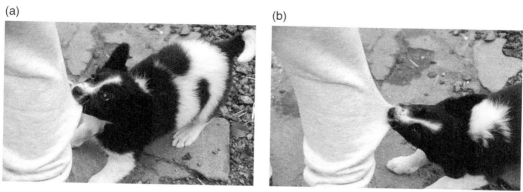

Figure 5.28 (a, b) Nipping can also include pulling on clothing. Valeriy Volkonskiy/Adobe Stock Photos.

Table 5.7 Ways to stop nipping.

Description	Method
Redirecting attention	Change the puppy's focus from nipping to a different activity such as playing with a toy or chew.
Using toys	Utilize dog toys or chews as distractions to prevent the puppy from nipping at hands or clothes. A long tug toy is useful for this technique.
Training opportunities	Use training treats or kibble to redirect the puppy's behavior toward desirable behaviors like sitting or targeting.
Stopping play or interaction	Remove the puppy's desired interaction, such as play or attention, as a consequence for continued nipping. Do not wrestle or play with hands and feet.
Using a confinement area	If nipping persists, redirect the puppy into a designated area with a safe and appropriate toy to help them relax.
Providing appropriate chew toys	Offer the puppy suitable chew toys, especially during teething, to soothe their gums and redirect chewing behavior.
Mental enrichment	Engage the puppy in mentally stimulating activities to reduce excess energy and nipping behavior.

Jumping

Jumping on people is a common behavior problem in dogs. Traditional techniques for preventing or correcting this behavior, which often involve physical punishment, tend to be ineffective. Instead, teaching the dog to sit for greetings, an alternative "good" behavior, is a more successful approach to dissuading jumping, a "bad" behavior. This can be achieved through treat scatters on the floor at the dog's feet and games like SMART x 50 to build a repertoire of desired behaviors. When the dog chooses to sit instead of jump, rewarding this choice encourages sitting. Maintaining all four feet on the ground should also be heavily rewarded.

Alternatively, teaching the dog to go to a specific mat or platform for greetings and reinforcement can be an effective strategy, with a remote treat dispenser working well for this purpose. One of the primary reasons punishment-based training fails to stop jumping behavior is that the attention the dog, receives inadvertently rewards them for jumping. For many dogs, this attention is a stronger motivator than the consequences of physical punishment. Simply removing attention or ignoring the dog is not a solution either, as this approach can lead to frustration and "extinction bursts," during which the dog intensifies their efforts to jump and claw, even when ignored. However, with patience and consistent effort, training that uses positive reinforcement and encourages alternative behaviors can gradually reduce the unwanted habit of jumping.

Guarding Behavior

Many puppy caregivers are aware of food-related aggression and take steps to prevent or address this issue. However, some common techniques might inadvertently worsen the behavior. Actions such as removing the puppy's bowl while eating, especially if the puppy shows protest, touching the puppy or the bowl during meals, or feeding by hand one piece at a time can increase fear, anxiety, and frustration and ultimately result in aggression related to food.

Positive Association Training

Although it is often best to let puppies eat in peace, they can learn to associate the presence of humans around their food bowl with "good" things. This can be achieved by having the caregiver walk by and toss a special treat, such as cheese or hot dog pieces, into the bowl while the puppy eats. After a couple of weeks, if there is no sign of protective behavior, the caregiver can start occasionally reaching for the bowl or picking it up, always returning it with a special treat inside.

Disturbances during meals should be minimized and only done occasionally to avoid crossing into teasing or annoyance. Offering a spoon with canned food, squeeze cheese, peanut butter, or a similar item while the bowl is removed and then replaced can also be effective.

Trading Technique

A similar technique of trading for something of higher value can teach dogs to willingly give up items like rawhides or other treasures. Using phrases like "What ya got?" and "Do you want to trade?" in a "jolly" voice can keep emotional arousal and protective emotions to a minimum. Never chase the dog for an item. If the object is neither expensive nor dangerous, let them keep it, but always offer a higher-value item in exchange. If the puppy begins bringing items to trade, such as their food bowl or shoes, this should be considered a sign of successful training.

Addressing Underlying Health Issues

If a puppy exhibits signs of guarding food or consuming nonfood items, investigate and rule out underlying gastrointestinal issues, such as malabsorptive or maldigestive disorders, which are more prevalent than compulsive or anxiety-based behaviors. Similarly, guarding a specific person can be a sign of anxiety. If a dog guards their bed or resting area, this may suggest underlying pain, especially if quickly moving away is difficult for them. Also, consider the location of the guarded resting area. Moving it to a more open yet still low-traffic area could be advisable.

Counter Surfing

Counter surfing can be a normal behavior for dogs, who are naturally inclined to forage. When food is left on counters dogs are likely to find it, reinforcing this behavior. The behavior can become particularly persistent due to intermittent reinforcement. Even when food is not consistently present on the counters, the occasional discovery of food reinforces this behavior. Punishment, corrections, or stern demands such as "off" or "leave it" and physically moving the dog away from the counter tend to be ineffective for stopping this behavior and do not address the root cause for the behavior. A more effective strategy is to "puppy proof" the counters making sure no food items are left within the dog's reach. This preventative strategy removes the temptation and incentive for counter surfing, addressing the issue at its source.

Additionally, to prevent dogs from accessing the kitchen and food preparation areas, consider sectioning off these spaces with gates. Teaching dogs how to settle on a mat during food preparation and mealtimes gives an opportunity to reinforce an alternative behavior. A long-lasting food-dispensing or puzzle toy helps to keep them engaged. By conditioning dogs to relax on a mat and placing it in or near the kitchen, you can effectively encourage them to associate the mat with positive experiences and learn that food rewards come only when they are settled on their mat. This strategy addresses counter-surfing behavior and promotes a structured, positive way for dogs to participate in kitchen activities without engaging in unwanted behaviors.

Digging

Digging is another normal behavior for dogs, often used to stay cool or create a comfortable resting area. However, this behavior can frustrate caregivers, especially if it damages the yard. Dogs may also dig out of frustration or a lack of mental stimulation or the desire to hunt, explore smells, or investigate noises. To prevent excessive digging, dogs should not be left unsupervised outdoors.

Regardless of the underlying cause, it is important to make sure that the dog's basic needs are being met. These needs include adequate enrichment, positive interactions with humans and other animals, and proper shelter. Dogs also need to stay cool in hot weather and warm in colder conditions.

To minimize unwanted digging, a practical approach is to allocate a specific part of the yard for this activity while restricting access to areas where digging is undesirable. Creating a designated digging area helps channel a dog's natural digging instincts constructively (Figure 5.29). For example, setting up a kiddie pool filled with sand or sectioning off a part of the yard works well. Burying treats and toys in the area can attract the dog's attention and encourage them to focus their digging efforts there instead of other parts of the yard. This method not only helps prevent yard damage but also provides a stimulating and enjoyable activity for the dog. By accommodating their natural instincts in this controlled and safe setting, dogs can indulge in their digging behavior without disruption.

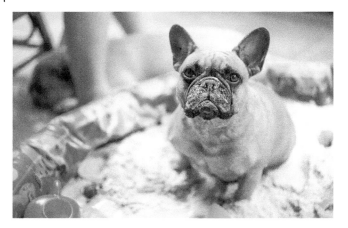

Figure 5.29 Providing a designated digging area can manage destructive behaviors and provide an opportunity for dogs to dig. *Source:* tienuskin/Adobe Stock Photos.

Pulling/Chewing on the Leash

Pulling and chewing on the leash often stems from frustration or anxiety (Figures 5.30 and 5.31). Such behavior may signal that the dog's basic needs for adequate exercise, mental stimulation, or a consistent routine are not being fully met. The use of aversive tools like prong, choke, and electronic collars can also contribute to this behavior.

Identifying and addressing underlying factors, such as insufficient sleep, overstimulation, or inconsistent interactions with the dog, are essential when managing this behavior. Introducing a tug toy can serve as an effective distraction and outlet. Another option is to use a second leash. When the dog starts tugging on one leash, you can drop it while still maintaining control with the second leash. This technique provides a way to manage the behavior without reinforcing it. Using longer leashes and engaging in games designed for teaching loose leash walking can also help reduce this behavior. These activities provide not only physical exercise but also mental stimulation, addressing the root causes of frustration or anxiety that contribute to leash chewing and pulling.

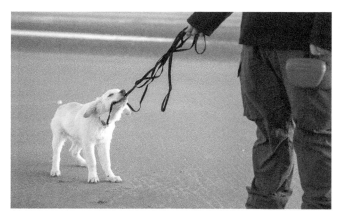

Figure 5.30 Pulling on a leash is a common but frustrating behavior in dogs. *Source:* stephm2506/Adobe Stock Photos.

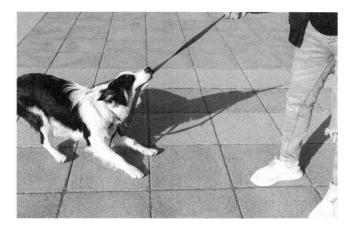

Figure 5.31 Pulling on a leash can be an anxiety-based behavior or the result of using aversive tools. *Source:* Alberto Cotilla/Adobe Stock Photos.

Conclusion

Understanding the developmental stages of dogs from the juvenile period through to social maturity is essential for any caregiver. Acknowledging and adapting to the changes in behavior and needs during these stages can significantly enhance the bond between caregivers and their pets. Through consistent training, socialization, and patience, caregivers can help their dogs navigate these formative years. This approach lays the groundwork for a well-adjusted, sociable, and behaviorally sound adult dog.

Caregivers should be aware that encountering problems such as the dog growling or lifting a lip requires them to immediately stop their current approach. In such instances, consulting a board-certified veterinary behaviorist might become necessary, as the situation could escalate from preventative training to a serious and potentially dangerous behavior problem.

References

Champagne, F.A. (2008). Epigenetic mechanisms and the transgenerational effects of maternal care. *Frontiers in Neuroendocrinology* 29 (3): 386–397.

Duxbury, M.M., Jackson, J.A., Line, S.W., and Anderson, R.K. (2003). Evaluation of association between retention in the home and attendance at puppy socialization classes. *Journal of the American Veterinary Medical Association* 223 (1): 61–66. https://doi.org/10.2460/javma.2003.223.61.

Foyer, P., Wilsson, E., and Jensen, P. (2016). Levels of maternal care in dogs affect adult offspring temperament. *Scientific Reports* 6 (1): 19253. https://doi.org/10.1038/srep19253.

Freedman, D.G., King, J.A., and Elliot, O. (1961). Critical period in the social development of dogs. *Science* 133 (3457): 1016–1017.

Gazzano, A., Mariti, C., Notari, L. et al. (2008). Effects of early gentling and early environment on emotional development of puppies. *Applied Animal Behaviour Science* 110 (3–4): 294–304. https://doi.org/10.1016/j.applanim.2007.05.007.

Godbout, M. and Frank, D. (2011). Persistence of puppy behaviors and signs of anxiety during adulthood. *Journal of Veterinary Behavior: Clinical Applications and Research* 1 (6): 92.

Houpt, K.A. (2018). *Domestic Animal Behavior for Veterinarians and Animal Scientists*. 6 Ames: IA Wiley.

Morrow, M., Ottobre, J., Ottobre, A. et al. (2015). Breed-dependent differences in the onset of fear-related avoidance behavior in puppies. *Journal of Veterinary Behavior* 10 (4): 286–294.

Pierantoni, L., Albertini, M., and Pirrone, F. (2011). Prevalence of owner-reported behaviours in dogs separated from the litter at two different ages. *Veterinary Record* 169 (18): 468–468. https://doi.org/10.1136/vr.d4967.

Rezvani, T., Shreyer, T., and Croney, C. (2021a). *At-A-Glance: Social Interactions: Dogs and Other Dogs*. Purdue University Canine Welfare Science https://caninewelfare.centers.purdue.edu/resource/at-a-glance-social-interactions-dogs-and-other-dogs-croney-research-group/ (accessed March 21, 2024).

Rezvani, T., Shreyer, T., and Croney, C. (2021b). *At-A-Glance: Social Interactions: Dogs and People*. Purdue University Canine Welfare Science https://caninewelfare.centers.purdue.edu/resource/at-a-glance-social-interactions-dogs-and-people-croney-research-group/ (accessed March 21, 2024).

Scott, J.P. and Fuller, J.L. (1965). *Genetics and the Social Behavior of the Dog*. Chicago, IL: University of Chicago Press.

Serpell, J. (ed.) (2017). *The Domestic Dog: Its Evolution, Behavior and Interactions with People*, vol. 2. Cambridge, Cambridge University Press.

Slabbert, J.M. and Rasa, O.A. (1993). The effect of early separation from the mother on pups in bonding to humans and pup health. *Journal of the South African Veterinary Association* 64 (1): 4–8.

Stepita, M.E., Bain, M.J., and Kass, P. (2013). Frequency of CPV infection in vaccinated puppies that attended puppy socialization classes. *Journal of the American Animal Hospital Association* 49 (2): 95–100. https://doi.org/10.5326/JAAHA-MS-5825.

6

Setting Kittens Up for Success

Raising a kitten into a well-adjusted, sociable, and happy adult cat involves a deep understanding of their specific behavioral, environmental, and developmental needs. Each stage of a kitten's growth requires attention to different aspects of care, from socialization to basic training and enrichment.

Developmental Periods of Behavior

Cats, like dogs, undergo stages of development, although these stages in cats may be less distinctly defined. The variation in individual development can be due to factors such as genetics, environmental influences including human interaction, and maternal conditions like stress and nutrition.

Neonatal Stage: (0–2 Weeks)

The neonatal period in kittens begins at birth and lasts until about 2 weeks of age. During this stage, kittens are completely dependent on their mother, often referred to as the queen (Figure 6.1). The queen's responsibilities include initiating nursing and aiding in the elimination process, as kittens need perineal stimulation for both urination and defecation during their first two weeks of life. Kittens are born blind, almost deaf, and with limited mobility, and they have an inability to regulate their body temperature (Figure 6.2).

In this initial phase, a kitten's main activities are eating and sleeping, with an average of about four hours a day spent suckling in the first week. Kittens primarily rely on their senses of smell and touch, as well as their ability to detect warmth to survive, as they are born with their eyes and ears closed (Figure 6.3). They purr when suckling and may cry out when experiencing physical discomfort, though their vocalizations are generally minimal. Despite their neurologic immaturity at birth, which limits their movement, kittens possess a prenatal righting reflex that allows them to reposition themselves if they are rolled onto their back.

As kittens progress through the neonatal period, their sensory capabilities begin to evolve. Their eyes and ears gradually open and become functional, marking a significant milestone in their sensory development. The development of sensory capabilities is influenced by various factors including the paternity of the kitten, the amount of light they are exposed to, the sex of the kitten, and the mother's age. For instance, kittens raised in dimmer light conditions tend to open their eyes earlier compared to those in standard lighting. Similarly, kittens born to younger mothers usually open their eyes sooner than those from older mothers. Additionally, female

Veterinary Guide to Preventing Behavior Problems in Dogs and Cats, First Edition. Christine D. Calder and Sarah C. Wright.
© 2025 John Wiley & Sons, Inc. Published 2025 by John Wiley & Sons, Inc.

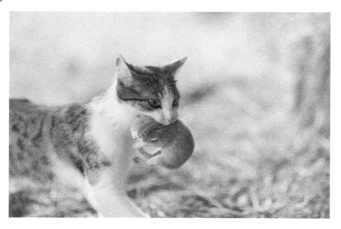

Figure 6.1   A mother cat carries her young kitten. *Source:* Cubodeluz/Adobe Stock Photos.

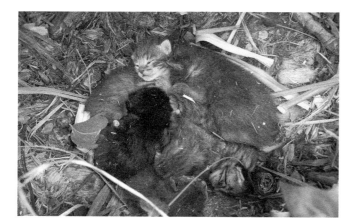

Figure 6.2   Newborn kittens huddle together for warmth. *Source:* CB_Stock/Adobe Stock Photos.

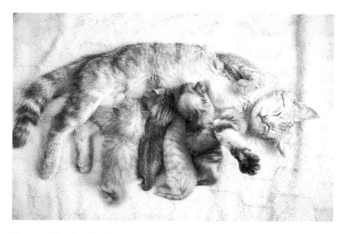

Figure 6.3   In the first two weeks of life kittens eat and sleep. They use their sense of touch and smell to find food. *Source:* bozhdb/Adobe Stock Photos.

kittens often develop their senses earlier than their male counterparts. These observations highlight the significant role of genetic and environmental elements in the early development of kittens (Turner and Bateson 2013).

Transitional Stage: (2–3 Weeks)

The transitional period in a kitten's development, occurring from the second to the third weeks of life, is marked by rapid physical and behavioral changes. During this phase kittens begin to gain some independence from their mother, featuring significant improvements in locomotor skills and a considerable enhancement of sensory capabilities. Kittens start to crawl and walk, though their movements may still be uncoordinated, and their eyes and ears become fully functional, marking a major milestone in their development (Figure 6.4).

Additionally, during this phase kittens experience the eruption of deciduous teeth and the full development of their sense of smell. Although they typically do not start consuming solid foods until around the age of 3 weeks, this developmental stage is marked by the maturation of their sensory abilities and coincides with a significant increase in social behavior. Kittens become more interactive with their littermates and begin to engage with humans, marking an important period for their social development and overall growth. At this time, active interaction with their environment helps shape their future behavioral patterns.

Kittens should remain with their mother and littermates for as long as possible. Research indicates that kittens separated from their mothers and hand-raised from 2 weeks of age often exhibit more fear and aggression toward humans and other cats (Chon 2005; Seitz 1959). Additionally, these kittens tend to be more sensitive to new stimuli, have poorer learning capabilities, and show underdeveloped social and parenting skills. However, these negative effects can be mitigated if kittens are hand-reared in a home with behaviorally normal and socially adept cats, allowing them to learn through observation (Turner and Bateson 2013). Observing their mother and interacting with siblings help kittens acquire appropriate social skills. Those raised without littermates typically acquire social skills more slowly than those raised in a normal social environment (Turner and Bateson 2013).

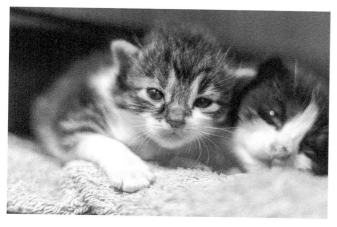

Figure 6.4 As kittens enter into the transitional phase their eyes and ears start to open. *Source:* Holger/ Adobe Stock Photos.

Socialization Stage: (3–9 Weeks)

In kittens the socialization period usually spans from the third to the seventh week of age, a phase often referred to as the "sensitive period." While this period is critical for their behavioral development, it can extend up to 9 weeks of age, depending on factors such as genetics, environmental influences, and individual experiences (Beaver 2003; Turner and Bateson 2013). In contrast to dogs, whose socialization period typically ends later, cats' socialization period is traditionally considered to end earlier. However, considering that kittens' social play often peaks between 9 and 14 weeks of age, the end of the socialization period in cats may not be as definitive as previously thought.

Importance of Socialization for Development

Socialization opportunities are needed for both neurologic and physical development, continuing throughout a cat's life beyond kittenhood. This period is ideal for forming social attachments not only to other cats but also to humans and other animals. The experiences kittens undergo during this time, both positive and negative, can have lasting impacts on their development, influencing their interactions with new individuals as adult cats.

Staying with Mother and Littermates

Kittens should ideally remain with their mother (queen) and littermates during this sensitive period (Beaver 2003; Turner and Bateson 2013). Early separation may lead to delayed social skills, especially in kittens without littermates. Therefore, the timing of adoption requires careful consideration to ensure kittens have the opportunity to gain early social experiences while benefiting from learning within their feline family.

Physical Development Milestones

This stage also coincides with significant physical developments. By 4 weeks of age kittens have fully functional hearing and can recognize their mother's sounds (Szenczi et al. 2016). Their depth perception is present, though visual acuity continues to improve until about 16 weeks of age. By 6 weeks of age kittens exhibit adult-like righting ability and full control over their elimination, demonstrating normal species-specific behaviors like digging and covering their waste. The gape response (flehmen) emerges around 5 weeks of age and resembles adult behavior by 7 weeks of age.

Play Behavior and Its Evolution

Play behavior, integral to development, starts when kittens are between 2 and 4 weeks old, primarily involving social interactions with littermates or, in the absence of littermates, their mother (Beaver 2003; Delgado and Hecht 2019; Turner and Bateson 2013). By 4 weeks of age interest in their littermates' movements is high, and by 6 weeks of age adult-like locomotion and eye–paw coordination develop (Beaver 2003; Delgado and Hecht 2019; Turner and Bateson 2013). Social play peaks around 9–14 weeks of age and includes a variety of ritualized sequences. These consist of motor activities such as leaping, pouncing, side stepping, and chasing, as well as specific postures. Kittens may present their underside, face off with a littermate, and then engage further by holding the other cat with their forelimbs, rolling, stalking, and playfully raking the playmate with their hind legs (Delgado and Hecht 2019). Object and locomotory play begins at 6 weeks of age and peaks around 16 weeks of age (Figure 6.5) (Beaver 2003; Delgado and Hecht 2019; Turner and Bateson 2013). After 14 weeks kittens transition to more object-oriented play and learn play fighting, with a shift from social and object to predatory play between 12 and 16 weeks of age (Beaver 2003; Delgado and Hecht 2019; Mendl 1988; Turner and Bateson 2013).

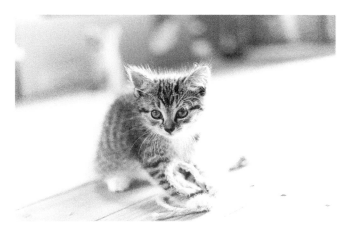

Figure 6.5 Object play peaks at about 16 weeks of age. *Source:* Jrn/Adobe Stock Photos.

Guiding Playful Behaviors

When playing with kittens, caregivers should guide them toward appropriate activities such as using toys that can be tossed, wand toys, and other toys that flitter, sparkle, and float to channel their playful instincts properly. Redirecting kittens from human hands and feet to these toys helps prevent them from developing inappropriate play behaviors with humans. Object and predatory play, which emerges around 7–8 weeks of age and peaks by 18 weeks of age, should be encouraged with a variety of toys (Overall et al. 2005). Kittens should be redirected away from human hands and feet to toys, without inducing conflict, fear, or arousal. Avoid positive punishment in the form of shouting or spraying water to stop rough play. Instead, focus on teaching acceptable play habits, ensuring the kittens grow into well-adjusted adult cats (Overall et al. 2005).

Predatory Behavior

Once the kittens are about 3 weeks old, mother cats begin teaching them the basics of predation (Caro 1980; Overall et al. 2005; Turner and Bateson 2013). By around 5 weeks old kittens start exhibiting predatory behaviors independently (Overall et al. 2005; Turner and Bateson 2013). This period also marks the beginning of their transition to solid food, often influenced by their mother's dietary choices, which shape their taste preferences (Overall et al. 2005; Turner and Bateson 2013). The timing of weaning plays a critical role in the development of these behaviors. Kittens weaned early, around 4 weeks of age, typically display predatory behaviors earlier than is usual (Barrett and Bateson 1978; Bateson et al. 1990; Martin and Bateson 1985; Overall et al. 2005; Tan and Counsilman 1985). On the other hand, those weaned later, at about 9 weeks of age, tend to experience a delay in the development of these behaviors and are less prone to engage in actual prey killing (Barrett and Bateson 1978; Bateson et al. 1990; Martin and Bateson 1985; Overall et al. 2005; Tan and Counsilman 1985).

Development of Fearful Reactions and Individual Differences

Fearful responses to threatening stimuli can emerge in kittens as early as 6 weeks old (Beaver 2003; Turner and Bateson 2013). However, due to their developing eyesight and limited recognition abilities, kittens are not able to respond to visual cues until they are at least 4 weeks old (Beaver 2003; Turner and Bateson 2013). Between 6 and 8 weeks of age they start to react to both visual and olfactory threats in a manner similar to adult cats (Beaver 2003; Turner and Bateson 2013). During their second month individual behavioral differences become more apparent (Beaver 2003; Turner and Bateson 2013). These variations are shaped by genetic factors and the diversity of their early environments. Increased handling, introducing a mild level of stress, seems to accelerate these developmental processes (Beaver 2003; Meier 1961).

Personality Types in Kittens

Researchers exploring cat personalities have identified a variety of personality types, yet there remains a lack of consensus in the field regarding the terminology, methods, and conclusions (Gartner and Weiss 2013). The development of a kitten's personality is influenced by several factors, including early socialization experiences, genetic background, and both social and observational influences. Recognizing the individual personalities and preferences of kittens is essential. By tailoring the socialization process to match the comfort level of each kitten, caregivers can ensure that each experience is a positive and engaging one.

Optimal Time for Socialization

The most receptive period for socializing kittens to humans and other species is between the ages of 2 and 9 weeks (Beaver 2003; Overall et al. 2005; Turner and Bateson 2013). Increased handling by people during this time significantly reduces the likelihood of kittens developing a fear of humans (Beaver 2003; Meier 1961; Overall et al. 2005; Turner and Bateson 2013). For kittens to become social pets, human contact before the age of 7 weeks is critical for the development of socially acceptable behaviors (Beaver 2003; Collard 1967; Overall et al. 2005; Turner and Bateson 2013). Kittens not handled by humans before reaching 14 weeks of age, especially before 9 weeks of age, are less likely to socialize with humans (Beaver 2003; Karsh and Turner 1988). Therefore it is advisable to practice regular, gentle handling such as picking up and holding before the kitten reaches 14 weeks of age, ideally starting as early as possible (Figures 6.6 and 6.7) (Karsh and Turner 1988; Lowe and Bradshaw 2002; Overall et al. 2005).

Positive Interactions and Exposure to Novel Stimuli

During this sensitive period, in addition to positive and gentle interactions with humans, kittens need to be exposed to a variety of novel stimuli in a nonthreatening manner (Overall et al. 2005; Rheingold and Eckerman 1971). Effective socialization involves providing kittens with choice and

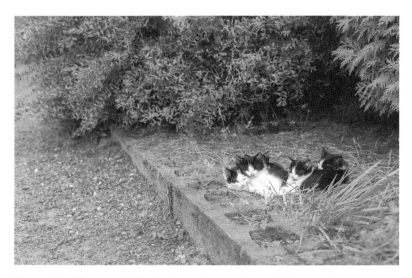

Figure 6.6　Kittens with limited to no interactions with humans from a young age are less likely to approach and interact with humans. *Source:* Александр Лебедько/Adobe Stock Photos.

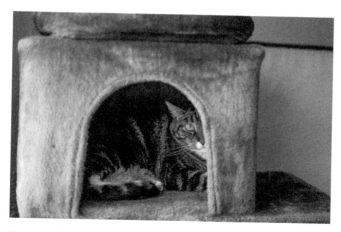

Figure 6.10 All cats need a safe place to hide. *Source:* seaseasyd/Adobe Stock Photos.

Description of a Safe Place

A safe place for a cat is a private and secure area that often provides a sense of enclosure, isolation, or seclusion. This can be an elevated space for some cats, while others may prefer lower hiding spots (Figure 6.11). It is a retreat where a cat can feel safe and protected, even if not entirely hidden (Figure 6.12). Additionally, when the cat is relaxed, this space doubles as a resting or sleeping area.

Methods to Provide a Safe Place

- **Hiding places:** Offer individual hiding spots such as cardboard boxes or cat carriers.
- **Perches and shelves:** Perches should be spacious enough for the cat to stretch fully. A hammock-style dip in the middle offers a sense of hiding (Figure 6.13).
- **Outdoor access:** The decision to keep cats indoors, allow outdoor access, or both depends on individual preferences, local laws, and safety. Outdoor enclosures, strollers, or leash walking (with positive reinforcement training) are safe options for outdoor access (Figures 6.14–6.16).
- **Multicat households:** In homes with multiple cats, safe places should have more than one entry to prevent blocking by another cat. There should be at least one safe spot per cat, and these areas should be separated from each other.
- **Accessibility for kittens and older cats:** For kittens and less mobile older cats, place boxes, perches, and shelves at lower heights or provide ramps for easy access.

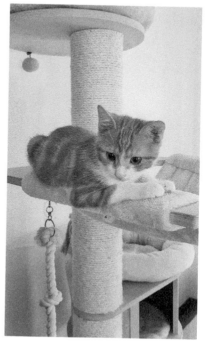

Figure 6.11 Cats prefer vertical spaces. *Source:* Jakel/Adobe Stock Photos.

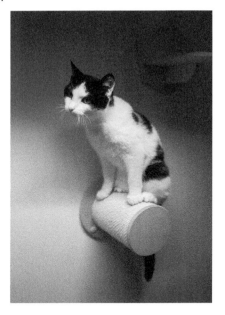

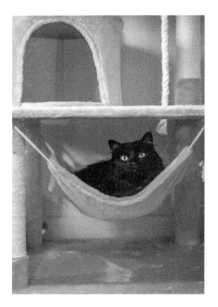

Figure 6.12   Cats prefer perches to feel safe and secure. *Source:* Евгений Вершинин/Adobe Stock Photos.

Figure 6.13   A hammock can provide a safe haven for many cats, helping them feel secure when partially hidden. *Source:* seaseasyd/Adobe Stock Photos.

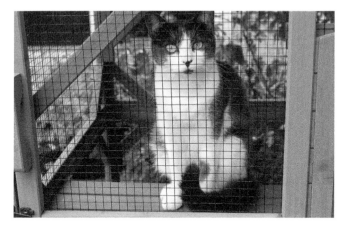

Figure 6.14   An outdoor catio can be a safe place for indoor cats to explore the outdoors. *Source:* Kellie/Adobe Stock Photos.

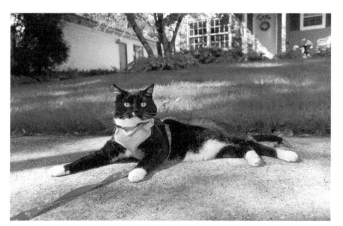

Figure 6.15   Cats can be trained to walk on a harness and leash for enrichment opportunities. *Source:* soupstock/Adobe Stock Photos.

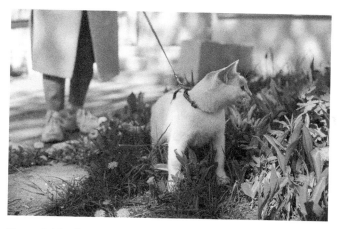

Figure 6.16   Some cats enjoy walks and opportunities to explore outside. *Source:* glebcallfives/Adobe Stock Photos.

Pillar 2: Providing Multiple and Separated Resources

Cats require access to essential resources, including areas for feeding, drinking, elimination, scratching, playing, and resting or sleeping. In multicat households distributing these resources across multiple locations minimizes stress and allows each cat access to essential resources without stress or competition. This is particularly important since cats selectively social and tend to be solitary when hunting or eating. Elimination areas, food and water bowls, play areas, resting spaces, and scratching posts should be positioned in separate locations within the living space (Figures 6.17–6.20). This separation not only enlarges the environment for the cats but also reduces the likelihood of resource competition. Providing a variety of options for each resource type such as multiple spots for resting and feeding further caters to the individual needs of each cat (Table 6.2).

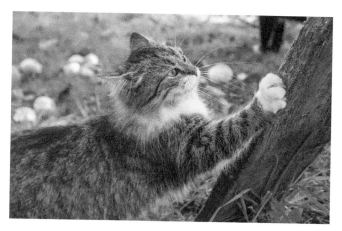

Figure 6.17   Scratching is a basic need of cats. *Source:* alenka2194/Adobe Stock Photos.

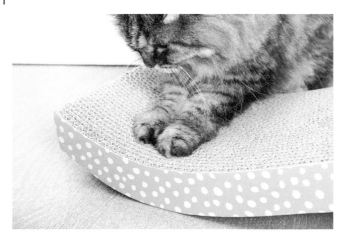

Figure 6.18 Cats should be provided with a variety of scratching surfaces. *Source:* Petra Richli/Adobe Stock Photos.

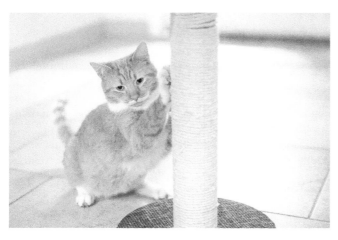

Figure 6.19 Scratching posts should be placed in high traffic areas of social importance. *Source:* Mary Swift/Adobe Stock Photos.

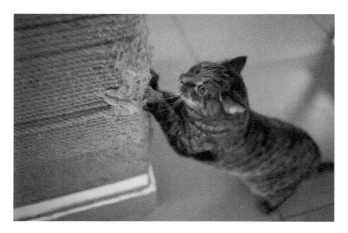

Figure 6.20 When they scratch, cats deposit pheromones for communication to other cats. *Source:* Евгений Вершинин/Adobe Stock Photos.

Table 6.2 Multicat households.

Consideration	Details
Resource allocation	Each cat or social group needs access to separate resources to prevent resource blocking and reduce stress.
Social groups identification	Identify social groups, as cats in the same group often share behaviors like allorubbing, allogrooming and playing. Provide separate resources for each group.
Feeding stations	Set up several feeding stations. Have a separate feeding and watering station. Each cat should have their own bowl and feeding location.
Resting areas	Provide plenty of safe places and resting areas in different locations, offering both privacy and outdoor visibility.
Elimination areas	Place litter boxes away from feeding and resting areas and make sure they are easily accessible to all cats.
Social dynamics	In multicat environments, consider social dynamics and ensure there are enough resources for all cats and their social groups.

Litter-Box Training

Litter-box training is an important aspect of kitten care, ensuring a clean living environment for both the kitten and their caregiver (Table 6.3). This training process involves familiarizing the kitten with the litter box and encouraging its use. Kittens instinctively look for a spot to dig and conceal their waste, which usually makes litter-box training a relatively easy and quick task for kittens.

For successful litter-box training consistency should be maintained. The litter box should be placed in an accessible location that also provides some privacy, away from the kitten's eating and sleeping areas. The litter box must remain clean because many cats, despite their tolerance, may eventually refuse to use a box that is not clean. This involves regular scooping and changing of the litter to ensure it remains fresh. The choice of litter is important, as is the cleaner used for the box. Kittens typically prefer a fine-grained, unscented litter that is gentle on their paws and not overwhelming to their sensitive noses.

Table 6.3 Key features and maintenance practices for litter boxes.

Feature/aspect	Preferred choice/action
Size of litter box	Larger boxes are generally preferred. Should be 1.5 times the cat's body length. The cat should be able to turn around without touching the sides.
Type of litter	Fine-grained, unscented, scoopable/clumping litter.
Use of liners	Avoid using liners.
Use of deodorizers	Avoid strong deodorizers.
Cleanliness	Daily scooping; weekly washing with mild detergent recommended.
Type of cleansers	Avoid strong cleansers like Pine-sol or bleach.
Replacement of box	Replace the box if it retains a strong odor.

Pillar 3: Encouraging Play and Predatory Behavior

Providing for Natural Behaviors

Encouraging cats to engage in hunting-like behaviors is necessary for their overall wellbeing (Table 6.4). Utilizing toys, interactive play with caregivers or other cats, and offering meals through food-dispensing and puzzle toys can all meet this need. Cats instinctively follow a predatory sequence that includes locating, stalking, chasing, pouncing, and "killing" their prey. This behavior is observed even in well-fed cats and is important for their physical activity and mental stimulation.

Consequences of Restricted Behavior

When cats do not have opportunities to engage in their natural predatory behaviors, it can lead to obesity and frustration. These issues may then result in behaviors like overgrooming, the development of stress-related diseases, or misdirected aggression.

Table 6.4 Methods to encourage play and predatory behaviors.

Method	Description
Hide food	Hide food in various locations and scatter-feed to simulate hunting.
Puzzle feeders	Use puzzle and timed feeders for small, frequent meals.
Play with toys	Use rod or wand toys with fur or feather attachments to mimic prey.
Rotate toys	Change toys regularly to maintain interest and prevent habituation.
Safe play	Avoid using hands or feet as toys to prevent injury.
Variety of toys	Provide toys that can be manipulated or contain food.
Outdoor play	Utilize outdoor space for interactive play (where safe).
Separate play in multicat homes	Provide separate toys and playtime to avoid competition among cats.
Adjust for age	Modify play for older cats and kittens based on their physical abilities.
Safe storage	Store toys with strings or small parts away to prevent ingestion.
Special considerations	For confined or convalescent cats, provide suitable play options and consistent caregivers.

Pillar 4: Positive, Consistent, and Predictable Human–Cat Interaction

Importance of Social Interaction

Regular, friendly, and predictable interaction with humans is beneficial for cats (Table 6.5). Positive and consistent handling from a young age helps reduce fear and stress and strengthens the bond between humans and their cats. However, cats' social preferences vary widely, influenced by genetics, early experiences, and living conditions. Many cats prefer frequent but low-intensity social contact, which gives them control over their interactions with humans. This allows them to initiate, moderate, and stop contact according to their comfort level (Ellis et al. 2013).

Table 6.5 Building relationships with cats.

Method for positive interaction	Description
Initiate contact	Allow cats to initiate human interactions.
Approach level	Approach cats at their level and avoid direct eye contact.
Comfort and stroking	Let cats sniff to become comfortable, then gently stroke heads and cheeks if they are relaxed and initiate contact.
Respect boundaries	Respect the cat's choice to end interactions; do not force further contact.
Understand preferences	Be aware of each cat's likes and dislikes regarding petting, grooming, play, being picked up, and lap sitting.
In multicat households	Provide individual attention to each cat, free from interference by other cats.

Affiliative Behaviors and Preferences

Cats exhibit affiliative behaviors toward their preferred humans, including head and body rubbing, sitting on laps, and sometimes grooming (see Figures 6.21 and 6.22 and Box 6.1). These preferences can vary significantly among individual cats and should be respected to prevent defensive behavior such as aggression toward other cats or humans, stress-related diseases, or urine marking behaviors (Ellis et al. 2013).

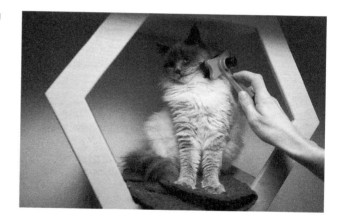

Figure 6.21 Some cats enjoy grooming as a way to interact with humans. *Source:* Евгений Вершинин/Adobe Stock Photos.

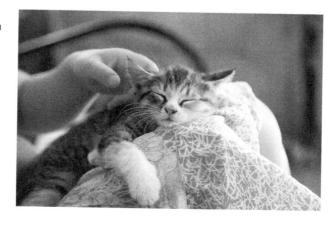

Figure 6.22 When relaxed kittens may close their eyes and hold their ears down slightly to the side. Their body should be relaxed and not tense. *Source:* Anna/ Adobe Stock Photos.

Box 6.1   Recognizing Signs of Relaxation and Willingness to Interact

Look for behaviors like slow blinking, purring, facial rubbing, attempts to climb onto laps, staying close, or pushing against a person.

Head bunting is a sign of attention seeking and depositing of pheromones; respond with gentle rubbing, massaging, or stroking around the temple area, as allowed by the cat.

Be cautious with a rollover and abdominal exposure, as many cats do not want a belly rub.

Training and Social Skills Development

Kitten kindergarten classes typically feature basic training that lays the foundation for desirable behavior patterns early in life. This training encompasses a range of skills, including how to use a scratching post, respond to their name, and engage in gentle play without using claws. Acquiring these skills early on helps prevent the onset of problematic behaviors such as inappropriate scratching or biting.

Training kittens and fostering their social skills are important in their integration into the human world. When done properly, this process not only significantly strengthens the bond between kittens and their caregivers but also promotes a peaceful living environment.

Importance of Positive Reinforcement Training

Positive reinforcement training is a highly effective method for teaching kittens desired behaviors (Figure 6.23). By emphasizing the reward of desirable actions, this method motivates the kitten to repeat those actions. The rewards can be varied, ranging from treats, praise, and petting to playtime, tailored to what the kitten finds most motivating. The effectiveness of positive reinforcement lies in its ability to build a strong association between the desired behavior and a pleasant outcome, thereby increasing the likelihood of the kitten repeating the behavior in the future.

Clicker Training and Clear Communication

Clicker training is a popular form of positive reinforcement training that uses a distinct sound, a "click," to mark the exact moment a desired behavior occurs. This clear form of communication

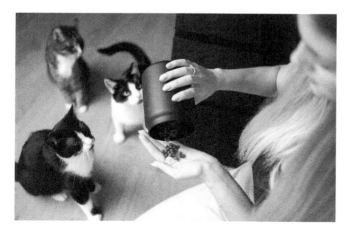

Figure 6.23   Positive reinforcement is a powerful tool for teaching new behaviors and provides mental enrichment. *Source:* FurryFritz/Adobe Stock Photos.

helps kittens understand exactly which behavior is being rewarded. The sound of the click becomes a predictor of a reward, helping to accelerate learning. As training progresses the click itself becomes a form of reward due to its association with food.

Teaching Basic Cues

Basic cues such as "come when called," "targeting" or "touch," and "stationing" or staying on a mat are all essential skills that enhance a kitten's comprehension of human expectations and improve their interaction with the environment. For example, training a kitten to come when called serves not only as a practical behavior but also as a safety measure. Targeting, which involves teaching a kitten to touch a specific object with their nose, lays the groundwork for more complex behaviors and aids in directing them in a specific location. Stationing on a mat teaches a kitten the appropriate places to rest or stay, which can help deter them from going to undesired places like on top of the kitchen counter or the dining table.

Example for Teaching Touch   Let us imagine training a kitten named Luna to target a finger using a clicker and chicken treats. The first step is to condition Luna to the clicker. This means clicking the clicker and immediately giving her a small piece of chicken. Repeat this process multiple times until Luna starts to look for the chicken in anticipation whenever she hears the clicker.

Once Luna understands that the clicker sound means a treat is coming, start the targeting exercise. Present your finger to Luna. The moment she sniffs your finger, click the clicker and give her a chicken treat. After several repetitions, wait until she actually touches her nose to your finger before you click and treat.

As Luna gets more consistent with touching her nose to your finger (doing it about 80% of the time you present your finger), start adding a verbal cue. Right before she touches your finger, say "touch." Click and treat after she does the action. Keep practicing this until she reliably touches your finger with her nose 80% of the time when you say "touch."

Now it is time to add some movement. Move your finger so Luna has to take a step or two to touch it. Click and treat each successful attempt. Gradually increase the distance she has to move, working up to the point where Luna will come running across the room to touch your finger when you say "touch."

Finally, incorporate vertical spaces into your training. Ask Luna to "touch" your finger as she jumps on and off different surfaces like the couch, ottoman, or chair. Each time she successfully touches your finger, click and treat. This not only helps reinforce the targeting behavior but also encourages her to explore and interact with various elements in her environment.

Building Important Life Skills

Training kittens in these behaviors is about more than just teaching tricks; it is about building essential life skills. For example, teaching a kitten to station on a mat helps them understand boundaries within the home (Figure 6.24). This skill is useful for managing a kitten's behavior in various scenarios such as during mealtimes, when administering medications, or when introducing new cats into the household.

Gentle Play and Social Behavior

Encouraging gentle play without using hands or feet as toys is another important aspect of training. This approach helps kittens learn appropriate play behavior with humans, which reduces the likelihood of rough play as they grow. Social skills such as respecting boundaries and understanding gentle interactions are just as important as learning new behaviors for the development of a well-behaved and sociable cat.

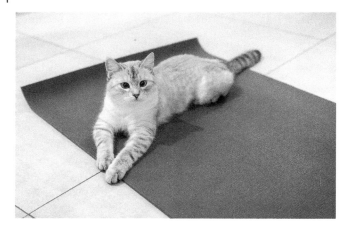

Figure 6.24 Teaching cats to go to a mat is a foundational behavior that has many benefits. *Source:* Sergei Gorin/Adobe Stock Photos.

Drawbacks of Punishment and Negative Reinforcement in Kitten Training

Understanding the negative effects of punishment, especially positive punishment, is essential in kitten training. Positive punishment involves adding an unpleasant stimulus to reduce the frequency of an undesired behavior, for example yelling at a kitten or spraying them with water to discourage them from jumping on the counter. These actions can have detrimental effects on the kitten's emotional wellbeing and may damage the bond between the kitten and their caregiver.

Positive Punishment   One of the significant issues with positive punishment is its potential to induce fear, anxiety, frustration, and even aggression in kittens. This outcome is especially likely when the punishment is harsh or applied inconsistently. Instead of learning the desired behavior, kittens may begin to associate their caregiver or the training process itself with negative experiences. Such associations can hinder their overall learning and development, potentially resulting in long-term behavioral issues and a diminished level of trust.

Negative Reinforcement   Negative reinforcement, distinct from positive punishment, can also present challenges. It involves removing an unpleasant stimulus to increase the likelihood of a behavior being repeated. For instance, using a loud noise to discourage a kitten from jumping on he counter and stopping the noise once the kitten gets down is an example of negative reinforcement. This method aims to encourage the desired behavior by eliminating something unpleasant, unlike positive punishment, which introduces something unpleasant to discourage a behavior. Both methods can be aversive, although their end goals differ: reinforcement aims to increase the frequency of a behavior, while punishment seeks to decrease it.

Counter Surfing Smokey   Let us consider a kitten named Smokey who has a habit of jumping on the kitchen counter. His caregiver, Tom, noticed that Smokey particularly liked to jump onto the counter to watch birds from the shelf over the sink, where the bird feeder was visible.

Tom's first step was to remove any food from the counter to ensure it was not attracting Smokey. He then bought a new cat tree, placed it near the window at the end of the counter, and added Smokey's favorite bed and occasional treats on it. Although Tom moved the bird feeder, Smokey continued to jump on the counter.

Tom next tried to discourage this behavior by making a noise every time Smokey jumped up, stopping the noise when Smokey jumped off. However, in the long run this negative reinforcement did not work well; in fact, Smokey started avoiding Tom in the kitchen. Frustrated, Tom resorted to spraying Smokey with water (positive punishment) whenever he found him on the counter. While Smokey would jump down at the sight of the water bottle, he continued to jump onto the counter when Tom was not around.

Realizing that his approach might be causing fear and anxiety, Tom educated himself about positive reinforcement and clicker training. He decided to teach Smokey to station to a mat using the cat's favorite treats and a clicker. He started by shaping Smokey to first look at, then place one paw, then two, and eventually all four paws onto a nonslip bathmat, eventually sitting down on it. Tom added the cue "mat" and reinforced Smokey each time he went to the mat on cue.

When Smokey was ready, Tom placed the mat on the cat tree and started the training all over again in this new location. Now, every time they entered the kitchen Smokey would run to the mat on the cat tree, knowing he would receive his favorite chicken treats. Tom successfully replaced the counter-jumping behavior with the stationing behavior using positive reinforcement training, and this time it stuck!

Side Effects of Punishment Both positive punishment and negative reinforcement can have detrimental effects. For instance, using a water spray bottle to deter a kitten from jumping on the counter (a form of positive punishment) may yield temporary results, but it fails to teach the desired behavior. Moreover, it can instill fear or distrust toward the caregiver.

Positive Reinforcement Training

In contrast to the previously mentioned training methods, positive reinforcement training is more humane and effective. Through the rewarding of desired behaviors, a foundation of trust and willingness to learn is established. Because there is no guess about what earns a reward stress is kept to a minimum, and therefore the learning environment leads to a more predictable behavioral outcome and strengthens the relationship between caregiver and kitten. Understanding the differences between the four quadrants and the benefits of positive reinforcement training is key to a successful and positive training experience for all.

Pillar 5: Respecting the Cat's Sense of Smell

Understanding Olfactory and Chemical Signals

Cats use their sense of smell and chemical cues, like pheromones, to make sense of their environment and feel safe (see Box 6.2). They have a special organ, the vomeronasal organ, which helps them detect these pheromones. Cats mark their territory and communicate with other cats by rubbing their faces and bodies on surfaces, leaving behind their scent. If their scent marking is disrupted, they might exhibit stress-related behaviors such as urine marking and scratching (Figures 6.25 and 6.26 and Table 6.6).

Avoid using strong-smelling products that could disrupt the cat's sensory perception.

Introduce new items to the cat's scent profile using a cloth rubbed with the cat's scent or synthetic feline pheromone.

Provide scratching areas for scent deposition through glands in the cat's paws.

Maintain "olfactory continuity" by washing bedding on a rotation basis, keeping some items scented with the cat's smell (Ellis et al. 2013).

Use synthetic pheromones to reduce anxiety and promote positive behaviors.

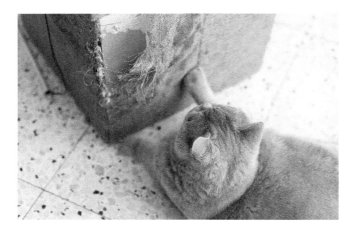

Figure 6.25 Where a cat scratches has social significance. During the scratching process, pheromones are deposited on surfaces. *Source:* Inna/ Adobe Stock Photos.

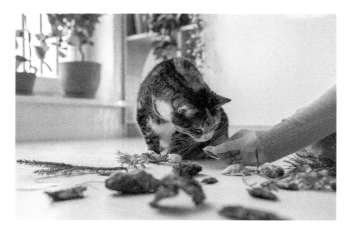

Figure 6.26 Olfactory enrichment. DimaBerlin/Adobe Stock Photos.

Table 6.6 Ways to reduce overstimulating scents in the environment.

Scent exposure	Description
Punishment of scent marking	Do not punish scent marking or house-soiling.
Scent marking opportunities	Ensure each cat or group has chances to scent mark their environment.
Reintroduction after veterinary visits	Use pheromone diffusers when reintroducing a cat post-veterinary visit to maintain scent harmony.
Minimizing human involvement	Reduce human interference during reintroduction in multicat homes.
Early scent exposure	Expose kittens to a variety of scents early on to build tolerance to new smells.

Veterinarians can provide guidance to help caregivers identify normal species-specific behaviors. Understanding what normal cat and dog behaviors are helps them to recognize and distinguish what is abnormal.

Perceptions of Pet Behavior

Some behaviors, while normal, may be undesirable or challenging for caregivers. The way a caregiver perceives a behavior does not always mean that it is an abnormal behavior or that there is an underlying problem with the animal. Such behaviors could be due to inadequate or inappropriate training or not meeting a pet's basic needs, rather than being a primary behavioral problem.

Behavior and Medical Conditions

Some behavioral problems in pets may stem from underlying medical conditions, therefore a thorough physical examination is necessary, along with a complete medical workup that includes a minimum of a complete blood count, serum biochemistry, urinalysis, and endocrine testing. However, the distinction between medical and behavioral problems is often not clear-cut. The presence of underlying medical problems does not necessarily mean that they are the sole cause of or even related to the animal's behavior. Moreover, medical conditions are not always completely ruled out through screening tests alone, and thus they may contribute to an animal's behavior without their definitive diagnosis (Demontigny-Bédard and Frank 2018; Landsberg et al. 2013; Siracusa 2024; Stelow 2018).

Intervention and Behavior Problems

Intervention becomes necessary when abnormal behaviors significantly impact the pet's quality of life or the caregiver's ability to manage and enjoy their pet. The diagnosis of behavior problems is always specific to the individual animal and their environment (Odendaal 1997). Veterinarians can offer valuable insights into when and how to intervene, which may involve a combination of behavior modification techniques, training, and, in some cases, medication (Demontigny-Bédard and Frank 2018). Through their support and guidance, caregivers can effectively manage and address pet behavior issues.

Common Behavior Problems in Dogs

Behavior problems in dogs can vary widely and often present challenges for their caregivers. It is essential to understand and address these issues in order to promote the wellbeing of both the dog and the human family members. Regardless of the problem behavior, recognizing the underlying emotional state and motivation for the behavior will help lead to an effective management and treatment plan. It is also important to recognize that many behavior problems cannot be cured, although improvement is possible in many cases.

Aggression

Aggression has many definitions, and this behavior can be expressed differently depending on the environment or context of the situation. To gain a better understanding of the dog's motivation, the triggers for the behavior first need to be identified. Dogs may exhibit aggression toward familiar people, unfamiliar individuals, other dogs, or different animals. Additionally, aggression can surface in the stressful environment of a veterinary hospital. Because aggression can appear in multiple forms and poses such a risk to both human and animal health, it is the most common reason for dogs being referred to a board-certified veterinary behaviorist (Bamberger and Houpt 2006).

Root Cause of Aggression

Veterinarians can help caregivers by identifying the root causes of aggression and developing strategies to manage and modify this behavior, ensuring the safety of all involved. First, it is important to rule out underlying medical causes that may be contributing to aggression. For example, the pain associated with arthritis can play a role in an animal's aggressive behavior. Therefore, it is important to perform a complete physical exam and screening lab work to identify potential diseases that may affect the animal's behavior. However, it is equally important to understand that an underlying medical disease may not entirely account for the aggressive behavior on its own.

Management in Aggression Cases

Despite the underlying cause leading to aggressive behavior, the primary goal of any treatment and management plan should be to ensure human and animal safety as much as possible. Safety can be achieved through management, improved communications, discontinuation of punishment, and the use of aversive tools, in addition to training and behavior modification.

Management Strategies and Tools

The focus of management is to alter the environment in such a way that there is decreased arousal and limited potential for dogs to practice aggressive behavior. The management strategies that are effective for one case will vary from those that are effective for another due to the individuality of each dog's behavior. Some examples of management include:

- Helping caregivers understand triggers for their pet's aggressive behavior in order to minimize exposure to those triggers as much as possible. For example, this may mean walking at different times of the day in order to avoid other dogs that are out at a similar time or no longer having guests over to the house to prevent exposure to new people.
- Creating a safe space to separate pets from visitors, other household animals, and small children is an effective strategy for managing interactions. This separation minimizes the risk of injury to both the pet and individuals but also provides the pet with a retreat to avoid situations and environments that may induce anxiety, fear, or frustration. This approach is beneficial for maintaining peace and safety within the home.
- Muzzle training is recommended for all dogs that pose a bite risk. This process requires time and patience to properly condition them to wear a muzzle comfortably. Given that any dog can potentially bite, especially when experiencing protective emotions, muzzle training should be considered a foundational skill for all puppies, even if they are not displaying aggressive behaviors at the time. Muzzles are never punishment; they are a safety tool for protective contact.

Education

Clear communication regarding client expectations is critical for long-term success in managing dogs that use aggression. Clients should understand that progress can be slow and nonlinear, so patience and consistency are imperative. Equally valuable is the recognition that aggression is a normal part of a dog's behavioral repertoire and thus will never be fully eliminated or "cured." Instead, aggressive behavior can be well managed to promote the long-term safety and happiness of both the client and the dog.

Additionally, educating clients about dog body language is important. While overt signs of aggression such as growling, lunging, and snarling are often easily recognized, more subtle signs are equally, if not more, important to identify. Recognizing these signs helps prevent the escalation of the behavior by allowing the dog to be removed from the situation.

Clients can further set themselves and their dogs up for success by engaging in open, honest conversations about their dog's behavior with individuals likely to interact with the dog such as children, close family friends, and so on. These discussions should cover the dog's sensitivities and strategies for safe interaction, should any interactions occur.

See Table 7.3 for approaches to other behavior problems in dogs.

Table 7.3 Other behavior problems in dogs.

Behavior	Description/examples	Underlying causes/results	Approach
Anxiety	Can take the form of generalized anxiety, situational anxiety, or separation-related disorders. Recognizing the symptoms and triggers is vital for caregivers.	Generalized anxiety may cause excessive restlessness, poor sleep, and an increase in reactivity, while separation-related disorders often result in distress when the dog is home alone.	Behavior modification techniques and, when needed, the use of medications to reduce anxiety and enhance the dog's quality of life.
Barking	Excessive barking can be disruptive and challenging for both caregivers and their neighbors.	Fear, anxiety, frustration, alerting, or attention seeking.	Addressing the root cause through positive reinforcement training, strategic management, environmental enrichment, and behavior modification.
Cognitive dysfunction syndrome (CDS)	Similar to dementia in humans, prevalent in elderly dogs.	Medical co-morbidities are common and need to be differentiated first.	Support to enhance quality of life.
Compulsive behaviors	Tail chasing, shadow/light chasing, circling, barking, and licking, which can negatively impact a dog's wellbeing.	Anxiety, conflict, frustration, or stress; there may also be an underlying medical component or pathological cause.	Identify triggers and develop strategies to interrupt and redirect these behaviors.
Destructive behaviors	Chewing furniture or digging can be destructive to the home and frustrating for caregivers.	Frustration, anxiety, or a need for mental stimulation.	Provide appropriate chew toys and engage the dog in mentally stimulating activities to redirect and manage this behavior.
Fear-based behaviors	Cowering, hiding, bolting, and avoidance of environments, people, dogs, and objects Some dogs will bark, lunge, snap, and bite as part of the fear response.	Inadequate socialization, a traumatic event, genetics, and prenatal influences.	Initial management strategies to keep the dog feeling safe. Positive reinforcement training establishes foundational behaviors in preparation for behavior modification, to equip the dog with better coping skills and modify their behavior.

(Continued)

Table 7.3 (Continued)

Behavior	Description/examples	Underlying causes/results	Approach
House-soiling	Toileting in inappropriate areas.	Medical issues and behavioral concerns.	Rule out medical causes, then veterinarian can provide guidance on housetraining and behavior modification strategies.
Noise phobias	Fear of thunderstorms or fireworks.	Genetics, traumatic events, musculoskeletal pain.	Reduce exposure to noises through ear coverings and establishing a safe space. In situations where the specific noise cannot be identified or managed, medications may be necessary.
Nuisance and unruly behaviors	Jumping up on guests or grabbing and pulling on the leash.	Fear, anxiety, or frustration.	Teach foundational behaviors that are incompatible with jumping, as well as using foundational tools such as a front clip harness and a standard 4–6-foot leash. Training and behavior modification strategies may also be required.
Predatory behaviors	Chasing small animals.	Genetics – can be a normal species-specific behavior.	Training and management to ensure safety of both dog and potential prey.

Common Behavior Problems in Cats

Cats have their own unique set of behavior problems that may be challenging for their caregivers (Table 7.4).

Training Problems versus Emotional Issues

Understanding the difference between behavior problems that are primarily related to training and those stemming from emotional or psychological factors allows for the customization of intervention strategies to specifically address the needs of the pet, greatly improving the chances of successful behavior modification and promoting the animal's overall wellbeing. This distinction guides the selection of the most appropriate approach for intervention and treatment.

Training Problems

Training problems typically involve behaviors that can be addressed through teaching the pet new skills or reinforcing desirable behaviors. Examples of training issues include teaching social skills, foundational behaviors, leash manners, and basic housetraining. These problems are often rooted

Table 7.4 Common behavior problems in cats.

Behavior	Description/examples	Underlying causes/results	Approach
Aggression	Aggression toward familiar people, unfamiliar individuals, other cats, or various animals (Ley 2021).	Unfamiliarity or stressful environment such as veterinary hospital.	Identify triggers and implement strategies to manage and modify aggressive behaviors to ensure safety.
Anxiety	Increased vocalizations and separation-related behaviors; destructive behaviors and elimination disorders when cat is left alone (de Souza Machado et al. 2020).	Inadequate socialization, genetics, fear conditioning, traumatic event.	Identify sources of anxiety and develop behavior modification plans to alleviate cat's distress.
Cognitive dysfunction syndrome (CDS)	Disorientation, changes in sleep patterns, and altered interactions with caregivers.	Many medical co-mobidities possible. Pain and hypertension should be high on the differential list.	Support to improve quality of life.
Compulsive behaviors	Excessive grooming, vocalizations or tail-chasing.	Environmental stressors lead to conflict, anxiety, or frustration. If left untreated, these behaviors can result in or be caused by dermatological conditions, pain, or other health issues.	Recognize compulsive behaviors and implement strategies to manage and redirect these actions.
Destructive behaviors	Scratching furniture or pica.	Often normal behavior, but investigate medical conditions such as gastrointestinal disease when issues like chewing and food stealing occur.	Evaluate the environment to understand the reasons behind the behaviors, enabling development of a plan to meet the basic needs outlined in the 5 Pillars of a Healthy Feline Environment (Ellis et al. 2013) and provide outlets to channel and redirect these behaviors.
Fear-based behaviors	Skittishness and avoidance behaviors.	Underlying fears may be related to specific situations or general anxiety.	Develop management and specific behavior modification plans to reduce fear of a particular stimulus in a controlled and positive manner.
House-soiling	Toileting in inappropriate areas and urine marking.	Often has an underlying medical component, or can be a primary behavior problem.	Rule out health problems Adopt multimodal enrichment and behavior modification strategies. For urine marking, identify the triggers and implement environmental management to reduce stress and conflict between cats; medications may help.
Noise phobias	Loud or sudden sounds like thunderstorms or fireworks.	Inadequate socialization, a traumatic event, musculoskeletal pain.	Management strategies such as creating safe spaces or using medication to reduce anxiety.
Nuisance and unruly behaviors	Jumping on counters, knocking objects off shelves.	Often normal species-specific behaviors, but caregivers may find them disruptive.	Environmental management, multimodal enrichment, training on stationing to a mat, and behavior modification.

in a lack of understanding or communication between the caregiver and the pet. With consistent training and positive reinforcement techniques, training problems can be addressed effectively.

Emotional Issues

On the other hand, emotional or psychological issues are behavior problems rooted in deeper underlying emotional causes such as fear, anxiety, frustration, or past trauma. These behaviors may manifest as aggression, destructive behaviors, or severe anxiety disorders. Identifying emotional or psychological issues requires a more in-depth evaluation, including a comprehensive review of the pet's behavior history, identification of specific triggers for the behavior, and an assessment of the pet's overall physical and emotional health. Addressing these problems often involves a multifaceted approach, including management strategies, training, behavior modification techniques, medications, and creating a supportive environment to assist the pet in coping with and overcoming their emotional challenges.

How to Approach Behavior Problems in Practice

Addressing behavior problems in dogs and cats requires a comprehensive approach that encompasses various aspects of their wellbeing (Table 7.5). Veterinarians play an important role in guiding caregivers through the process of managing and modifying behavior problems (Strickler 2018).

One aspect of this approach is **management and safety**. Caregivers should be educated on how to create a safe environment for their pets and prevent situations that trigger problematic behaviors. This may include using crates, baby gates, or leash management to control the pet's access and interactions. Safety measures not only protect the caregivers and others but also help reduce the pet's stress and anxiety. They also slow down the progression of the behavior.

Meeting the **basic needs** of pets is another fundamental component. This involves ensuring they have proper nutrition, exercise, mental stimulation, and a comfortable living environment. Meeting these needs can significantly impact a pet's behavior. Consider a dog with a tendency to chew furniture or dig holes in the yard. Providing proper mental enrichment through puzzle toys, interactive feeders, or positive reinforcement training sessions can engage their cognitive abilities, reduce frustration, and effectively reduce anxiety. By meeting their behavioral needs, caregivers can create a more fulfilling environment for their companions, which is instrumental in addressing and preventing common behavior problems.

Improving **communication** with pets is key to understanding their needs and addressing behavior problems effectively. Veterinarians can educate caregivers about reading their pet's body language and recognizing signs of stress or discomfort. This knowledge helps caregivers identify triggers and respond appropriately to prevent escalation of problematic behaviors.

Positive reinforcement training is a valuable tool in behavior modification. It involves rewarding desirable behaviors with treats or toys, increasing the frequency of those behaviors. Veterinarians can guide caregivers on using positive reinforcement techniques to reinforce good behavior and replace undesirable actions with more acceptable ones. They can also outline the pitfalls of punishment and potential side effects that come from the use of aversive tools, positive punishment, and negative reinforcement training techniques.

In some cases **medications** may be necessary to help manage behavior problems, especially when they are rooted in anxiety, fear, or compulsive disorders. Veterinarians can provide insights

Table 7.5   Treatment of behavior problems.

Category	Details
Preliminary steps	• Rule out medical conditions. • Obtain a more detailed behavioral history. • Determine behavioral diagnosis. • Safety and management. • Meet basic needs.
Improving communication	• Understand body language. • Positive reinforcement training. • Avoid all forms of punishment.

Tools	• Appropriate tools for management:
	  – Muzzle training.
	  – Front clip harnesses.
	  – 4–6 ft nonretractable leashes.
	  – Baby gates.

Medications	• Identify triggers for the behaviors. Can they be avoided or managed? • Maintenance medication. • Situational medication. • Nutritional supplementation. • Pheromones.
Behavior modification techniques	• Control the antecedents. • Positive reinforcement training. • Response substitution (DRA/DRI). • Desensitization and counterconditioning.
Not recommended for behavior modification	• Positive punishment. • Negative punishment. • Negative reinforcement. • Flooding. • Extinction.

DRA, differential reinforcement of an alternative behavior; DRI, differential reinforcement of an incompatible behavior.

into when medications are appropriate, whether as situational aids for specific triggers or as long-term maintenance to address chronic issues.

Furthermore, **behavior modification** techniques can be employed to help pets overcome their behavior problems gradually. This may involve desensitization and counterconditioning to change the pet's response to triggering stimuli or the training and differential reinforcement of alternative or incompatible behaviors.

Medications

Addressing behavior problems in dogs and cats may require the use of medications in specific situations.

When to Medicate

Identifying the right time to introduce medication is important (Table 7.6). Medication may be considered when caregivers can identify triggers for problematic behaviors but struggle to manage them effectively. For example, a dog with severe thunderstorm phobia may display extreme anxiety during storms despite attempts at management and desensitization and counterconditioning (DS/CC). In such cases medication can provide relief and reduce distress.

Table 7.6   When to prescribe.

Scenario	Guidelines
Immediate need	Prescribe medication during the initial assessment for severe cases (e.g., intense separation-related behaviors, extreme fear). Integrate medication into the overall behavior management plan.
Delayed need	If the behavior plan involves significant management changes without immediate need for medication and the pet has a good quality of life, consider postponing medication until a follow-up visit. Medication may not always be necessary.
Adjunct to behavior modification	For pets undergoing behavior modification but not progressing, introducing medication might be beneficial. Medications can improve the learning process and help facilitate behavior modification.

Maintenance versus Situational Medication

Information gathered from a comprehensive behavioral history helps to determine when medications are needed and which medication to choose. Maintenance medications are utilized in cases where the stimuli triggering the behavior cannot be adequately identified or managed. Examples of such situations include a dog that must stay home alone daily, a cat that engages in urine marking, or a dog with noise phobia where the specific sounds causing the behavior are difficult to pinpoint. On the other hand, situational medications are suitable for instances where the triggers for the behavior are identifiable and predictable yet not effectively managed, such as during thunderstorms, fireworks, car rides, or veterinary visits (Table 7.7).

When prescribing medications each animal should be approached as an individual, and medication choices should be made based on the behavioral diagnosis. Make sure clients have realistic expectations and do not compromise the safety of either the animal or humans in the home.

Table 7.7   Differences between situational and maintenance medications.

Medication type	Trigger identification	Time to effectiveness	Duration of effect	Dosage
Maintenance medications	Cannot identify or control the trigger for the behavior.	Several weeks to months.	Long-lasting, with mild to moderate effects.	Consistent dose regardless of behavior intensity.
Situational medications	Can identify but cannot manage or avoid the trigger for the behavior.	Hours to minutes.	Short period, requires redosing.	Adjusted based on trial dosage; given before the stimulus occurs.

Along with medication, a comprehensive treatment plan including management, training, and behavior modification will still be needed to successfully change the pet's behavior.

Time to Effect

When prescribing maintenance medications for behavior issues, it generally takes a minimum of 4–6 weeks to observe an improvement in the animal's behavior. Allow sufficient time before considering changes in dosage for these medications. In contrast, situational medications typically show effectiveness within 1–2 hours. Finding the most beneficial dosage for situational medications often involves trial and error. Therefore, conduct a trial dose of these medications in advance of when they are needed. This trial helps in determining the time it takes for a medication to become effective, its duration of effect, and any potential side effects, allowing for necessary adjustments.

Medications in Young Animals

Most medications do not have an age restriction. Starting medication earlier in the treatment process can be beneficial, often before the animal has extensively rehearsed the problematic behavior. Most medications prescribed for behavioral problems are safe for young animals, making early intervention a priority. This approach ensures timely and effective management of behavior issues in younger pets.

Polypharmacy

In some cases polypharmacy may be needed. These medications target neurotransmitters, each of which has a different effect on the modulation of behavior. Knowing the mechanism of action of the prescribed medication can help determine if medications can be combined for maximum efficacy.

Caution When Prescribing

Most medications used for treating behavioral conditions in animals are formulated for humans and are often prescribed off-label. It is essential to obtain informed consent from the client before prescribing. This includes informing them about potential side effects. Additionally, when prescribing these medications veterinarians should base their decision on their own diagnosis and treatment plan, rather than relying on recommendations from nonveterinarians. Regular follow-up should be required, and annual blood work is recommended for patients who continue with the medication over the long term.

Situational Medications

There are various medications available for specific situational use (Table 7.8). These include trazodone, which can help alleviate anxiety and stress in dogs during events like fireworks or travel. Clonidine is another option that can be useful for managing fear and anxiety-related behaviors. Sileo®, often used for noise phobias, is administered transmucosally to help calm dogs during stressful situations. Gabapentin, pregabalin, and benzodiazepines may also be prescribed to manage anxiety and fear in certain circumstances.

Table 7.8 Common situational medications.

Medication	Use	Dose	Side effects
Trazodone	Alleviates anxiety and stress during events like fireworks or travel.	3–8 mg/kg Q 8–24 h (dog) 25–50 mg per cat 1.5–2 h before veterinary visit.	Increase in anxiety Sedation Vomiting Increase in aggression (cats)
Clonidine	Useful for managing fear and anxiety-related behaviors.	0.01–0.05 mg/kg Q 8–12 h (dogs only).	Sedation Dry mouth Increased urine output
Sileo®	Administered transmucosally for noise phobias; helps calm dogs during stressful situations.	Label dose.	Sedation
Gabapentin	Prescribed to manage anxiety and fear in certain circumstances.	10–50 mg/kg 2 h prior to veterinary visit (dog) 50–100 mg *per cat* prior to veterinary visits. Decrease dose by 50% in cats with renal disease.	Sedation Ataxia
Pregabalin	Prescribed to manage anxiety and fear in certain circumstances. Neuropathic pain.	5 mg/kg Q 12 h (dog) 5 mg/kg 2 h before veterinary visit (cat).	Sedation Ataxia
Benzodiazepines	Used for managing anxiety and fear in certain situations. True anxiolytic and sometimes chosen for its amnesia effects.	Varied based on choice.	Agitation Ataxia Aggression Polyphagia Sedation

Maintenance Medications

For behavior problems with an ongoing or chronic nature, maintenance medications may be necessary (Table 7.9). These include selective serotonin reuptake inhibitors (SSRIs) like fluoxetine (Reconcile®, Pegasus Laboratories, Inc., Pensacola, FL), paroxetine, and sertraline, which can help manage anxiety and compulsive disorders over the long term. Tricyclic antidepressants (TCAs) such as clomipramine and amitriptyline may be prescribed for similar purposes. Additionally, serotonin-norepinephrine reuptake inhibitors (SNRIs) like venlafaxine and other medications like buspirone may be considered to address specific behavioral issues (Dantas and Ogata 2024; Maffeo et al. 2023; Metz et al. 2022). Selegiline (Anipryl®, Zoetis Inc., Florham Park, NJ) is a monoamine oxidase inhibitor (MAOI) approved for treatment of canine CDS or senile dementia.

In cases where behavior problems persist despite diligent behavior modification efforts, the introduction of medication can often make a substantial difference. Veterinarians can assess the individual needs of each pet, carefully weigh the potential benefits and risks of medication, and work collaboratively with caregivers to develop a comprehensive treatment plan. This approach, incorporating behavior modification and medications when necessary, ensures the best possible outcome for pets facing behavior challenges and helps caregivers keep their pets feeling safe.

Table 7.9 Common maintenance medications.

Medication class	Examples	Use	Dose	Side effects
Selective serotonin reuptake inhibitors (SSRIs)	Fluoxetine (Reconcile®), paroxetine, sertraline	Manage anxiety and compulsive disorders over the long term	Fluoxetine 0.5–2 mg/kg PO Q 24 h Paroxetine 1 mg/kg PO Q 24 h Sertraline 1–3 mg/kg PO Q 12–24 h	Agitation/increased anxiety Inappetence, vomiting, diarrhea Lower seizure threshold (fluoxetine least likely to affect seizure threshold) Sedation Tremors
Tricyclic antidepressants (TCAs)	Clomipramine, amitriptyline	Prescribed for similar purposes as SSRIs	Clomipramine 1–3 mg/kg Q 12 h (dog) 0.25–1 mg/kg Q 12–24 h (cat) Amitriptyline 1–4 mg/kg PO Q 12 h (dog) 0.5–1 mg/kg Q 24 h (cat)	Constipation Decreased appetite Dry mouth/dry eyes Increased anxiety Lower seizure threshold Sedation Tachycardia/tachyarrhythmia Urine retention
Serotonin-norepinephrine reuptake inhibitors (SNRIs)	Venlafaxine	Helps address specific behavioral issues. Used frequently to treat urine marking in cats. May be beneficial when there is a pain component to the behavior	0.5–2 mg/kg Q 12 h (dogs) 1 mg/kg Q 24 h (cats)	Decrease in appetite Sedation Urinary retention
Azapirone	Buspirone	Used in cats with intercat aggression (victim cat), noise phobias, and generalized anxiety	1–2 mg/kg PO Q 8–24 h (dog) 5–7.5 mg per cat Q 12 h	Aggression disinhibition Increased anxiety
Monoamine oxidase inhibitor (MAOI)	Selegiline	Cognitive decline	0.25–1 mg/kg PO Q 24 h	Agitation Disorientation Vomiting/diarrhea

Table 7.10 Expected changes on medications.

Expected changes	Description
Increased comfort and confidence	Pets become more comfortable and confident in their environment.
Learning and habits	Pets are more capable of learning new behaviors and habits, enabling more activities.
Reduction in undesirable behaviors	Noticeable reduction in the intensity, frequency, or duration of reactions or behaviors.
Recovery post reactions	Pets recover more quickly from episodes, reactions, or stressful events.

How to Know if Medications Are Working

When pets are prescribed medication for behavioral issues, certain changes in their behavior are expected (Table 7.10). Most often pets become comfortable, engaged, and more confident and cope better in their environment. They also become more capable of learning new behaviors and habits, enabling more activities. Additionally, there should be a noticeable reduction in the intensity, frequency, or duration of the pet's reactions or behaviors. Pets typically recover more quickly from episodes, reactions, or stressful events than they did before the medication.

Conclusion

Understanding and addressing behavior problems in dogs and cats form an essential aspect of veterinary practice. By differentiating between normal and abnormal behaviors and comprehensively exploring common behavior problems, veterinarians can provide lifesaving guidance and support to pet caregivers. With the right knowledge and strategies, these behavior issues can be managed effectively, improving the wellbeing of both pets and their human companions.

References

Bamberger, M. and Houpt, K.A. (2006). Signalment factors, comorbidity, and trends in behavior diagnoses in dogs: 1644 cases (1991–2001). *Journal of the American Veterinary Medical Association* 229: 1591–1601.

Dantas, L.M. and Ogata, N. (2024). Veterinary psychopharmacology. *Veterinary Clinics of North America, Small Animal Practice* 54 (1): 195–205.

Demontigny-Bédard, I. and Frank, D. (2018). Developing a plan to treat behavior disorders. *Veterinary Clinics of North America, Small Animal Practice* 48 (3): 351–365.

Ellis, S.L.H., Rodan, I., Carney, H.C. et al. (2013). AAFP and ISFM feline environmental needs guidelines. *Journal of Feline Medicine and Surgery* 15 (3): 219–230.

Landsberg, G., Hunthausen, W., and Ackerman, L. (2013). *Behavior Problems of the Dog and Cat*. Philadelphia, PA: Saunders Elsevier.

Ley, J. (2021). Aggression-cats. In: *Small Animal Veterinary Psychiatry* (ed. S. Denenberg), 180–190. Wallingford, UK: CABI.

Maffeo, N.N., Springer, C.M., and Albright, J.D. (2023). A retrospective study on the clinical use and owner perception of venlafaxine efficacy as part of a multimodal treatment for canine fear, anxiety, and aggression. *Journal of Veterinary Behavior* 64–65: 54–59.

Metz, D., Medam, T., and Masson, S. (2022). Double-blind, placebo-controlled trial of venlafaxine to treat behavioural disorders in cats: a pilot study. *Journal of Feline Medicine and Surgery* 24 (6): 539–549.

Odendaal, J.S.J. (1997). A diagnostic classification of problem behavior in dogs and cats. *Veterinary Clinics of North America, Small Animal Practice* 27 (3): 427–443.

Siracusa, C. (2024). The false dichotomy between medical and behavioral problems Veterinary Clinics of North America, Small Animal. *Practice* 54 (1): xiii–xiv.

de Souza Machado, D., Oliveira, P.M.B., Machado, J.C. et al. (2020). Identification of separation-related problems in domestic cats: a questionnaire survey. *PLoS One* 15 (4): e0230999.

Stelow, E. (2018). Diagnosing behavior problems: a guide for practitioners. *Veterinary Clinics of North America, Small Animal Practice* 48 (3): 339–350.

Strickler, B.G. (2018). Helping pet owners change pet behaviors: an overview of the science. *Veterinary Clinics of North America, Small Animal Practice* 48 (3): 419–431.

8

Pet Selection

Selecting the right pet is a significant decision that can have a lasting impact on a person's life. Caregivers must carefully consider various factors to ensure that their new companion is a good fit for their lifestyle, preferences, and needs. This chapter is dedicated to guiding caregivers through the process of pet selection. The options for acquiring a pet include animal shelters, rescue organizations, and breeders, each with its advantages and considerations.

Pet Selection Counseling

Pet selection counseling is the first step in preventing behavioral problems. Given the unique nature of each caregiver, animal, and situation, providing specific advice on pet selection is challenging (McBride 2005). Nonetheless, individuals looking to adopt a new pet can utilize various resources to guide their choice. Veterinarians should be prepared to offer this service to their clients (Bergman and Gaskins 2008), especially since many caregivers turn to alternative sources such as the internet for behavioral advice (Bergman et al. 2002).

In the pet selection process a questionnaire can be helpful. The consultant's role, however, is not to choose a specific breed, age, or sex for a family (Landsberg et al. 2013b). Rather, their job is to discuss the advantages and disadvantages of each breed and guide the family in selecting the sex, age, and particular dog or cat (Landsberg et al. 2013b). The selection consultation also offers an opportunity to provide the family with important information on health, feeding, housing, and especially on behavior and training (Landsberg et al. 2013b). Setting realistic expectations and offering behavioral advice during each visit with a puppy or kitten can help to lower the risk of future relinquishment (Table 8.1).

Genetics and Behavior

Significant research has been conducted into the genetics associated with behavior and behavior problems (Landsberg et al. 2013b). It is widely recognized that genetics play a role in various behavioral traits (Saetre et al. 2006; Scott and Fuller 1965; Wayne and Ostrander 2007). The potential for inheriting certain behavioral traits has partly influenced the development of specific dog breeds (Turcsan et al. 2011). Dogs have been selectively bred over generations for abilities such as retrieving, tracking, hunting, and guarding. However, undesirable traits can also be passed down through lineages. This does not imply that all behavior problems are genetic; many issues are related to poor socialization and other early life experiences (Turcsan et al. 2011).

Veterinary Guide to Preventing Behavior Problems in Dogs and Cats, First Edition. Christine D. Calder and Sarah C. Wright.
© 2025 John Wiley & Sons, Inc. Published 2025 by John Wiley & Sons, Inc.

Table 8.1 Factors to consider when selecting a pet.

Category	Considerations
Species and breed	Dog or cat Purebred or mixed breed Show or pet quality Breed traits (function, temperament, etc.)
Age and physical characteristics	Puppy/kitten or adult Appearance, size, hair coat
Sex and reproductive status	Male or female Neutered or intact
Financial commitment	Costs for food, housing, veterinary care, grooming, training/enrichment, etc.
Family and lifestyle	Family allergies/disabilities Daily routines, time at home Past pet experiences
Environment	Home type, location, fencing Restrictions (landlord, laws)
Long-term commitment	Pet's life expectancy Future living situation changes Care plans for absences and longevity
Pet's needs and caregiver's availability	Attention requirements Work hours Travel frequency
Interaction with existing pets	Compatibility with current pets Consultation with veterinarian
Personal preferences	Desired pet qualities (e.g., companionship, ease of care) Caregiver's experience and availability

Merely having a genetic predisposition for certain behavioral traits does not guarantee their expression, nor does it mean that all animals with the same genetic variations will exhibit these traits to the same degree. Protein structure, protein interactions, and environmental factors all influence the behaviors of individual animals (Nicholas 2010). The complexity of behavioral genetics is further increased by the fact that multiple mutations can affect a single behavioral trait. For instance, variation exists within the English Cocker Spaniel breed regarding levels of aggression in individual dogs (Podberscek and Serpell 1996). Additionally, due to selective breeding pressures, the specific mutations affecting behavior in one breed may differ from those in another breed.

Consequently, when determining the likelihood of specific behaviors or behavior problems in a given individual, consider not only the individual animal's breed but also their familial history and early life experiences. Behavior is a complex phenomenon and no single factor can fully explain the underlying reasons for a particular behavior problem.

Choosing Between Shelter, Rescue, and Breeders

The main options for acquiring a pet are animal shelters, rescue organizations, pet stores, and breeders, each offering distinct advantages and considerations (Table 8.2).

Table 8.2   Sources of pets.

Aspect	Shelter	Breeder	Rescue organization	Pet store
Adoption saves lives	✓ Many animals in need	✓ Ethical breeders	✓ Rescues at-risk pets	✓ Availability of puppies
Lower cost	✓ Lower adoption fees	✗ Can be expensive	✓ Reasonable fees	✗ May be costly up front
Vet care included	✓ Often spayed/ neutered	✓ Health guarantees	✓ Health checks	✗ Varies by store
Variety of breeds	✗ Varies by shelter; many are mixed breeds	✓ Specific breed choice	✗ Varies by rescue	✓ Wide variety of breeds
Supporting causes	✓ Supports animal welfare	✗ Supports breeding, which may or may not be ethical; significant individual variation	✓ Supports rescue	✗ Commercial interests
Uncertain history	✓ Unknown background	✗ Potential breed-specific/hereditary health issues	✗ Varies by rescue	✗ Limited transparency
Breed-specific traits	✗ Limited predictability	✓ Predictable traits	✗ Varies by rescue	✗ Predictable traits

✓, Pros; ✗, Cons

Behavioral issues are the primary reason dogs and cats are surrendered to shelters, rehomed, or euthanized, as noted by Patronek et al. (1996) and Salman et al. (2000). Providing preventative behavioral services offers an opportunity to educate caregivers about normal animal behaviors and to address common behavioral challenges; doing so helps keep pets in their homes.

For puppies and kittens, starting off on the right foot involves first choosing the appropriate pet, followed by socialization, attending puppy and kitten kindergarten classes, and learning basic behaviors. Shelter dogs and cats often have unknown backgrounds and may require behavior modification before adoption. Addressing these issues early on is easier than treating any behavior problems that may develop later.

Importance of Transparency

When adopting an animal, whether from a shelter or a rescue group, transparency is important. This means the organization should be open about the animal's overall health and behavioral needs while in their care. Medical records should be included in the adoption process, along with information about any known previous homes. Similarly, a good breeder should be transparent, inviting questions and being able to provide references. Shelters, rescue groups, and breeders should be willing to serve as a resource as pets transition into their new homes.

Animal Shelters

Animal shelters are typically operated by municipal or nonprofit organizations and often house a variety of pets, including dogs, cats, and occasionally other animals such as rabbits, guinea pigs, or birds. They provide an opportunity to give a second chance to animals in need, offering homes to pets that may have been abandoned or surrendered by previous caregivers. Shelters are an excellent choice for individuals looking to provide a new home to a pet while also supporting the ethical treatment of animals.

Rescue Organizations

Rescue organizations are typically nonprofit groups dedicated to rescuing and rehoming specific breeds or types of animals. These organizations often have a thorough screening process for potential adopters and may require a commitment to breed-specific care. Choosing a rescue organization allows caregivers to adopt a pet with a known background and potentially a better understanding of the animal's behavior and health history.

Abandoned and Orphaned Animals

Stray and homeless dogs and cats are a widespread issue globally (Sandoe et al. 2019). These animals might be abandoned intentionally, lost, or born in the wild. The problem is exacerbated by the attitude of some people who view animals as "disposable," leading them to stop caring for pets they once adopted (Robertson 2008).

Although many animals live in feral or semi-feral states, people still provide a considerable level of care for them. In the United States about 25% of households feed outdoor cats, even if they do not personally own them (Levy et al. 2003; Slater 2005). Some communities extend their support by offering basic veterinary care and spay/neuter services for these feral animals (Centonze and Levy 2002). Additionally, a notable number of households choose to adopt stray or feral cats, and to a lesser extent dogs, as pets (APPA 2018).

Breeders

Breeders are individuals or organizations that specialize in producing specific breeds of animals. Reputable breeders adhere to ethical breeding practices, prioritize the health and wellbeing of their animals, and provide proper socialization and early care. They should be willing to show their kennels and the animals under their care to prospective buyers. Genetic screening tests should be performed on all breeding animals, with particular attention given to known breed dispositions. The results of these tests should be available for prospective buyers to review. Caregivers seeking a particular breed with specific characteristics may opt for a responsible breeder. However, it is essential to thoroughly research and choose a breeder with a strong reputation to ensure the welfare of the animals. Clients should be directed to evaluate references from the breeder, including veterinarians and previous buyers.

As opposed to reputable breeders, pet stores, puppy mills, and breeding farms often produce animals with more behavioral and health problems. There is a higher frequency of inbreeding and a lower frequency of health screening. Medical histories and lineages are often unavailable. Because parental information is unknown, it is much harder to predict an individual animal's behavior and potential health problems that may arise.

Puppy Culture

Puppy Culture, created by Jane Messineo Lindquist, a professional dog trainer and breeder, is a comprehensive online program designed to assist breeders in training and socializing puppies from birth through their early socialization phase (https://shoppuppyculture.com/pages/about-puppy-culture). This program provides breeders with an in-depth understanding of puppy

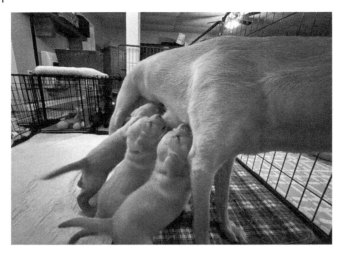

Figure 8.1 Puppy Culture is a breeder program that helps to give puppies an ideal start at life. Breeders who use this program tend to produce higher-quality, well-adjusted puppies. Courtesy of Rachel Thornton.

development and behavior, establishing a strong foundation for the puppies' continual learning and adaptation. Puppies raised with Puppy Culture are more likely to be well adjusted, confident, and exhibit fewer behavioral issues, thus facilitating a smoother transition to a new home (Figure 8.1).

Puppy Culture presents a structured approach to breeding and raising puppies, focusing on enhancing both their physical and mental development. Grounded in the latest scientific research, the program highlights the significance of early learning experiences and socialization opportunities. It ensures puppies receive a diverse range of experiences and skills, supporting their growth into confident and well-balanced adult dogs. This includes exposing puppies to various environments, people, and situations, as well as teaching them basic social skills.

The activities within Puppy Culture may involve acquainting puppies with different textures, sounds, and visuals; providing opportunities for play and exploration; and teaching basic behaviors like "sit" and "touch." The program also educates breeders and caregivers in canine behavior and development and offers guidance on appropriate socialization and care for puppies as they transition from the breeder to their new homes.

Breed and Breed Type

When selecting a specific breed, caregivers should be informed about the breed's history, purpose, and potential genetic and health concerns. The temperament and behavioral needs can vary significantly between breeds (Landsberg et al. 2013b). Clients should understand how these traits may affect whether an animal is suitable for their lifestyle. Additionally, caregivers should be prepared to address the grooming needs of their chosen breed. Veterinarians can assist clients in selecting groomers and ensuring that the animal's health is maintained through proper coat management.

Realistic Expectations and Desired Traits

Once the source of the pet has been established, caregivers need to set realistic expectations and identify the desired traits they seek in their new companion. It is important for caregivers to consider factors such as their living situation, available space, activity level, and the amount of time they can dedicate to pet care (Marder and Duxbury 2008).

Age of Adoption

Clients considering animal adoption need to understand the benefits and challenges of adopting pets at different ages to make the best choice for their situation. While there is no consensus on the best age for adopting puppies and kittens, some guidelines can help. Kittens should generally be adopted around 7 weeks of age, after they have had enough human interaction. If breeders keep kittens longer, it is important they still interact with people. For puppies, the usual advice is to adopt them at 8–10 weeks of age (McMillan 2017). However, if their early environment is not ideal and a new caregiver can provide better socialization, adopting at 6–7 weeks might be advisable. It is important to note, though, that puppies adopted before 8 weeks of age have shown an increased likelihood of later exhibiting aggression and separation-related behaviors (McMillan 2017). Understanding these details helps to increase the chances of a successful, permanent adoption (Powell et al. 2021b).

Young Animals

Both puppies and kittens can relatively easily adapt to new environments and stimuli during their socialization periods, as long as the experiences are perceived as positive (Casey and Bradshaw 2008). However, these young animals require considerable time and effort. They need regular, positive interactions with various people, animals, and environments for proper socialization. Additionally, they often demand significant energy for training (Powell et al. 2018). Clients seeking to adopt young animals should be encouraged to work with positive reinforcement-based trainers in order to help their new pets gain the skills and confidence they need to develop appropriate social skills and adapt to their new home environment.

Adult Animals

Compared to puppies and kittens, adult animals have different needs and often exhibit more mature behaviors. For example, they usually understand basic behavioral cues, are accustomed to longer periods without their caregiver, are familiar with leash walks, and understand feeding schedules. However, these traits are not guaranteed in every adult animal (Landsberg et al. 2013b). One notable advantage of adult animals is that they tend to be gentler during play, exhibiting less nipping, chewing, and scratching behaviors compared to younger animals (Graff and Gaultier 2002).
    Despite these positive traits, adopting adult animals comes with its own set of challenges. Adult dogs and cats are more likely to be returned to shelters after adoption than younger animals, which increases their risk of being euthanized (Powell et al. 2021b). This higher return rate may be attributed to a greater incidence of behavioral problems in adult animals. Being past their socialization period, they often find it more difficult to adapt to new environments and cope with their past experiences (Landsberg et al. 2013b). The older an animal is at the time of adoption, the more likely it is that they will exhibit problematic behaviors such as resource guarding or destructiveness (Martinez et al. 2011; McGreevy and Masters 2008). In the case of cats, there is a noted decrease in human interaction as they age, which can lead to challenges in forming a strong human–animal bond, resulting in a higher likelihood of the cat being returned (Brown and Stephan 2020; Hart et al. 2018).

Gender

When selecting a new pet, consider the differences in size and behavior between male and female animals. Intact male dogs often have a higher tendency toward aggression, and neutering does not always reduce this behavior. Compared to females, male cats are more prone to urine marking, though females can also exhibit this behavior. Male dogs may show less interest in greeting unfamiliar men. Moreover, in some breeds there may be behavioral differences between males and females.

Spaying or neutering an animal can have significant effects on both behavior and physical health. This is due to the removal of sex hormones that influence behavior (Giammanco et al. 2005; Hart and Eckstein 1997; Hart and Hart 2021). Although certain changes in behavior are commonly seen after these procedures, the extent and nature of these changes can vary widely among individual animals (Palestrini et al. 2021).

Since multiple factors influence behaviors like aggression, the effect of spaying or neutering is not the same for every animal (Urfer and Kaeberlein 2019). Therefore the decision to spay or neuter should be carefully considered, taking into account the specific circumstances of each animal. Deciding whether to spay or neuter an animal should be based on individual circumstances, and there should be a clear discussion with the caregiver about the risks, benefits, and limitations of current scientific understanding (Houlihan 2017).

Spaying or neutering an animal primarily impacts reproductive-related behaviors, as it involves the removal of sex hormones like testosterone, estrogen, and progesterone. This can result in notable changes in both behavior and physical health. For example, neutering male dogs typically reduces behaviors such as roaming, mounting, and urine marking (Neilson et al. 1997). In male cats, early neutering often leads to a decrease in aggression, sexual behaviors, and urine spraying (Howe 2015). However, these behavioral changes can vary widely among individual animals after spaying or neutering (Giammanco et al. 2005; Hart and Eckstein 1997; Hart and Hart 2021; Palestrini et al. 2021).

While many undesirable behaviors decrease after spaying or neutering, some behaviors may actually increase following these procedures. Neutering male dogs, for instance, might lead to increased aggression, with less than 33% showing a significant decrease in such behavior (Hart and Hart 2021; Neilson et al. 1997). Additionally, neutered male dogs are more prone to showing fearful and anxious behaviors (Kaufman et al. 2017). Similarly, early spaying or neutering in cats can result in increased fearful behavior (Moons et al. 2018; Spain et al. 2004).

Temperament Testing and Behavioral Evaluation

Temperament testing in shelters, often used to assist potential adopters, faces significant challenges. The interpretation of these tests is difficult and there is a high risk of mislabeling animals, leading to poor adoption outcomes and sometimes euthanasia (Patronek et al. 2019). The reliability of these tests is questionable, as the false-positive rate in shelter settings exceeds 50% (Mornement et al. 2014; Patronek et al. 2019). Additionally, the effectiveness of the tests is often compromised by the experience level of the evaluators. Some shelters rely on volunteers for behavioral assessments (Mornement et al. 2014), and when conducted by inexperienced staff or volunteers the accuracy of the results is diminished (Mornement et al. 2010). Although accuracy improves with increased experience and training (Diesel et al. 2008), shelters often struggle with a high personnel turnover; more experienced individuals can be difficult to retain due to limited resources (Duffy and Serpell 2012).

The evaluations in shelters typically focus on behaviors like aggression. Granted, an individual animal's reaction to other animals, children, and other stimuli is important information for a potential adopter to know. However, the methods used are not always reliable for accurately assessing such behaviors (Barnard et al. 2012; Shabelansky et al. 2015). Furthermore, defining specific behaviors and temperament traits is challenging due to varying definitions and behaviors associated with a single trait, leading to confusing test results (Lockwood 2016). Fear-based behaviors, often exacerbated in shelter environments, can result in misidentifying and misunderstanding animals (Patronek et al. 2019).

Completed caregiver assessments have their own limitations. Often caregivers under-report problem behaviors when surrendering pets (Segurson et al. 2005), with surveys showing nearly 70% of caregivers claiming no behavior problems (Dinwoodie et al. 2019; Powell et al. 2021a; Salman et al. 2000). Despite this, caregiver surveys can provide valuable supplementary information for shelter staff (Duffy et al. 2014) and assist in guiding post-adoption training and rehabilitation (Stephen and Ledger 2007).

Shelter stress can significantly affect an animal's behavior during temperament testing (Mornement et al. 2014). Factors like unfamiliar surroundings and the absence of familiar companions can increase stress levels (Shiverdecker et al. 2013), and behaviors observed during tests conducted soon after admission may not reflect the animal's typical behavior in a home setting (Mornement et al. 2014).

For young puppies, temperament testing often does not predict adult behavior, except in cases of excessive fear. As pets mature, the effects of early handling, socialization, learning, and maturation can make temperament testing more predictive (Palestrini et al. 2021). Kittens, with a sensitive period waning by 9 weeks of age, may have more accurate temperament assessments than puppies. Adult cats tested for reactions to various stimuli can be categorized into groups, with the most positive responses suggesting a likely positive adjustment to a new home.

The validation of temperament testing protocols, especially those used for pet adoption, is often uncertain. These tests typically assess traits such as responsiveness to training, reactivity, fearfulness, sociability, and aggression (Duffy and Serpell 2012). However, broadly applying the results of these tests to pets may not be accurate. While current tests concentrate on evaluating fearfulness, reactivity, sociability, and trainability using a range of methods, it is important to note that there is no standardized or universally accepted method for testing fear in animals.

Living Situation and Space

Consider the caregiver's living situation. Is the caregiver living in an apartment or a house with a yard? Are there any pet ownership restrictions imposed by the landlord or homeowners' association? The size and type of the living space, along with any related restrictions, play a significant role in determining the most appropriate type and size of pet for that environment.

Activity Level and Time Commitment

Caregivers need to assess their activity level and daily schedule when considering pet ownership. Pets vary in their needs; for example, high-energy dog breeds often require more exercise and mental stimulation. It is important for caregivers to reflect on whether they have the necessary time and commitment to meet these needs. Additionally, they should consider how a pet will integrate into their daily routine, including the responsibilities of feeding, grooming, and veterinary care.

Desired Traits and Compatibility

Caregivers should identify the specific traits they desire in a pet such as temperament, size, breed, age and consider compatibility with their lifestyle and family dynamics. For example, families with small children may prefer a pet known for their gentle disposition, while an active individual may seek a pet that can keep up with outdoor activities.

Introducing Pets

Veterinarians can serve as an important resource for clients introducing new pets to existing pets within a household (Bergman and Gaskins 2008). Many pet-to-pet introductions result in aggressive interactions, which can persist beyond the initial interaction and even worsen over time (Horwitz and Neilson 2007; Levine et al. 2005). Therefore, veterinarians should be well informed to guide caregivers on safe introductions (Figure 8.2). Further, veterinarians should advise caregivers to proceed with caution and seek the guidance of a veterinary behaviorist if introducing animals with a known history of aggression (Bergman and Gaskins 2008).

Canine Introductions

There are multiple ways to promote positive dog-to-dog introductions. Before new dogs are introduced, they need to have an engaging relationship with their caregiver and be able to respond to basic cues amid distractions. These cues include touch (nose to hand) and recall (coming when called), both taught using positive reinforcement. Caregivers should be able to safely handle their

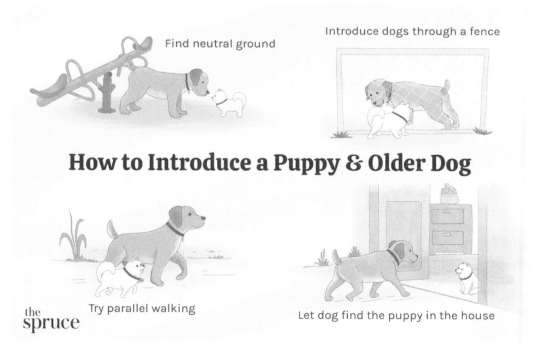

Figure 8.2 Steps for introducing a puppy and older dog. *Source:* Dotdash Meredith / https://www.thesprucepets.com/introducing-dogs-and-puppies-2805078 (accessed February 3, 2024).

dog both on and off the leash and in the presence of various distractions. Observation and interpretation of body language help caregivers to quickly intervene if needed to ensure each dog is engaged and comfortable with the introduction. The Shelter Playgroup Alliance is an excellent resource for interpreting body language during dog–dog interactions (www.shelterdogplay.org).

Ideally dogs should be introduced in a "neutral" territory or with a barrier such as a fence or gate for safety (Table 8.3). Introductions are best conducted in open spaces away from a dog's home to minimize the chance of fighting (Bradshaw and Lea 1992; Houpt 1991; Shyan et al. 2003) and to give each dog space to move away if they feel uncomfortable. Interactions should not be forced, and food and toys should be absent to reduce the risk of resource guarding. Keeping arousal levels low is important, and frequent check-ins (voluntary eye contact) along with calm and relaxed behaviors should be encouraged and reinforced through the use of positive reinforcement (Horwitz and Neilson 2007; Sherman 1996).

Table 8.3 Conducting dog-to-dog introductions.

Aspect	Details
Relationship with caregiver	Before introduction, both dogs should have an engaging relationship with their caregiver. Dogs should know basic behaviors such as touch, come, and settle on a mat, and caregivers need to be comfortable handling their dog both on and off leash safely.
Reading body language	Caregivers should be observant and skilled at reading dog body language and be prepared to intervene if necessary.
Location of introduction	Introduce dogs in "neutral" territory. Open spaces away from a dog's home are ideal. Alternatives include parallel walks and the use of gates or fences for safety.
Minimizing aggression triggers	Avoid triggers like free access to food and toys during initial interactions, and keep arousals to a minimum.
Rewarding behavior	Use positive reinforcement techniques to reward desirable behaviors such as frequent check-ins, touch, and active engagement with the caregiver.

Feline Introductions

Cat-to-cat introductions, like those with dogs, should be managed through a variety of strategies (Table 8.4). The introduction should be gradual, progressing only if both cats are comfortable (Figure 8.3). Initially it is best to separate the cats in their own core territories or spaces (Ley 2020). This separation allows them to smell and hear each other through a solid, opaque barrier, preventing the overarousal that can lead to protective emotions and defensive behaviors (Beaver 2003; Bergman and Gaskins 2008; Heath 2018). Each area should include all basic needs and resources like a litter box, resting area, vertical and hiding spaces, as well as feeding and water stations.

Room rotation and rubbing each cat with the same cloth can facilitate scent transfer, aiding in their assimilation (Landsberg et al. 2013a). Additionally, a common space should be set up where the cats can spend time independently, equipped with key resources such as resting, vertical, and hiding areas. This allows them to become familiar with each other's scents and deposit their own pheromones.

When the cats show comfort with this setup and no signs of arousal from the other's scent or sound, supervised time in the communal area can begin (Figure 8.4). Feeding them on opposite sides of the room is advisable. During introductions, all cats should always have the option to retreat to their core spaces. Teaching behaviors such as touch (nose to target or hand), coming

Table 8.4 Cat-to-cat introductions.

Step	Description
Understanding cat groups	Household and neighborhood cats often form stable groups with overlapping territories. New cats are not usually readily accepted into these groups.
Initial introduction	New cats should be confined to a specific area that becomes their core territory, away from the other cats. This should be equipped with all basic needs and resources (litter box, resting area, vertical spaces, food, and water dish). The household cats should have their own space and then there should be a community space.
Scent familiarization	Give the existing cats an opportunity to smell the new cat under the door, but avoid direct visual contact at first. If this is stressful for either cat, block the scent transfer under the door with a towel.
Space sharing	Time-share the community space between the new and existing cats to familiarize them with each other's scents. This is done individually at first.
Exploration	When the cats are comfortable in the communal space and can readily relax, it is time to start supervised meetings.
Supervised meeting	Give the cats access to the communal area, keeping them as far apart as possible, ideally during feeding or play. Foundational behaviors such as stationing on a mat, nose targeting, and coming when called help to manage the cats, if they need to be redirected back into their safe space. Pattern games can also be used.
Monitoring interaction	If the cats remain relaxed and there is no evidence of defensive behaviors (staring, hissing, growling), gradually increase their supervised time together. Provide escape routes to safe areas for any uncomfortable cat.
Handling aggression	If aggression occurs, separate the cats and return to the previous steps.
Using pheromones	Feline-appeasing pheromones (spray or diffuser) can aid in integrating a new cat.
Timeframe for integration	The process can sometimes take several months or longer before the cats are comfortable around each other. It is important not to rush this process.

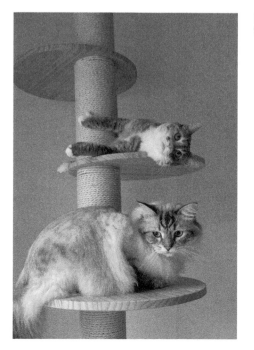

Figure 8.3 Introducing a new cat into an existing home takes time and patience. *Source:* Jasmine Pang / Pexels.

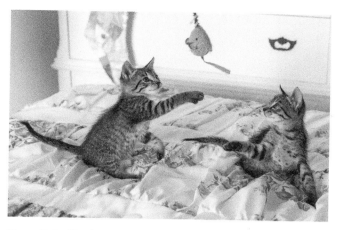

Figure 8.4 Play is a great way to build relationships between cats. *Source:* Michelle_Raponi / Pixabay.

when called, and stationing on a mat using positive reinforcement can help maintain relaxation and facilitate redirection and removal if needed. The caregiver should closely monitor the cats' body language and intervene if necessary.

If the cats continue to be comfortable with each other's proximity, they can spend more time together in the communal room, though they should always have the option to retreat. If fearful or aggressive behavior occurs, the process should be slowed and the interaction level adjusted to avoid such responses. This process can take weeks or even months, and rushing it is not advisable.

Introducing Cats and Dogs

Introducing a new dog to a home with a resident cat, or a new cat to a home with a resident dog, requires patience and time. This process can be challenging, and safety should always be the priority. Initially keep the new pet separated from the resident pet. Allow both animals to become comfortable and engaged in their own spaces. To facilitate familiarity without direct interaction, use closed doors as a safety measure to prevent accidental encounters. Utilize a common area, giving each pet time to become comfortable with the other's scent.

If, after a few days, both pets seem relaxed and comfortable, the introduction process can begin (Figure 8.5 and Table 8.5). Before this introduction both the dog and the cat should ideally be familiar with basic behaviors for easier management, such as coming when called and nose-to-hand targeting. In homes with multiple cats, introduce the dog to each cat separately. The same approach applies if there are multiple dogs: introduce each dog to the new cat individually. If the dog struggles to engage with people, pause the introductions until they learn foundational behaviors, or consider getting help from a qualified professional.

Start the introductions briefly, possibly behind a gate, allowing the cat and dog to sniff and explore each other at their own pace. Ensure that each animal has the option to leave if they wish. If the first meeting results in defensive or fearful behavior such as hissing, growling, or cowering from the cat or barking, lunging, or snarling from the dog, stop the introduction immediately. In such cases it is advisable to consult a board-certified veterinary behaviorist.

If the introductions proceed well, remove the gate to allow more free interaction. However, do not force these interactions. Continuously supervise and observe their body language to ensure both pets are comfortable with each other. Over time, less supervision may be needed. Avoid letting

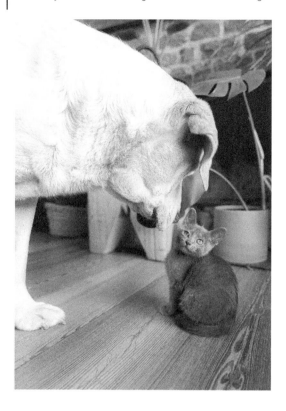

Figure 8.5 When introduced properly, cats and dogs can form harmonious relationships. *Source:* belen capello / Pexels.

Table 8.5 Dog and cat introductions.

Stage	Description
Initial separation	Keep the new pet separated from the resident pet. Allow both animals to become comfortable and engaged in their own spaces.
Facilitating familiarity	Use closed doors as a safety measure to prevent accidental encounters. Utilize a common area, giving each pet time to become comfortable with the other's scent and presence.
Beginning introduction	After a few days, if both pets seem relaxed and comfortable, the introduction process can begin. The dog and the cat should be familiar with basic behaviors such as coming when called and nose-to-hand targeting. For multiple pets, introduce each one individually.
Managing first interactions	If the dog struggles to focus and engage with people, pause the introductions until they learn foundational behaviors or get help from a professional. Start the introductions briefly, possibly behind a gate, allowing them to sniff and explore each other at their own pace.
Progressing interaction	If the first meeting results in defensive or fearful behavior, stop the introduction immediately and consider consulting a board-certified veterinary behaviorist. If introductions go well, remove the gate to allow more free interaction.
Observation and supervision	Do not force interactions. Continuously supervise and observe their body language to ensure comfort. Avoid letting the dog continually bark at the cat or maintain a fixed stare. Be aware that cats running away can trigger a chase response in dogs.

the dog continually bark at the cat or maintain a fixed stare, as this can be intimidating and cause fear in the cat. Additionally, be aware that cats running away can trigger a chase response in dogs.

Conclusion

The process of selecting a pet is a significant decision that requires careful consideration of various factors. Caregivers should carefully weigh the options of adopting from a shelter, a rescue organization, or a breeder, taking into account the ethical and practical implications of each choice. Having realistic expectations and a clear understanding of the desired traits in a pet is essential for a successful match. Veterinarians and pet professionals, by guiding caregivers through this process, can help individuals make informed decisions that lead to fulfilling and lasting relationships between pets and their caregivers. A well-thought-out pet selection process lays the foundation for a harmonious and happy life together.

References

APPA (2018). *2017–2018 National Pet Caregivers Survey*. Stamford, CT: American Pet Products Association.

Barnard, S., Siracusa, C., Reisner, I. et al. (2012). Validity of model devices used to assess canine temperament in behavioral tests. *Applied Animal Behaviour Science* 138: 79–87.

Beaver, B.V. (2003). Feline social behavior. In: *Feline Behavior: A Guide for Veterinarians, 2* (ed. B.V. Beaver), 127–163. Philadelphia, PA: Saunders.

Bergman, L. and Gaskins, L. (2008). Expanding families: preparing for and introducing dogs and cats to infants, children, and new pets. *Veterinary Clinics of North America, Small Animal Practice* 38 (5): 1043–1063.

Bergman, L., Hart, B.L., Bain, M., and Cliff, K. (2002). Evaluation of urine marking by cats as a model for understanding veterinary diagnostic and treatment approaches and client attitudes. *Journal of the American Veterinary Medical Association* 221 (9): 1282–1286.

Bradshaw, J.W.S. and Lea, A.M. (1992). Dyadic interactions between domestic dogs. *Anthrozoös* 5 (4): 245–253.

Brown, W.P. and Stephan, V.L. (2020). The influence of degree of socialization and age on length of stay of shelter cats. *Journal of Applied Animal Welfare Science* 24 (3): 238–245.

Casey, R.A. and Bradshaw, J.W.S. (2008). The effects of additional socialisation for kittens in a rescue centre on their behaviour and suitability as a pet. *Applied Animal Behaviour Science* 114: 196–205.

Centonze, L.A. and Levy, J.K. (2002). Characteristics of free-roaming cats and their caretakers. *Journal of the American Veterinary Medical Association* 220: 1627–1633.

Diesel, G., Brodbelt, D., and Pfeiffer, D.U. (2008). Reliability of assessment of dogs' behavioural responses by staff working at a welfare charity in the UK. *Applied Animal Behaviour Science* 115: 171–181.

Dinwoodie, I.R., Dwyer, B., Zottola, V. et al. (2019). Demographics and comorbidity of behavior problems in dogs. *Journal of Veterinary Behavior* 32: 62–71.

Duffy, D.L., Kruger, K.A., and Serpell, J.A. (2014). Evaluation of a behavioral assessment tool for dogs relinquished to shelters. *Preventive Veterinary Medicine* 117: 601–609.

Duffy, D.L. and Serpell, J.A. (2012). Predictive validity of a method for evaluating temperament in young guide and service dogs. *Applied Animal Behaviour Science* 138: 99–109.

Giammanco, M., Tabacchi, G., Giammanco, S. et al. (2005). Testosterone and aggressiveness. *Medical Science Monitor* 11 (4): RA136–RA145.

Graff, E. and Gaultier, E. (2002). Adaptation of adopted cats to their homes – a retrospective study. *Proceedings of the AVSAB/ACVB Scientific Session* 33–36.

Hart, B.L. and Eckstein, R.A. (1997). The role of gonadal hormones in the occurrence of objectionable behaviours in dogs and cats. *Applied Animal Behaviour Science* 52 (3–4): 331–344.

Hart, L.A. and Hart, B.L. (2021). An ancient practice but a new paradigm: personal choice for the age to spay or neuter a dog. *Frontiers in Veterinary Science* 8: 603257.

Hart, L.A., Hart, B.L., Thigpen, A.P. et al. (2018). Compatibility of cats with children in the family. *Frontiers in Veterinary Science* 5: 278.

Heath, S. (2018). Understanding feline emotions … and their role in problem behaviours. *Journal of Feline Medicine and Surgery* 20 (5): 437–444.

Horwitz, D.F. and Neilson, J.C. (2007). Aggression/canine: interdog/familiar dogs. In: *Blackwell's Five-Minute Veterinary Consult: Canine and Feline Behavior* (ed. D.F. Horwitz), 63–70. Oxford: Blackwell Publishing.

Houlihan, K.E. (2017). A literature review on the welfare implications of gonadectomy of dogs. *Journal of the American Veterinary Medical Association* 250 (10): 1155–1166.

Houpt, K.A. (1991). Aggression and social structure. In: *Domestic Animal Behavior for Veterinarians and Animal Scientists*, vol. 2 (ed. K.A. Houpt), 34–74. Ames, IA: Iowa State University Press.

Howe, L.M. (2015). Current perspectives on the optimal age to spay/castrate dogs and cats. *Veterinary Medicine: Research and Reports* 6: 171–180.

Jokinen, O., Appleby, D., Sandbacka-Saxén, S. et al. (2017). Homing age influences the prevalence of aggressive and avoidance-related behaviour in adult dogs. *Applied Animal Behaviour Science* 195: 87–92.

Kaufman, C.A., Forndran, S., Stauber, C. et al. (2017). The social behaviour of neutered male dogs compared to intact dogs (*Canis lupus familiaris*): video analyses, questionnaires and case studies. *Open Journal of Veterinary Medicine* 2 (1): 22–37.

Landsberg, G., Hunthausen, W., Ackerman, L. (2013a). Feline aggression. In: Handbook of Behavior Problems of the Dog and Cat, 3., (eds. G. Landsberg, W. Hunthausen, and L. Ackerman), *pp.* 327–343. Philadelphia, PA: Saunders.

Landsberg, G., Hunthausen, W., Ackerman, L. (2013b). Pet selection and the genetics of behavior. In: Handbook of Behavior Problems of the Dog and Cat, 3., (eds. G. Landsberg, W. Hunthausen, and L. Ackerman), *pp.* 29–37. Philadelphia, PA: Saunders.

Levine, E., Perry, P., Scarlett, J., and Houpt, K.A. (2005). Intercat aggression in households following the introduction of a new cat. *Applied Animal Behaviour Science* 90: 325–336.

Levy, J.K., Woods, J.E., Turick, S.L., and Etheridge, D.L. (2003). Number of unowned free-roaming cats in a college community in the southern United States and characteristics of community residents who feed them. *Journal of the American Veterinary Medical Association* 223: 202–205.

Ley, J. (2020). Aggression in cats. In: *Small Animal Veterinary Psychiatry* (ed. S. Denenberg), 180–190. Wallingford: CABI.

Lockwood, R. (2016). Ethology, ecology and epidemiology of canine aggression. In: *The Domestic Dog: Its Evolution, Behavior, and Interactions with People*, vol. 2 (ed. J. Serpell), 160–181. Cambridge: Cambridge University Press.

Marder, A. and Duxbury, M.M. (2008). Obtaining a pet: realistic expectations. *Veterinary Clinics of North America, Small Animal Practice* 38 (5): 1145–1162.

Martinez, A.G., Pernas, G.S., Casalta, F.J.D. et al. (2011). Risk factors associated with behavioral problems in dogs. *Journal of Veterinary Behavior* 6: 225–231.

Table 9.1 The difference between fear, anxiety, and phobia.

	Fear	Anxiety	Phobia
Definition	A normal response to real or perceived threats, often with identifiable stimuli	Typically lacks a distinct fearful stimulus and is considered maladaptive or abnormal	An extreme, irrational fear response
Stimulus	Identifiable and real or perceived threat	Often lacks a distinct or specific stimulus	Specific object or situation, often irrational
Response	Usually proportional to the threat	Disproportionate to or without a clear threat	Excessive and unreasonable to the stimulus
Progression	Adaptive and protective Normal behavior	Maladaptive, can be chronic Abnormal behavior	Irrational and overwhelming Abnormal behavior

Approaches to Severe Cases

In extreme cases, where welfare is a concern, medications might be necessary to aid dogs in adapting to their new homes. Signs of severe anxiety include a lack of interaction with humans in the household or bolting behavior. These dogs may be flight risks, necessitating safety measures like martingale collars, harnesses, microchips, GPS collars, and long lines.

Handling Mild Cases

For milder cases, management, training, behavior modification, and time could suffice (Table 9.2). These dogs need to be monitored for any progression in behavior. Some dogs with generalized anxiety may resort to defensive aggression when they feel threatened.

Table 9.2 General treatment plan for fear and anxiety.

	Strategies and tools
Encouraging eating	Use of medications as needed. Food-dispensing toys. Puzzle toys.
Creating a safe space	Personalized safe area (crate, room, exercise pen). Warm blankets. Bluetooth speaker for calming music. Pheromone diffuser. Variety of food-dispensing toys. Cover for the area for added security (if needed).
Use of food-dispensing and puzzle toys	Encourages exploration of the environment. Builds confidence.
Positive reinforcement training	Teaching "touch" to build trust and predictability. Chin rest behavior for communication and relaxation. Leash skills for engaging walks. Relaxation exercises. "Touch" for guiding and redirecting the dog around fearful stimuli.

Table 9.3 General treatment plan for car ride anxiety.

Strategy	Description
Positive association with cars	Make sure the car consistently predicts positive experiences.
Secure transportation	Use an impact-resistant crate or a harness with a seat belt for safety during rides.
Medication	Administer antinausea medications like Cerenia® (Zoetis Services LLC, Parsipanny, NJ) for dogs prone to motion sickness. Antianxiety medications may be needed.
Engaging activities	Provide long-lasting food-dispensing or puzzle toys to keep the dog occupied during the ride and to help condition a positive emotional response. A remote treat dispenser can be helpful.
Gradual exposure	Begin with short trips to enjoyable destinations such as for coffee (human) and treats (dog) or hiking to build positive associations.
Relaxation exercises	Implement relaxation techniques transferable to the car environment.
Use of calming aids	Employ tools like calming caps or ear muffs to reduce visual and auditory stimuli that may worsen the dog's fear and anxiety.

Car Ride Anxiety

Many dogs from shelters experience anxiety during car rides. This may stem from various factors, including limited exposure to car rides in their previous homes, associating cars with danger due to survival instincts from living on the streets, or traumatic experiences like long transports in cramped conditions. Car ride anxiety can significantly impact the quality of life for both the dog and their human companion (Figure 9.2 and Table 9.3).

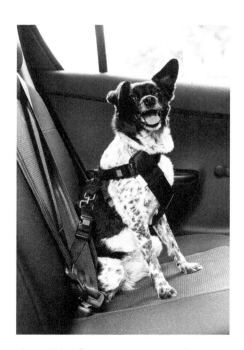

Figure 9.2 Car ride anxiety can affect the quality of life for both the dog and their caregiver. *Source:* Andrey Popov/Adobe Stock Photos.

Aggression

Aggression can be displayed through a range of behaviors such as barking, growling, lunging, snapping, biting, direct staring, stiffening of the body, raising of the fur (piloerection), and leaning toward an individual or object. It is not considered a diagnosis but often a clinical sign of underlying diseases, which can be physical (such as pain, endocrine, metabolic, neurologic, or dermatologic conditions) or emotional (like fear, anxiety, or frustration). In certain cases, aggression may be a normal behavior such as maternal aggression or resource guarding (Table 9.4).

Frustration

Frustration is recognized as a negative emotional state that can lead to various behavioral issues in dogs including aggression and separation-related behaviors (McPeake et al. 2021). This frustration often occurs

Table 9.4 General treatment plan for aggression in dogs.

Step	Description
Identifying underlying causes	Determine the root cause and identify specific triggers for aggressive behavior.
Management and avoidance of triggers	Avoid known triggers and stop the progression of the behavior to prevent further incidents.
Teaching alternative behaviors	Teach dogs new ways to communicate distress, like moving to a mat or room, offering eye contact, or a chin rest.
Behavior modification	Focus on changing the dog's emotional state associated with aggression after establishing alternative behaviors.
Avoiding certain training methods	Avoid positive punishment, negative reinforcement, and negative punishment when modifying aggressive behavior, as these techniques suppress the behavior temporarily without addressing the root emotional cause.
Using positive reinforcement	Use positive reinforcement to strengthen the human–animal bond and to teach foundational behaviors in preparation for behavior modification.
Professional assistance	Aggression is due to emotional arousal and therefore treatment will require behavior modification and not just training.
	Seek the help of qualified professionals, including a board-certified veterinary behaviorist, for successful management and treatment of aggression.

when dogs are unable to obtain something they desire (Lenkei et al. 2018; Mills et al. 2012; Notari 2009). Such desires can be social, like wanting to interact with people or other dogs, or non-social, like chasing prey, accessing food, or playing with toys (Mills and Zulch 2010).

Physical barriers, like doors or being on a leash, can prevent dogs from reaching these desired things, leading to frustration (Lenkei et al. 2021). When restrained by a leash, dogs may show redirected aggression due to being unable to reach their target (Figure 9.3). Similarly, if a dog cannot access a resource they expect or need, this can cause stress and result in aggressive behavior (Hargrove 2015).

Frustration in dogs can often stem from fear, particularly when they are prevented from reaching a perceived safe space (Lenkei et al. 2018; Mills and Zulch 2010). This frustration may occur in scenarios where a dog's expectations go unmet, such as when an anticipated reward is not

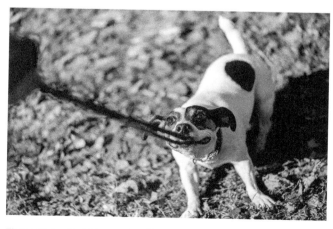

Figure 9.3 Grabbing and pulling on the leash can be a sign of frustration. *Source:* alexei_tm/Adobe Stock.

provided or if they feel their personal space is being invaded (Hargrave 2015). Specific triggers can include the absence, reduction, or delay of rewards. Dogs value their personal space and may become frustrated if they perceive an encroachment on their territory. Furthermore, frustration can also arise from being restrained or confined in a manner that restricts their ability to escape from an unwelcome situation (Yin 2009).

In addition to aggression, frustration is a significant factor in separation-related problems in dogs, where they become stressed due to being separated from their caregivers. It has also been linked to the development of repetitive and compulsive behaviors (Lenkei et al. 2021; Luescher 2009). In many of these scenarios, a lack of control over their environment is a common trigger for frustration (Panksepp 2004).

House-Soiling and Housetraining

Housetraining is often one of the primary challenges faced by caregivers of shelter dogs, particularly for dogs that may not have lived in a home environment before. The process requires patience, consistency, and a structured approach to help these dogs learn and adapt (Figure 9.4 and Table 9.5).

Supervision and Management

One effective house training strategy is to manage the dog's environment. Start by restricting the dog's access to the entire house using baby gates, closed doors, or exercise pens. Set up designated areas for elimination, sleeping (using a bed or an open crate), and eating (at a feeding station). This structured approach helps the dog learn the routine more easily and prevents them from feeling overwhelmed by too much space too soon.

Establishing and Maintaining a Schedule

Establishing a consistent schedule is key for successful housetraining. Consistent feeding times help regulate the dog's digestive system, making it easier to predict when they will need to eliminate. Regular bathroom breaks, ideally at the same time each day, also help the dog learn when and where it is appropriate to urinate and defecate. Keeping a log can be beneficial in determining the dog's natural schedule and adjusting the routine accordingly. This log should track feeding times, elimination times, and any accidents, providing valuable insights into the dog's patterns and needs.

Positive Reinforcement and Cleaning Up Accidents

Using positive reinforcement is essential when housetraining shelter dogs. Promptly rewarding the dog with a treat, fun game, or toy after they successfully eliminate outside reinforces the desired behavior. This approach encourages the dog to repeat the action, fostering a positive association between eliminating outdoors and receiving rewards.

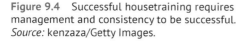

Figure 9.4 Successful housetraining requires management and consistency to be successful. *Source:* kenzaza/Getty Images.

Table 9.5 Steps to housetraining.

	Description
Creating a controlled environment	Limit the dog's access within the home using baby gates or exercise pens.
	Designate specific areas for elimination, sleeping, and eating.
	Helps the dog understand and learn the routine.
Establishing and maintaining a schedule	Consistent feeding times to regulate digestion and predict elimination.
	Regular elimination breaks at similar times each day.
	Keep a log of feeding, elimination times, and accidents to identify the dog's patterns.
Positive reinforcement	Reward the dog with treats for successful outdoor elimination.
	Reinforces the behavior in the desired location and encourages repetition.
	Associates elimination outside with positive outcomes.
Avoiding punishment for accidents	Avoid punishing indoor accidents as it is ineffective and damages the dog–caregiver relationship.
	Punishment can cause fear and lead to the dog hiding when needing to eliminate.
	Can create distrust, frustration, and anxiety.
Addressing indoor accidents	Clean accidents indoors promptly with an enzyme-based cleaner.
	Effectively removes odors to prevent the dog from returning to the spot.
	Important to clean without displaying frustration or anger toward the dog.

Avoiding Punishment for Accidents

Punishing dogs for indoor accidents is not only ineffective but can also damage the relationship between the dog and the caregiver. Punishment may make the dog fearful and cause them to hide when they need to eliminate, further complicating the housetraining process. Such an approach can result in distrust, frustration, and anxiety.

Addressing Indoor Accidents

If an accident happens indoors, it should be addressed by promptly cleaning the area with an enzyme-based cleaner. These cleaners are effective in removing odors and discourage the dog from returning to the same spot for future elimination. It is important to clean up without showing frustration or anger toward the dog.

Separation-Related Disorder

Separation-related disorder, once known as separation anxiety, is common among dogs and can be complex (De Assi et al. 2020). Often this disorder is multifactorial (Figure 9.5). Separation-related behaviors may be due to various factors such as frustration, generalized anxiety, isolation distress, confinement anxiety, noise or storm phobia, fear-related aggression, territorial behaviors, or an underlying medical condition (Lenkei et al. 2018). While hyperattachment may play a role, it is not necessarily indicative of a separation-related disorder (Fagen 2023). For shelter dogs, past experiences can contribute to heightened sensitivity to being left alone, along with frustration. Additionally, the confinement often required during the shelter transport system can exacerbate this anxiety, potentially leading to confinement anxiety.

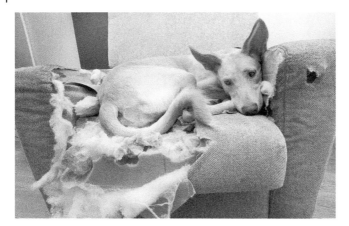

Figure 9.5 Separation-related disorders are common in dogs. This behavior is often complex and multifaceted. *Source:* Sandra/Adobe Stock.

Clinical Signs

The behaviors exhibited by dogs suffering from a separation-related disorder can vary, but they typically include excessive barking, destructiveness, and house-soiling (De Assis et al. 2020; Lund and Jørgensen 1999). Destructive behaviors might include chewing on furniture, scratching at doors, or other actions that could be misinterpreted as disobedience or spite. However, it is important to recognize that these behaviors are often manifestations of the stress and anxiety the dog feels when separated from their caregiver. In some instances, these behaviors may not stem from anxiety at all (Denenberg 2021).

Managing Separation-Related Behaviors

Managing separation-related behaviors in dogs involves several steps. First, identify the root cause or motivation behind the behavior and any comorbidities they may have. For dogs with confinement anxiety, simply allowing them to stay out of the crate or confinement may resolve the behavior. Training foundational behaviors and using positive reinforcement can reduce frustration and anxiety, making interactions with humans more predictable. Independence exercises are also beneficial, teaching dogs to relax away from their caregivers, whether they are present or not. Providing enrichment items and puzzle toys can keep dogs occupied, especially if they tend to pace when home alone, by engaging them in foraging, licking, and sniffing activities, which can lower arousal levels.

Behavior Modification

Initial Phase: Safe Haven Training Establishing a safe haven in the home is the first step in any behavioral treatment plan. This space should be a designated area where the dog feels secure and comfortable and should include their bed, favorite toys, and an item carrying the caregiver's scent. The dog should learn to be comfortable spending time in this space, both in the presence and absence of the caregiver. Establish a routine where the dog receives a special food-dispensing or puzzle toy daily in this area (this can also be the spot where the dog is fed). Frozen puzzle toys, Kong® wobblers, and lickable mats work well. A remote treat dispenser can also be utilized during this phase.

Short, Frequent Departures   Start with the caregiver being at home but out of the dog's immediate sight to help the dog adjust to not always having their caregiver close by. As the dog becomes more comfortable with these brief absences within the home, the caregiver can begin to leave the house for short periods. Start with just a few minutes and gradually increase the duration. During these times, provide the dog with enrichment items and food-finding activities. Using remote treat dispensers, interactive toys, and treat-dispensing puzzles not only distracts the dog but also promotes behaviors such as snuffling, sniffing, licking, chewing, and foraging. This method helps redirect the dog's focus from anxiety to engaging activities, fostering a positive association with being alone.

Alternative Plan   Dogs that exhibit a high level of frustration when confined or left home alone may respond better to a modified version of this treatment plan. Initially, video recording the dog is necessary to observe their behavior. The next step involves identifying a range of food-dispensing and puzzle toys that the dog enjoys and engages with, accompanied by a variety of food treats, including shredded cheese, spreadable items, frozen treats, and even their own kibble. Then observe and record the dog's preferred food items and toys. After ranking the food and toys based on the dog's preference, they should be arranged in a decompression loop. This loop should place higher-value toys (those the dog engages with most) and higher-value food in the location where the dog is likely to first go after their caregiver leaves. Subsequently, arrange the food-dispensing and puzzle toys in the areas the dog is likely to visit next, leading toward the safe space, an open crate, or an area where the dog is most relaxed such as a couch, bed, or rug. A large chenille mat can be effective here, serving a dual purpose as a snuffle mat.

Prepare the decompression loop before leaving and dismantle it after returning home. The objective is to gradually reduce the number of stations as the dog becomes quicker to engage and settle over time. Adjustments should be based on video monitoring. If the dog refuses to eat, consider medications or modifications to current medication.

Departures and Arrivals

Another key aspect of managing separation-related behaviors is to make departures and arrivals low-key, without ignoring the dog. Excessive attention during these times can heighten a dog's anxiety. Instead, teach alternative behaviors to reinforce such as keeping all four feet on the floor or targeting for greetings. Establishing routines offers predictability and consistency. In severe cases, it may be necessary to seek professional help from a board-certified veterinary behaviorist.

Dangers of Punishment

Overcoming separation-related behaviors takes time and patience. Punishing the dog for anxious and destructive behaviors is counterproductive and can make the problem worse. Instead, a compassionate, gradual, and systematic approach, focusing on building the dog's confidence and comfort with being alone, is key to helping a dog overcome this behavior.

Unruly Behaviors

Unruly behaviors in shelter dogs, including jumping on people, mouthing, chewing inappropriate items, counter surfing, and leash pulling, present common challenges for new caregivers. While these behaviors are often normal, they can also be expressions of fear, anxiety, and frustration. The first step in addressing these issues is make sure that the dog's basic needs are being met, including positive human interaction, social and physical exercise, enrichment opportunities, and undisturbed rest and sleep. If these behaviors are identified as normal yet problematic, many can be effectively managed and modified using positive reinforcement techniques.

Jumping and Mouthing

Jumping and mouthing are common behaviors in dogs, typically driven by excitement or a desire for attention. These behaviors, although normal, can be challenging in a home environment, especially with shelter dogs who may not have received prior training. There are effective strategies to modify these behaviors by reinforcing alternative, acceptable actions.

Addressing Jumping

Jumping on people is usually a dog's method of greeting or seeking attention (Figure 9.6). The initial step in managing this behavior involves using a safe space or gated area to restrict access to the door when people enter and exit. To modify this behavior, one effective strategy is to reward the dog with treats when all four feet are on the ground. If the dog jumps the caregiver should refrain from giving verbal reprimands, as even these can be interpreted as a form of attention. Instead, wait until the dog has all four feet on the ground, then immediately mark and reward this behavior with attention or treats. This approach teaches the dog that keeping all feet on the floor is a more rewarding way to receive attention.

Teaching the dog to station on a mat or platform offers an effective alternative to jumping, as these two behaviors are incompatible – the dog cannot jump up and remain on the mat at the same time. Training the dog to go to the mat when someone enters the room and rewarding them for staying put can effectively redirect their behavior from jumping to stationing. Incorporating a remote treat dispenser as part of the training and behavior modification plan can further facilitate this behavior change.

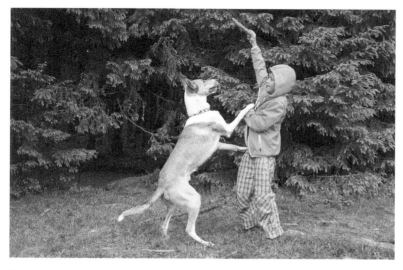

Figure 9.6 Jumping is a common, normal behavior that often is reinforced. *Source:* Petr Bonek/Adobe Stock Photos.

Managing Mouthing

Mouthing, where a dog gently bites or chews on hands or clothing, is often a playful or exploratory behavior. To address mouthing, redirection toward appropriate chew toys is the key. When the dog begins to mouth, gently redirect them to a chew toy and then positively reinforce their interaction with the toy. This teaches them that chewing toys is more acceptable and rewarding than mouthing people. Nose targeting is an alternative strategy to teach a dog that noses touch hands but teeth do not.

Addressing Chewing and Counter Surfing in Dogs

Chewing and counter surfing are behaviors commonly seen in dogs (Figure 9.7), especially those who may not have been taught boundaries in a home setting, like many shelter dogs. These behaviors, although natural, can be problematic and even dangerous. Addressing them effectively involves a combination of management, training, and redirection. Be sure to evaluate these dogs for underlying gastrointestinal disease, as this can also be a cause for this behavior.

Managing Inappropriate Chewing

Dogs naturally tend to chew, a behavior that serves both as a form of play and a means of exploring their environment. To manage chewing effectively, provide the dog with appropriate chew toys and actively teach them which items are acceptable to chew. This can be done by positively reinforcing the dog when they choose to chew on appropriate items. Acknowledging and rewarding the dog's choice of an appropriate chew toy with praise and treats encourage the behavior. Consistent reinforcement helps the dog learn which items are theirs to chew on. Excessive or abnormal chewing can also signal gastrointestinal disease or oral pain, and the dog should be evaluated if this behavior is abnormal or excessive such as ingesting foreign objects.

Preventing Counter Surfing

Counter surfing, where dogs jump up onto kitchen counters to scavenge for food or items, requires a proactive approach. Prevention is key in managing this behavior. Making sure that counters and

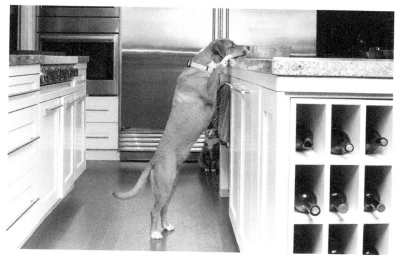

Figure 9.7 Counter surfing is a common behavior in dogs. *Source:* Yurikr/Getty Images.

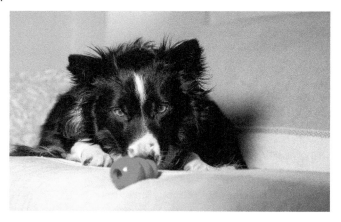

Figure 9.8 Food-dispensing and puzzle toys facilitate relaxation, provide distractions, and help with problem-solving skills. *Source:* Tepepa79/Getty Images.

accessible surfaces are clear of food and other temptations is the first step. This reduces the likelihood of the dog being rewarded for counter surfing by finding something to eat or play with on the counter.

Teaching "Trade Up"

Another effective strategy for managing chewing and counter surfing is to teach the dog the "trade up" technique. If the dog grabs an item they should not have, avoid chasing or forcefully retrieving the item. Instead, offer them something more appealing in exchange such as a treat or their favorite toy (Figure 9.8). This approach teaches the dog that relinquishing items leads to receiving something even better, thereby avoiding any confrontational scenarios.

Relaxation: Differential Reinforcement of an Incompatible Behavior (DRI) or Alternative Behavior (DRA)

Shaping relaxation on a mat, especially in the kitchen or dining areas, can be highly effective for preventing counter surfing. Teaching the dog that being on and relaxing on their mat, particularly when food is present, is rewarding introduces an alternative behavior that is incompatible with counter surfing. This strategy deters the unwanted behavior and curbs begging tendencies.

Managing Leash Pulling in Dogs

Leash pulling is a common challenge faced by many dog caregivers, especially with shelter dogs who might not have had previous leash training. This behavior can turn walks into more stressful and less enjoyable outings. However, with appropriate tools and training techniques, leash pulling can be effectively managed, making walks enjoyable experiences for both the dog and the caregiver.

Utilizing the Right Equipment

Managing leash pulling is significantly aided by the use of proper walking equipment. A front clip harness serves as an excellent tool for this purpose. Unlike traditional collars or back clip harnesses, a front clip harness redirects the dog's movement toward the caregiver when they begin to pull, making it easier to capture their attention and reduce pulling. Using a standard 4–6 ft leash, rather than a retractable leash, provides more control and consistency during training. This type of leash ensures that the dog does not get mixed messages about how far they can go. For caregivers who need their hands free, a waist leash can be a practical option, allowing for more relaxed movements and freeing up the hands for distributing treats and encouraging engagement.

Training Techniques and Engagement

Training the dog to walk calmly on a leash starts with teaching foundational behaviors for engagement such as offered eye contact and hand targeting. During training, the caregiver needs to be more captivating than the surrounding environment. Carrying toys (like squeaky balls, a ball on a rope, or a flirt pole) and food rewards (such as peanut butter in a pouch or squeeze cheese) can increase the dog's interest, making the caregiver the exciting part of the walk, especially when there are distractions. Rewarding the dog for keeping a loose leash or for offering attention during walks reinforces calm walking and encourages frequent check-ins.

Positive Reinforcement Training

Positive reinforcement training is an effective and humane method for teaching a dog new behaviors and social skills. This approach emphasizes rewarding desired behaviors, thereby encouraging dogs to repeat them. Social skills such as walking politely on a leash, not jumping on people, responding when called, and settling on a mat despite distractions give dogs the opportunity to learn how to interact comfortably with humans and adapt to living in the human world. Focusing on these skills not only helps to develop behaviorally sound dogs but also fosters a positive and engaging relationship between dogs and their human companions (Table 9.6).

Capturing

Capturing is a technique used in positive reinforcement training that involves observing and rewarding natural behaviors dogs exhibit without prompting or forcing. This method builds a dog's repertoire of default (freely offered) behaviors.

Understanding Capturing and Its Benefits

Leveraging natural behaviors that dogs exhibit in their daily routines and reinforcing these behaviors with capturing techniques is an effective and enjoyable training method. By marking spontaneous actions like sitting, lying down, or looking at the caregiver with a clicker or a verbal cue like "yes" and then rewarding them, dogs gradually learn that these behaviors yield desirable outcomes, thereby increasing their frequency.

Capturing's primary benefit lies in its capacity to cultivate default behaviors – actions a dog instinctively performs in certain situations without explicit instruction. For instance, a dog may learn that sitting calmly results in receiving attention and treats, leading them to sit by default when seeking attention. These default behaviors play a key role in managing and redirecting undesirable ones (e.g., sitting instead of jumping).

The Role of Shaping in Training

Shaping complements capturing in dog training by focusing on gradually developing more complex behaviors through successive steps. This method breaks down a desired behavior into

Table 9.6 Pros and cons of the four contingencies.

Contingency	Pros	Cons
Positive reinforcement	Builds trust and encourages learning. Focuses on rewarding desired behaviors. Creates an ideal learning environment. Enhances communication between dog and caregiver.	Requires consistency and patience. May take longer to see results compared to some punishment methods.
Negative reinforcement	Can be effective for teaching certain behaviors. Increases the frequency of a behavior by removing an unpleasant stimulus.	Can cause confusion and frustration. Dogs may not understand why discomfort is applied. Can harm the relationship between the dog and caregiver. Potential for increased stress and anxiety.
Positive punishment	Can yield quick results in stopping unwanted behavior, although often temporarily.	Can lead to fear, anxiety, frustration, and breakdown in trust. Dogs may associate punishment with the trainer or environment. Can exacerbate the unwanted behaviors. Does not guide toward desired behavior.
Negative punishment	In some cases can be used to extinguish behavior.	Can cause frustration or confusion. May lead to increased anxiety or unwanted behaviors. Does not instruct the dog on the desired behavior. Requires consistent and clear communication for effectiveness.

smaller, manageable parts, rewarding the dog at each progression. For instance, in teaching a dog to fetch the process might start with rewarding interest in a toy, followed by touching, picking it up, bringing it back, and finally handing it to the caregiver.

Benefits of Capturing and Shaping

Capturing and shaping facilitate teaching desirable behaviors as well as enhance caregivers' training abilities. These techniques improve caregivers' skills in observation, timing, and understanding reinforcement strategies. Such skills are essential for creating a positive and communicative relationship with the dog.

Punishment and Negative Reinforcement

Positive Punishment

Positive punishment involves the addition of a stimulus to reduce the frequency of a behavior, such as using a shock collar to stop barking or jerking on the leash to prevent pulling (Figure 9.9). Although it might yield quick results, this method often leads to unintended consequences like fear, anxiety, frustration, pain, and injury. A significant issue with positive punishment is that it does not guide the dog toward the desired behavior but instead focuses on penalizing the undesired one. Consequently, dogs may associate the punishment with the trainer or the training

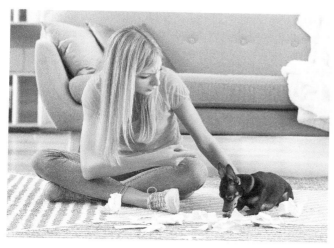

Figure 9.9   The goal of positive punishment is to decrease the frequency of behavior; however, it tends to be overused, and the potential for undesirable emotional side effects is high. *Source:* Pixel-Shot/Adobe Stock Photos.

environment rather than with their own behavior. This association can damage the trust between the dog and their caregiver.

Positive punishment is considered inappropriate for training or behavior modification. In contrast, positive reinforcement training, the more humane and effective method that utilizes adding a stimulus to increase the frequency of a behavior, is preferred. This method builds engagement, encourages learning, and is less stressful for the dog.

Understanding Negative Reinforcement in Dog Training

Negative reinforcement involves the removal of a stimulus to increase the frequency of a desired behavior. For example, applying continuous pressure on a dog's hindquarters until they sit results in the pressure release serving as the reward for sitting. While effective for teaching specific behaviors, this method has significant downsides.

A major issue with negative reinforcement is its potential to cause confusion and frustration in dogs. They might not understand why they are experiencing discomfort or which specific behavior will end it. This confusion can make dogs stressed and anxious, possibly leading to unpredictable behavior.

Just as with positive punishment, negative reinforcement can damage the relationship between the dog and their caregiver. Dogs may begin to associate their caregiver with unpleasant experiences, weakening their bond.

The Role of Negative Punishment in Dog Training

Negative punishment involves the removal of stimulus to reduce the frequency of a behavior. For example, if a dog jumps on someone for attention, the person might turn away or exit the room, effectively taking away the attention the dog seeks. This technique can effectively teach dogs that certain actions will lead to losing something they value.

However, negative punishment comes with drawbacks. It may cause frustration or confusion in dogs, especially if they fail to immediately understand the connection between their behavior and the loss of a reward. This lack of understanding can result in increased anxiety, frustration, or even further unwanted behaviors as the dog tries to regain the lost attention or reward.

Like other forms of punishment, negative punishment does not teach the dog what behavior is desired. Instead, it only signals that their current behavior is not producing the expected outcome. Therefore, maintaining consistent and clear communication is essential to ensure dogs comprehend the reason behind the reward's removal and what behavior is expected. This approach should be used with caution and is not generally appropriate for training or behavior modification.

Pattern Games for Dog Training

Overview

Leslie McDevitt's Control Unleashed® introduces pattern games such as 1-2-3 Game, Up and Down, Ping Pong, Whiplash Turn, Look at That, Give Me a Break, LATTE, and Superbowls, providing enjoyable and engaging activities for animals of all species (McDevitt 2019). These games are not only mentally stimulating but also establish predictable patterns, helping animals maintain focus in distracting, overstimulating, and overwhelming environments (Table 9.7). Designed to create a structured and predictable framework, these games enable animals to better process and adapt to their surroundings through repetitive sequences (Figure 9.10). This approach effectively manages arousal in stressful situations, and the animal is more likely to eat even when distractions are present, reducing the need for distance in the behavior modification process (McDevitt 2019).

Empowerment Through Start-Button Behaviors

A key component of pattern games is their use of "start-button" behaviors, which empower animals to initiate the game sequence on their own. This demonstrates their readiness to participate, even amid distractions. A common example of such behavior is offering eye contact. For example, the Up and Down game is especially useful in confined spaces, like a veterinary hospital's examination room. Here, the dog alternates their gaze between a treat on the floor and the trainer, effectively maintaining engagement despite any distractions. Pattern games not only provide clear guidelines and promote a sense of choice and control for the dog but also act as effective

Table 9.7 Types of pattern games and their general use.

Pattern game	Description
1-2-3 Game	The dog learns to expect a treat on the third word of a sequence. This game helps the dog stay engaged and follow the caregiver, adapting to various transitions within the environment and obstacles. This game has many uses, including teaching loose leash walking, reducing reactivity on the leash, transitioning from the car into buildings, walking down stairs, and building up duration.
Give Me a Break Game	Teaches a dog they have the option to move away and seek out their caregiver, reducing fear, anxiety, and frustration. This is frequently used to reduce barking out the window and to give the dog agency.
Look At That (LAT) and Mat Work	LAT teaches dogs to glance at an object, person, or animal, then return their gaze to their caregiver for a reward. No interaction is ever expected and this game gives the dog an opportunity to point out things in the environment that make the dog uncomfortable without reacting.
	Mat work involves teaching dogs to seek out a designated area for relaxation and safety. LAT is often used as the final step in mat work for scenarios like visitor arrival or meal times.

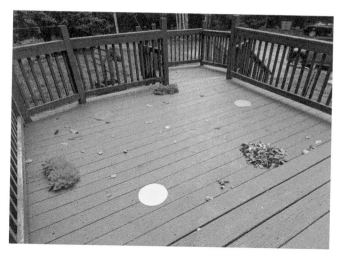

Figure 9.10 LATTE is a pattern game that uses a decompression loop of enrichment items (stations). The dog moves through the stations and food is sprinkled into each station. A fearful stimulus can be located in the distance (person, dog, object). The dog controls how close they move toward the stimulus by offering eye contact to move to the next station. This game is a useful tool for behavior modification. *Source:* Christine Calder (book author).

communication tools. They improve a dog's adaptability and behavior while significantly enhancing the bond between dogs and their caregivers.

Dog-to-Dog Introductions for Shelter Dogs

When introducing a shelter dog to other dogs, it is essential to follow a careful and structured approach for the safety and comfort of all animals involved. The introductions should initially take place in a neutral environment, away from areas familiar to either dog, to minimize defensive behaviors.

Starting with Parallel Walking

Begin by engaging in parallel walking at a safe distance, allowing the dogs to become aware of each other's presence without direct interaction. This approach can help reduce tension and lets the dogs acclimatize to one another. During these initial walks, each dog should be on a leash and handled by a separate person, ensuring they have enough space to retreat if they feel uncomfortable. While walking, the use of the 1-2-3 Game helps keep engagement around distractions and arousal to a minimum.

Observing Body Language

Caregivers should closely observe the dogs' body language during introductions. Look out for signs of protective emotions and defensive behaviors such as stiff posture, prolonged staring, growling, or raised hackles. On the other hand, engaging behaviors that indicate a positive response include relaxed body language, playful bows, and tails wagging at mid-level.

Gradually Decreasing Distance

If engaging behaviors are observed, handlers can cautiously reduce the distance between the dogs, while slowly bringing them within close proximity. Should either dog show signs of discomfort or protective emotions, calmly separate them and consider trying again later, after more parallel walking sessions or utilizing an alternative strategy (Tooley and Heath 2023).

Understanding Individuality in Dog-to-Dog Introductions

Each dog is unique, and this is especially true for shelter dogs who may have past experiences influencing their social behavior; therefore patience and persistence are necessary during this process. If the initial meetings between dogs are successful, subsequent interactions can gradually allow for more direct contact, always under close supervision.

Using Treats and Pattern Games

Using treats to build a positive conditioned emotional response (CER+) in the presence of another dog can be very effective. Implementing pattern games such as the 1-2-3 Game, Superbowls, or LATTE, as discussed earlier, can be extremely helpful in facilitating these introductions as part of the behavior modification process (McDevitt 2019).

Introducing a Shelter Dog to Other Household Animals

When introducing a shelter dog to other pets such as cats, take a step-by-step approach (Figure 9.11). Start with management strategies like using gates or keeping the dog on a leash, allowing the other pet to have an escape route or a safe space to retreat to if they feel threatened or overwhelmed. Both animals should be familiar with foundational behaviors such as targeting, voluntary eye contact, and relaxation exercises. Additionally, for dogs, muzzle training can enhance safety for everyone involved in the introduction process.

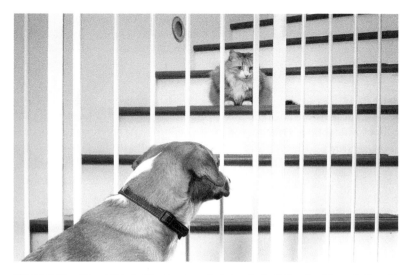

Figure 9.11   How introductions are made is key to building healthy relationships between dogs and other pets in the home. *Source:* Petra Richli/Adobe Stock Images.

Monitoring Body Language

During introductions, closely observe the body language of both the dog and the other animal. In dogs, signs of stress or aggression include growling, stiffening, and intense staring. Cats may show stress by hissing, arching their back, or flattening their ears. Relaxed body postures and curiosity without aggression are positive signs.

Managing Initial Interactions

Start with short interactions and gradually increase their length as the animals become more comfortable with each other. Engage each animal separately during this process. Two adult caregivers may be needed for safety reasons. If the dog hyperfixates or shows excessive interest toward the other pet, intervene calmly and redirect the dog's attention.

In some cases, particularly with prey-driven dogs or very fearful cats, full integration may not be possible. This process can take time, and success depends largely on the behavior and past experiences of the animals involved. However, with patience and careful monitoring, many dogs can learn to live harmoniously with other pets in the home.

Conclusion

Adopting a shelter dog is a journey filled with challenges and rewards. Understanding their unique needs, addressing common behavioral issues, and employing positive reinforcement training are key to helping these dogs adjust to their new homes. With patience, love, and proper care, shelter dogs can make wonderful, loyal companions. Their transformation and growth in a new home can be a deeply rewarding experience for both the dog and their human companions.

References

De Assis, L.S., Matos, R., Pike, T.W. et al. (2020). Developing diagnostic frameworks in veterinary behavioral medicine: disambiguating separation related problems in dogs. *Frontiers in Veterinary Science* 6: 499.

Denenberg, S. (2021). Affective disorders in cats and dogs. In: *Small Animal Veterinary Psychiatry* (ed. S. Denenberg), 207–226. Wallingford: CABI.

Fagen, A. (2023). Separation-related disorders. In: *Behavior Problems of the Dog and Cat* (ed. G. Landsberg, L. Radosta, and L. Ackerman), 297. Philadelphia, PA: Elsevier Health Sciences.

Hargrave, C. (2015). Anxiety, fear, frustration and stress in cats and dogs — implications for the welfare of companion animals and practice finances. *Companion Animal* 20 (3): 136–141.

Lenkei, R., Gomez, S.A., and Pongrácz, P. (2018). Fear vs. frustration–possible factors behind canine separation related behaviour. *Behavioural Processes* 157: 115–124.

Lenkei, R., Faragó, T., Bakos, V., and Pongrácz, P. (2021). Separation-related behavior of dogs shows association with their reactions to everyday situations that may elicit frustration or fear. *Scientific Reports* 11 (1): 19207.

Luescher, A.U. (2009). Repetitive and compulsive behaviour in dogs and cats. In: *BSAVA Manual of Canine and Feline Behavioural Medicine* (ed. D.F. Horwitz and D.S. Mills), 236–244. Quedgeley: BSAVA Library.

Lund, J.D. and Jørgensen, M.C. (1999). Behaviour patterns and time course of activity in dogs with separation problems. *Applied Animal Behaviour Science* 63 (3): 219–236.

McDevitt, L. (2019). *Control Unleashed: Reactive to Relaxed*. South Hadley, MA: Clean Run.

McPeake, K.J., Collins, L.M., Zulch, H., and Mills, D.S. (2021). Behavioural and physiological correlates of the canine frustration questionnaire. *Animals* 11 (12): 3346.

Mills, D. and Zulch, H. (2010). Appreciating the role of fear and anxiety in aggressive behavior by dogs. *Veterinary Focus* 20 (1): 44–49.

Mills, D.S., Dube, M.B., and Zulch, H. (2012). *Stress and Pheromonatherapy in Small Animal Clinical Behaviour*. Chichester: Wiley.

Notari, L. (2009). Stress in veterinary behavioural medicine. In: *BSAVA Manual of Canine and Feline Behavioural Medicine* (ed. D.F. Horwitz and D.S. Mills), 136–145. Quedgeley: BSAVA Library.

Panksepp, J. (2004). *Affective Neuroscience: The Foundations of Human and Animal Emotions*. Oxford: Oxford University Press.

Tooley, C. and Heath, S.E. (2023). Emotional arousal impacts physical health in dogs: a review of factors influencing arousal, with exemplary case and framework. *Animals* 13 (3): 465.

Yin, S.A. (2009). *Low Stress Handling, Restraint and Behavior Modification of Dogs & Cats*. Davis, CA: CattleDog Publishing.

10

The Shelter Cat

In animal shelters and rescue organizations, cats are among the most frequently rehomed pets. Many cats end up in these environments due to behavioral issues, changes in their caregivers' living situations, or the arrival of a new family member. A substantial number of these cats are either stray or feral (Figure 10.1). Annually, approximately two million cats are adopted from shelters, accounting for about 25% of all cat adoptions (ASPCA 2024; New et al. 2004; Patronek et al. 1997).

Research indicates that factors such as temperament, personality, appearance, behavior with people, and age play significant roles in the adoption of both dogs and cats (Podbersek and Blackshaw 1988; Weiss et al. 2012). For kittens, personality and playfulness are influential factors, whereas for adult cats, their behavior with people is more influential (Dybdall and Strasser 2011; Fantuzzi et al. 2010; Gourkow and Fraser 2006; Weiss et al. 2012). Ultimately, in selecting a cat, programs like the American Society for the Prevention of Cruelty to Animals' (ASPCA) Meet Your Match® Feline-ality program and FeBarq can assist potential adopters in finding adult cats that best align with their lifestyle, needs, and interests (Duffy et al. 2017).

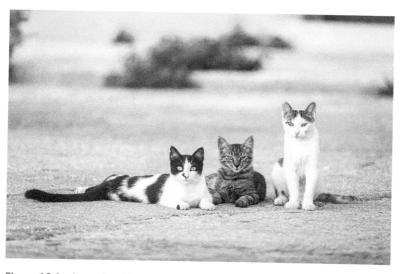

Figure 10.1 It can be difficult to distinguish feral cats in the shelter environment. Making this distinction is needed when reaching outcome decisions. *Source:* Tim Raack / Pexels.

Unique Needs for Rehomed and Shelter Cats

Cats transitioning to new homes from shelters face distinct challenges, differing from those raised in stable environments. A primary challenge for these cats is the stress associated with relocation and adapting to new, unfamiliar surroundings. As creatures of habit, cats may find abrupt changes disorienting and anxiety inducing. To facilitate a smoother transition, adopters need to create a secure and welcoming space. This space should include hiding spots and vertical areas where the cat can feel safe. Additionally, adopters must exercise patience while acclimating a shelter cat to their new home. Allowing the cat to explore and adjust at their own pace helps them acclimate faster.

Selecting a New Cat

Cats are naturally selectively social, solitary hunters, and often territorial. They typically do not favor the company of other cats, making the introduction of a new kitten or cat into a cat-free household often more straightforward. However, it is possible for cats to form strong social bonds with others, though this can take time and is not always guaranteed.

New kittens, while energetic and requiring certain adjustments like kitten-proofing the home and basic training (such as carrier tolerance and nail trims), offer a lot of joy with their playfulness and curiosity. On the other hand, adult and senior cats from shelters or rescues might be better suited for those seeking a calmer and more independent companion such as new cat owners or elderly individuals. If there is already a dog in the home, selecting a cat that has had positive experience with dogs previously can help make the transition smoother (Figure 10.2).

Selecting a New Cat in Multicat Households

Introducing a new cat into a home with existing cats can be a delicate process, especially considering the age and temperament of the resident cats. Adult cats may adapt more easily to new kittens than to other adult cats. Older, geriatric cats often get along better with new companions who are

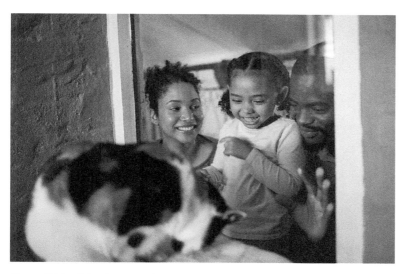

Figure 10.2 Adopting a cat from the shelter has many benefits. How cats are selected depends on individual preferences. *Source:* S Fanti/peopleimages.com/Adobe Stock.

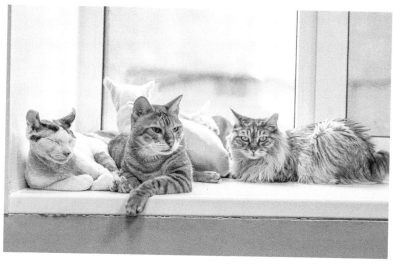

Figure 10.3 When introducing a new cat into the household, the appropriate number of resources helps to reduce environmental stress. *Source:* svetlanais/Adobe Stock.

of a similar age and temperament. The sex of neutered cats typically does not significantly affect their ability to bond, although neutered males are generally more accepting.

The number of available resources significantly influences the size of a cat colony. When introducing a new cat, having adequate resources such as litter boxes and feeding stations to minimize conflicts is a necessity (Figure 10.3). For those considering multiple cats, adopting littermates, a bonded adult pair, or compatible kittens of the same age is typically the best approach. This method helps alleviate territorial stress and reduces conflicts that might occur when a new cat enters the environment of an existing cat.

Assessing Shelter Cat Behavior

Understanding the specific behavior and temperament of each cat is essential for effectively matching shelter cats with potential adoptive homes. A cat's behavior can be influenced by various factors, including the shelter environment. Therefore, it is beneficial to gather information from multiple sources and, where available, insights from previous owners can be particularly valuable (Janeczko 2015). This comprehensive understanding not only aids in finding suitable homes for the cats but also helps in providing appropriate care while they remain in the shelter.

Previous Caregiver Interviews

Interviewing the previous caregiver when a cat is surrendered to a shelter provides invaluable insights. Collecting intake information from these caregivers allows for a deeper understanding of the cat's needs, behavior in a familiar home environment, and the reasons for surrender. Having this knowledge before the cat encounters the inherent stress of the shelter environment is beneficial.

Sheltering can be extremely stressful for almost all cats, with some taking months to adapt to the shelter environment and others never fully adjusting during their entire stay (Broadley et al. 2014; Kessler and Turner 1997; Rochlitz et al. 1998). This stress significantly affects behavior, often leading to unexpected actions (Janeczko 2015) and posing health and safety risks for both the animals and staff. It also complicates the accurate assessment of an animal's typical behavior. Furthermore, cats experiencing higher stress levels are less likely to be adopted (Dybdall et al. 2007; Fantuzzi et al. 2010), resulting in prolonged shelter stays and increased stress, which further diminish their chances of future adoption. Therefore, it is critical to identify and address stress in shelter animals as soon as possible.

Shelter Observations

Daily interactions between shelter staff and cats can yield a wealth of information about each individual cat's behavior. Staff should record and analyze these observations to reveal a cat's preferences and assist in matching them to a suitable home. This also gives an opportunity for staff to learn the preferred handling methods of the cats, their level of sociability, and housing preferences (Janeczko 2015).

Additionally, these observations can alert staff as to when problems may be developing. Changes in behavior often signal illness, and attentive observation enables staff to intervene early when medical issues arise (Camps et al. 2019). Providing prompt medical treatment reduces the stress experienced by the animals, promoting more positive welfare. This not only benefits their health but also increases their chances of being adopted.

The Role of Formal Behavior Evaluations in Shelters

When assessing cats, formal behavior evaluations measure consistent behaviors and enable comparisons in similar circumstances over time, providing insights into an individual animal's behavior (Ellis 2022; Mendl and Harcourt 2000). However, it is important to recognize the potential unreliability of these evaluations due to several factors (Mornement et al. 2014; Patronek et al. 2019). The stress from the shelter environment significantly impacts a cat's behavior during evaluations, especially if they are conducted shortly after the cat's arrival (Broadley et al. 2014; Kessler and Turner 1997; Rochlitz et al. 1998), necessitating a minimum of three days for cats to acclimate to the shelter before being evaluated. During this acclimation period, stress-minimizing efforts are crucial, including the use of Low Stress Handling® techniques, spot cleaning, and careful observation of the cat's body language (Griffin 2022).

Because these evaluations capture behavior at a specific moment, they might not accurately reflect an animal's behavior in various settings such as a home environment (Newbury et al. 2010). Additionally, variability in results can arise from the differing education and training levels of the staff and volunteers conducting these evaluations (Mornement et al. 2010). Therefore, a thorough evaluation should encompass additional sources of information, including the cat's history from previous caregivers and observations by shelter staff, to aid in effectively matching a cat with a new home (Janeczko 2015).

Behavior Assessment Tools

ASPCA Meet Your Match Feline-ality

The ASPCA's Meet Your Match Feline-ality program is one type of behavior assessment designed to pair shelter cats with the most compatible potential adoptive homes, taking into account not only the cat's behavior but also the preferences and goals of the adopter. The outcome of the evaluation places each cat into one of nine "feline-alities":

1) Private Investigator
2) Secret Admirer
3) Love Bug
4) The Executive
5) Sidekick
6) Personal Assistant
7) MVP (Most Valuable Pussycat)
8) Party Animal
9) Leader of the Band

For each of these feline-alities there is a description available on the ASPCA Meet Your Match website (https://aspcameetyourmatch.org/feline-alities). These descriptions provide potential adopters with a better understanding of what to expect from a cat with a particular feline-ality, including likely behaviors and traits.

Matching Adopters with Cats

The ASPCA's Meet Your Match Feline-ality program also categorizes the nine feline-alities into three major adopter groups. These groups are determined based on survey results completed by potential adopters:

- **Purple** (corresponding to feline-alities 1–3).
- **Orange** (corresponding to feline-alities 4–6).
- **Green** (corresponding to feline-alities 7–9).

This classification system considers the personality and lifestyle of the adopter, along with their expectations and desires for a feline companion. By using this tailored pairing system, potential adopters can more accurately select a shelter cat that will fit well into their home environment.

Should adopters be interested in a cat from a different color group than their survey suggests, shelter staff can offer additional education and information. This advice focuses on the specific needs, preferences, and behaviors of the selected cat, thus increasing the chances of a successful adoption (ASPCA 2008).

Common Behavior Problems in Shelter Cats

Shelter cats frequently display behavior problems, which can stem from past experiences or the stress of the shelter environment. It is important to recognize and address these issues to give these cats the best opportunity for a successful and compatible life in a new home. Aggression and house-soiling are among the most common behavior problems seen in shelter cats.

Aggression in Shelter Cats: Types and Management

There are different types of aggression in cats, each requiring a different approach for management and treatment (Table 10.1).

Play Aggression

Commonly seen in kittens and young adult cats, play aggression involves overly excited behaviors during play such as biting or scratching. Though not typically malicious, it can be painful or

Table 10.1 Different types of feline aggression and their management strategies.

Type of aggression	Description
Play aggression	Common in kittens and young adult cats, involves biting or scratching during play. Mitigated by providing interactive toys and play sessions.
Aggression toward other cats	Cats may become aggressive in close quarters with unfamiliar cats, showing hissing, growling, or physical altercations. Gradual introductions are recommended.
Fear-based aggression	Stress in the shelter can lead to fear-based aggression. Important to distinguish if aggression is due to stress or if the cat is feral. Practices vary among shelters. Common at the veterinary hospital.
Petting-induced aggression	Unexpected aggression during petting, possibly due to overstimulation or pain. Signs include dilated pupils and tail lashing. Gentle, brief stroking is advised.
Redirected aggression	Occurs when a cat cannot respond to a stimulus and redirects aggression. Common triggers are loud noises or the sight of stray cats. Minimize exposure to these triggers.
Pain-induced aggression	Occurs in response to pain, leading to aggression to avoid touch or movement. Management includes avoiding touching painful areas and effective pain control.
Territorial aggression	Cats defend their territories and may show aggression toward new or returning cats. Slow introductions and creating separate spaces can help.
Maternal aggression	Queens nursing kittens may show aggression. Providing a quiet, low-stress environment and limiting visitor contact helps in managing this behavior.

frightening for humans. Recognizing signs of play aggression and providing appropriate outlets for a cat's energy, like interactive toys and "hands free" play sessions, can help reduce and manage this behavior.

Aggression Toward Other Cats

As territorial animals, cats can become aggressive when housed in close quarters with unfamiliar cats. Aggressive behaviors may range from hissing and growling to physical altercations. Adopters should introduce cats to each other gradually, allowing them to become familiar with each other's scent and presence before attempting direct interactions.

Fear-Based Aggression

On entering a shelter many cats undergo significant stress, which can trigger fear-based aggression (Janeczko 2015). Identifying whether this aggression stems from the stress of the shelter environment or if the cat is feral and lacks socialization is crucial, as it affects decisions regarding the cat's future. This distinction aids shelter staff in determining whether the cat's behavior might improve with time or if the cat would thrive in a different type of home. However, there is no universally accepted method for making this distinction, leading to considerable variability in shelter practices (Alberthsen et al. 2013). Only about 15% of shelters have formal guidelines to help staff and volunteers make these critical decisions. The lack of such guidelines may increase variability in how cats are handled, leading to inconsistencies and the potential for misclassifying cats (Slater et al. 2010).

Petting-Induced Aggression

Some cats may unexpectedly display aggression during petting, for reasons that are not entirely clear. This behavior could be due to overstimulation or pain. Oftentimes their body language is

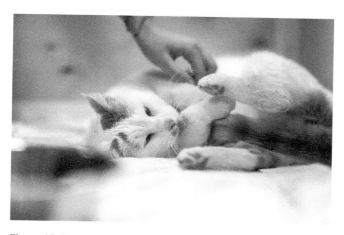

Figure 10.4 Cats with petting-induced aggression often demonstrate conflicted behaviors. They approach, roll over, or otherwise solicit petting, then bite or scratch once petting begins. *Source:* svetlanais/Adobe Stock.

conflicted: they may solicit attention and ask to sit on laps before suddenly lashing out and biting or scratching (Figure 10.4). Typically a cat will exhibit signs such as dilated pupils, tail lashing, and ears positioned backward before becoming aggressive.

Cats displaying petting-induced aggression should be evaluated for pain. To manage this behavior, caregivers should avoid handling or petting the cat without their consent and should refrain from using physical punishment or forced restraint. Never force interactions or attempt to pick up or interact with the cat while they are eating. Instead, caregivers can offer food while applying brief, gentle strokes, preferably around the face and neck and avoiding stroking down the cat's back. They can gradually increase the duration of stroking over time. However, if any signs of arousal is observed, they should immediately stop petting and avoid physical contact until the cat is relaxed again.

Redirected Aggression

When a cat becomes excited by a stimulus but cannot respond directly to it, the cat may redirect aggression toward a human or another animal. Redirected aggression is commonly triggered by stimuli such as loud noises, the sight of an outdoor or stray cat through a window, or an altercation with another cat in the house. In some cases a human may become the target of aggression following an aggressive interaction between indoor cats.

The most effective way to prevent redirected aggression is to eliminate or minimize exposure to these triggers. This can be done by pulling down window shades, window film, using deterrents to keep stray cats away from windows, or addressing underlying environmental stressors and agonistic interactions among indoor cats.

Pain-Induced Aggression

Cats experiencing pain may display aggression toward people or other pets, often as a way to avoid touch, movement, or activities that could exacerbate their discomfort. For instance, cats with osteoarthritis may react negatively to having their joints touched or manipulated, possibly responding with hissing, biting, or scratching. In some rare cases cats might continue to exhibit aggressive behaviors even after the painful areas have healed, likely as a defensive mechanism to avoid anticipated pain.

Managing pain-induced aggression involves avoidance of touching the cat's painful areas and an effective pain management plan. Cats inherently hide pain, so it can be difficult to diagnose. Videos from home and questionnaires can help with the diagnosis. Proper therapeutic strategies can significantly reduce pain and improve the cat's quality of life, thereby reducing instances of aggression.

Territorial Aggression

Cats are known to establish and defend their territories. They may exhibit aggression toward newly introduced cats and occasionally toward other animals or people who encroach on their established domain. In some cases cats might even show aggression toward resident cats that were previously accepted but have been away from home, like during a hospital stay. This aggression typically manifests as swatting, chasing, and attacking the newcomer. Slow introductions as described in Chapter 8 can help facilitate these introductions and build more harmonious relationships over time.

Maternal Aggression

Queens who have recently given birth and are nursing their kittens may display aggression toward anyone approaching them. This is normal behavior. To manage this, caregivers should create a quiet and low-stress environment for the queen and her kittens, limit the number of visitors, and refrain from contact if they notice any aggressive behavior. Typically, maternal aggression subsides as the kittens grow older and become more independent.

House-Soiling

House-soiling, or an elimination disorder, is another common behavior problem in shelter cats. Cats may urinate or defecate outside of the litter box for various reasons, including stress, illness, or a history of inconsistent litter box usage. Patience and a systematic approach are important when addressing house-soiling issues. Providing a clean and accessible litter box, identifying any potential stressors in the cat's environment, and ruling out medical causes are important steps in resolving this behavior.

Enrichment for the Shelter Environment

While cats are housed in a shelter, it is important to address all of their basic needs, including physical, mental, and emotional (Newbury et al. 2010). Providing enrichment can help care for their behavioral wellbeing, improving welfare and reducing current stress as well as limiting future stress (Fox et al. 2006; McMillan 2013). Stress reduction helps to promote physical health as well by lowering the risk of illness and improving brain health (Rosenzweig and Bennett 1996; Stella et al. 2013; Tanaka et al. 2012).

Enrichment also helps increase the likelihood that a given cat will be adopted. When cats are not comfortable in their environment, they are more likely to display fearful, defensive, or destructive behaviors, all of which make them less likely to be adopted (Gourkow and Fraser 2006; Weiss et al. 2012). In contrast, cats that are active, playful, approach people, and are housed in environments that facilitate adopter–cat interactions are more likely to be adopted (Dybdall and Strasser 2011; Fantuzzi et al. 2010; Weiss et al. 2012).

Enrichment should focus on multiple areas, including physical and social environments as well as mental enrichment (Table 10.2).

Table 10.2   Key aspects of the environment for shelter cats.

Aspect	Key points
Physical environment	Sufficient space for movement and play. Separate areas for litter, food, and rest. Access to hiding areas and elevated perches. Areas for scratching nails.
Social environment	Routine and structured interactions. Consideration for individual socialization preferences. Positive socialization for kittens. Compatible group housing based on age and health.
Mental enrichment	Use of food puzzles and a variety of toys. Consideration of individual preferences for toy types. Novelty to maintain interest. Training activities for mental stimulation.

Physical Environment

Cats should have enough space to freely move and play, and the distance between their litter box, food, and resting areas needs to be great enough to ensure these areas are functionally separate to allow cats to feel comfortable using them appropriately (Barry and Crowell-Davis 1999; Gouveia et al. 2011; Kessler and Turner 1999; Rochlitz 2002). They should also have access to hiding areas where they are able to obscure themselves from view (Figure 10.5). Hiding is an important way for cats to cope with the stress of the shelter environment, allowing them to feel more comfortable in their space and thus making them more likely to be adopted (Miller and Watts 2015). Similarly, cats feel more comfortable when able to access elevated perch areas to jump, climb, rest, and observe (Griffin and Hume 2006; Podberscek et al. 1991). Additionally, cats should have areas available to scratch their nails, a behavior that not only provides physical benefits such as stretching and removing nail sheaths but also allows for scent marking (Griffin and Hume 2006).

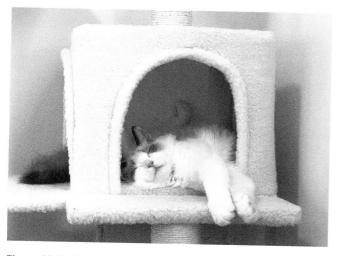

Figure 10.5   Cats need areas where they feel safe to reduce environmental stress. *Source:* David Yu / Pexels.

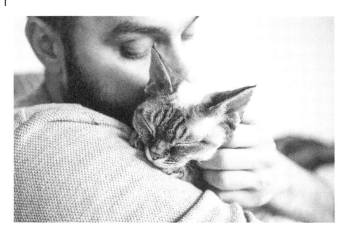

Figure 10.6 Social enrichment can be time spent with other cats or with humans. Each cat is an individual regarding what they prefer, and this needs to be taken into consideration when creating enrichment programs. *Source:* veera/Adobe Stock.

Social Environment

Cats thrive on routines, preferring consistent, structured interactions and schedules (Gourkow and Fraser 2006). Therefore, all human interactions should be positive and consistent from the cat's perspective to decrease stress and promote positive welfare. An individual cat's socialization level should be considered when planning human interactions; some cats may prefer to avoid direct contact, instead interacting through wand toys or simply just exist in close proximity (Figure 10.6). Efforts should be made to ensure positive socialization interactions for young kittens (2–7 weeks of age) in order to facilitate more successful adoptions (Miller and Watts 2015). Cats may be group housed so long as the groupings are composed of compatible, socialized individuals that are matched by age and health and the number of cats in one area does not create competition for resources (Kessler and Turner 1999; Newbury et al. 2010).

Mental Enrichment

Mental enrichment can be fulfilled in multiple ways (Figure 10.7). Variety in enrichment strategies can provide novelty within the environment, which encourages cats to explore and utilize all their senses (Mench 1998). One way to provide mental enrichment is through the use of food puzzles, stimulating a cat's instincts to hunt, bat, pounce, and grab (Young 2003). It is important to ensure that the cats are able to successfully utilize the puzzle feeders to avoid frustration. Cats' natural hunting tendencies can also be encouraged through the use of many types of toys (www.foodpuzzlesforcats.com). When deciding which toys to offer a cat, consider the type of behavior that individual prefers (e.g., chasing, swatting, jumping); novelty is also important with toys because many cats habituate to toys within 24 hours and begin to lose interest unless a new toy is introduced (Hall et al. 2002; Young 2003). Mental enrichment can also be promoted through training activities (see later).

Any enrichment program should be evaluated from the cat's perspective. Shelters will house cats with varied backgrounds, ages, and personalities, so enrichment programs should be tailored to meet their needs accordingly (Miller and Watts 2015).

more patience, progressing through desensitization and counterconditioning programs only as they are able to adjust to each new phase. The use of high-value treats such as Churu® or meat-flavored canned baby food can be helpful through this process, as kittens are often very hungry and will be more likely to approach people with food (Peterson 2008; Phillips 2005). Regardless of the kitten's age, subjecting the kitten to overwhelming or intense interactions with humans (flooding), such as being wrapped tightly in a "kitty purrito," should be avoided, as this could lead to protective emotions and emotional withdrawal or shutdown.

Adult cats also benefit from behavior modification techniques. Capturing and shaping techniques such as clicker training can promote positive welfare (Shreve and Udell 2015). For example, these techniques can be used to encourage cats to approach the front of their kennels, helping improve their adoption potential (Turner 2000). Particularly nervous cats may start very slowly and only emerge from their hiding space by a few inches, but with consistency and patience they can be encouraged to become more interactive (Bollen 2015). Desensitization and counterconditioning (DS/CC) can also be used to help cats become more comfortable with handling, grooming, and other care procedures (Sung and Berger 2022). These consistent, positive human interactions not only help cats who are fearful and stressed in the shelter but also help relatively well-adjusted cats become more adoptable by giving them skills to facilitate care in their new home such as the willingness to enter a carrier, have their nails trimmed, and take medications (Sung and Berger 2022).

Positive reinforcement-based training techniques are effective at reducing the stress experienced by shelter cats (Kogan et al. 2017; Sung and Berger 2022). Training sessions offer cats the opportunity to have choice and control over their environment, both of which are essential for allowing animals to cope with stress and maintain emotional and behavioral health (McMillan 2002; Rochlitz 2007).

Conclusion

Understanding the special needs and potential behavior problems of shelter cats is the first step in preparing them for their new home. Shelter staff can promote positive welfare for the cats in their care through careful attention to body language and recognizing the individuality of each cat. This understanding can increase the likelihood of successful adoption. Further, by addressing the issues of aggression, house-soiling, cat-to-cat introductions, introductions to other animals, and basic training and social skills, adopters can ensure that their shelter cat thrives in their newly adopted home.

References

Alberthsen, C., Rand, J.S., Paterson, M. et al. (2013). Cat admissions to RSPCA shelters in Queensland, Australia: description of cats and risk factors for euthanasia after entry. *Australian Veterinary Journal* 91 (1–2): 35–42.

ASPCA (2008). *Meet Your Match® Feline-Ality™ Manual and Training Guide*. Washington, DC: American Society for the Prevention of Cruelty to Animals.

ASPCA. (2024). Pet Statistics. https://www.aspca.org/helping-people-pets/shelter-intake-and-surrender/pet-statistics (accessed January 9, 2024).

Barry, K.J. and Crowell-Davis, S. (1999). Gender differences in the social behaviour of the neutered indoor-only domestic cat. *Applied Animal Behaviour Science* 64: 193–211.

Bollen, K. (2015). Training and behavior modification for shelter cats. In: *Animal Behavior for Shelter Veterinarians and Staff* (ed. E. Weiss, H. Mohan-Gibbons, and S. Zawistowski), 250–266. Hoboken, NJ: Wiley.

Broadley, H.M., McCobb, E.C., and Slater, M.R. (2014). Effect of single-cat versus multi-cat home history on perceived behavioral stress in domestic cats (*Felis silvestris*) in an animal shelter. *Journal of Feline Medicine and Surgery* 16 (2): 137–143.

Buffington, C.A.T., Westropp, J.L., Chew, D.J., and Bolus, R.R. (2006). Clinical evaluation of multimodal environmental modification (MEMO) in the management of cats with idiopathic cystitis. *Journal of Feline Medicine and Surgery* 8: 261–268.

Camps, T., Amat, M., and Manteca, X. (2019). A review of medical conditions and behavioral problems in dogs and cats. *Animals* 9 (12): 1133.

Dantas, L.M.S., Delgado, M.M., Johnson, I., and Buffington, C.A.T. (2016). Food puzzles for cats: feeding for physical and emotional wellbeing. *Journal of Feline Medicine and Surgery* 18: 723–732.

Duffy, D.L., de Moura, R.T.D., and Serpell, J.A. (2017). Development and evaluation of the Fe-BARQ: a new survey instrument for measuring behavior in domestic cats (*Felis s. catus*). *Behavioural Processes* 141: 329–341.

Dybdall, K., Strasser, R. (2011). Measuring attachment behavior and adoption time in shelter cats. In *Proceedings of the 20th Congress of the International Society of Anthrozoology*, Indianapolis, IN, USA, 4–6 August 2011, 65.

Dybdall, K., Strasser, R., and Katz, T. (2007). Behavioral differences between owner surrender and stray domestic cats after entering an animal shelter. *Applied Animal Behaviour Science* 104 (1): 85–94.

Ellis, J.J. (2022). Beyond "Doing Better": ordinal rating scales to monitor behavioural indicators of well-being in cats. *Animals* 12 (21): 2897.

Fantuzzi, J., Miller, K.A., and Weiss, E. (2010). Factors relevant to adoption of cats in an animal shelter. *Journal of Applied Animal Welfare Science* 13 (2): 174–179.

Fox, C., Merali, Z., and Harrison, C. (2006). Therapeutic and protective effect of environmental enrichment against psychogenic and neurogenic stress. *Behavioural Brain Research* 175 (1): 1–8.

Gourkow, N. and Fraser, D. (2006). The effect of housing and handling practices on the welfare, behavior, and selection of domestic cats (*Felis sylvestris* catus) by adopters in an animal shelter. *Animal Welfare* 15: 371–377.

Gouveia, K., Magalhaes, A., and De Sousa, L. (2011). The behaviour of domestic cats in a shelter: residence time, density and sex ratio. *Applied Animal Behaviour Science* 130 (1–2): 53–59.

Griffin, B. (2022). *Handling shelter cats. In Animal Behavior for Shelter Veterinarians and Staff* (ed. B.A. DiGangi, V.A. Cussen, P.J. Reid, and K.A. Collins), 349–383. Hoboken, NJ: Wiley.

Griffin, B. and Hume, K.R. (2006). Recognition and management of stress in housed cats. In: *Consultations in Feline Internal Medicine* (ed. J.R. August), 717–734. Philadelphia, PA: Saunders.

Hall, S.L., Bradshaw, J.W.S., and Robinson, I.H. (2002). Object play in adult domestic cats: the role of habituation and disinhibition. *Applied Animal Behaviour Science* 79: 263–271.

Janeczko, S. (2015). Feline intake and assessment. In: *Animal Behavior for Shelter Veterinarians and Staff* (ed. E. Weiss, H. Mohan-Gibbons, and S. Zawistowski), 191–217. Hoboken, NJ: Wiley.

Kessler, M.R. and Turner, D.C. (1997). Stress and adaptations of cats (*Felis silvestris catus*) housed singly, in pairs and in groups in boarding catteries. *Animal Welfare* 6 (3): 243–254.

Kessler, M.R. and Turner, D.C. (1999). Effects of density and cage size on stress in domestic cats (*Felis silvestris catus*) housed in animal shelters and boarding catteries. *Animal Welfare* 8: 259–267.

Kogan, L., Kolus, C., and Schoenfeld-Tacher, R. (2017). Assessment of clicker training for shelter cats. *Animals* 7 (10): 73.

McMillan, F.D. (2002). Development of a mental wellness program for animals. *Journal of the American Veterinary Medical Association* 220 (7): 965–972.

McMillan, F.D. (2013). Quality of life, stress, and emotional pain in shelter animals. In: *Shelter Medicine for Veterinarians and Staff, 2* (ed. L. Miller and S. Zawistowski), 83–92. Hoboken, NJ: Wiley.

Mench, J.A. (1998). Environmental enrichment and the importance of exploratory behavior. In: *Second Nature: Environmental Enrichment for Captive Animals* (ed. D.J. Shepherdson, J.D. Mellen, and M. Hutchins), 30–46. Washington, DC: Smithsonian Institute.

Mendl, M. and Harcourt, R. (2000). Individuality in the domestic cat: origins, development and stability. In: *The Domestic Cat: The Biology of Its Behavior (2)* (ed. D.C. Turner and P. Bateson), 47–64. Cambridge: Cambridge University Press.

Miller, K. and Watts, K. (2015). Environmental and behavioral enrichment for cats. In: *Animal Behavior for Shelter Veterinarians and Staff* (ed. E. Weiss, H. Mohan-Gibbons, and S. Zawistowski), 234–249. Hoboken, NJ: Wiley.

Mornement, K.M., Coleman, G.J., Toukhsati, S., and Bennett, P.C. (2010). A review of behavioural assessment protocols used by Australian animal shelters to determine the adoption suitability of dogs. *Journal of Applied Animal Welfare Science* 13: 314–329.

Mornement, K.M., Coleman, G.J., Toukhsati, S., and Bennett, P.C. (2014). Development of the behavioural assessment for re-homing K9's (B.A.R.K.) protocol. *Applied Animal Behaviour Science* 151: 75–83.

New, J.C., Kelch, W.J., Hutchison, J.M. et al. (2004). Birth and death rate estimates of cats and dogs in U.S. households and related factors. *Journal of Applied Animal Welfare Science* 7: 229–242. https://doi.org/10.1207/s15327604jaws0704_1.

Newbury, S., Blinn, M.K., Bushby, P.A. et al. (2010). *Guidelines for Standards of Care in Animal Shelters*. Apex, NC: Association of Shelter Veterinarians.

Patronek, G.J., Beck, A.M., and Glickman, T. (1997). Dynamics of dog and cat populations in a community. *Journal of the American Veterinary Medical Association* 210: 637–642.

Patronek, G.J., Bradley, J., and Arps, E. (2019). What is the evidence for reliability and validity of behavior evaluations for shelter dogs? A prequel to "No better than flipping a coin". *Journal of Veterinary Behavior* 31: 43–58.

Peterson, N. (2008). The way to tame a feral kitten's heart. A step-by-step approach to getting feral fur balls ready for adoption. *Animal Sheltering* November/December: 59–63.

Phillips, M. (2005). *Urban Cat League Guide to Socializing Feral Kittens*. New York: Urban Cat League.

Podberscek, A.L. and Blackshaw, J.K. (1988). Reasons for liking and choosing a cat as a pet. *Australian Veterinary Journal* 65: 332–333. https://doi.org/10.1111/j.1751-0813.1988.tb14523.x.

Podberscek, A.L., Blackshaw, J.K., and Beattie, A.W. (1991). The behaviour of laboratory colony cats and their reactions to a familiar and unfamiliar person. *Applied Animal Behaviour Science* 31: 119–130.

Pryor, K. (2002). *Clicking with cats in the shelter environment. In: Click! For Life, Clicker Training for the Shelter Environment, a Working Guide* (ed. K. Pryor), 30–35. Boston, MA: Karen Pryor Clicker Training.

Rochlitz, I. (2002). Comfortable quarters for cats in research institutions. In: *Comfortable Quarters for Laboratory Animals, 9* (ed. V. Reinhardt and A. Reinhardt), 50–55. Washington, DC: Animal Welfare Institute.

Rochlitz, I. (2007). Housing and welfare. In: *The Welfare of Cats* (ed. I. Rochlitz), 177–203. Dordrecht: Springer.

Rochlitz, I., Podberscek, A.L., and Broom, D.M. (1998). Welfare of cats in a quarantine cattery. *Veterinary Record* 143 (2): 35–39.

Rosenzweig, M.R. and Bennett, E.L. (1996). Psychobiology of plasticity: effects of training and experience on brain and behavior. *Behavioural Brain Research* 78 (1): 57–65.

Shreve, K.R.V. and Udell, M.A.R. (2015). What's inside your cat's head? A review of cat (*Felis silvestris catus*) cognition research past, present and future. *Animal Cognition* 18: 1195–1206.

Slater, M., Miller, K.A., Weiss, E. et al. (2010). A survey of the methods used in shelter and rescue programs to identify feral and frightened pet cats. *Journal of Feline Medicine and Surgery* 12 (8): 592–600.

Stella, J.C., Croney, C., and Buffington, T. (2013). Effects of stressors on the behaviour and physiology of domestic cats. *Applied Animal Behaviour Science* 143 (2–4): 157–163.

Sung, W. and Berger, J. (2022). *Training and behavior modification for shelter cats. Animal Behavior for Shelter Veterinarians and Staff* (ed. B.A. DiGangi, V.A. Cussen, P.J. Reid, and K.A. Collins), 445–475. Hoboken, NJ: Wiley.

Tanaka, A., Wagner, D.C., Kass, P.H., and Hurley, K.F. (2012). Associations among weight loss, stress and upper respiratory tract infection in shelter cats. *Journal of the American Veterinary Medical Association* 240 (5): 570–576.

Turner, D.C. (2000). The human-cat relationship. In: *The Domestic Cat: The Biology of Its Behaviour* (ed. D.C. Turner and P. Bateson), 193–206. Cambridge: Cambridge University Press.

Weiss, E., Miller, K., Mohan-Gibbons, H., and Vela, C. (2012). Why did you choose this pet?: adopters and pet selection preferences in five animal shelters in the United States. *Animals* 2 (2): 144–159.

Wells, D. and Hepper, P.G. (1992). The behaviour of dogs in a rescue shelter. *Animal Welfare* 1: 171–186.

Young, R.J. (2003). *Environmental Enrichment for Captive Animals*. Wheathampstead: Universities Federation for Animal Welfare.

11

Prevention and the Veterinary Hospital

Visiting a veterinary hospital can be a stressful and frightening experience for many pets (Figure 11.1). They may feel overwhelmed by the new environment, unfamiliar smells, and the possibility of undergoing medical procedures. This stress is often heightened if the pet is already ill or in pain (Lloyd 2017). Caregivers are sensitive to their pets' distress, which can negatively impact the perceived welfare of the animals during veterinary care (Mariti et al. 2016, 2017). In fact, the stress associated with veterinary visits is a substantial barrier to care, causing caregivers instead to turn first to the internet or friends for advice and information (Partners for Healthy Pets 2014).

Moreover, fearful and anxious pets present potential safety concerns for veterinary staff (Campbell 1985; Reimer 2020). Research has shown that nearly 33% of dogs display aggressive behaviors, and up to 10% of these dogs exhibit severe aggression (Edwards et al. 2019; Stellato et al. 2021). Animal-related injuries like bites and scratches not only cause physical harm but also pose the risk of transmitting zoonotic diseases (Campagna et al. 2023). In some cases, these injuries can be fatal (Epp and Waldner 2012). Dog bites alone constitute approximately 60–90% of animal bites leading to emergency room visits, and cat bites account for another 5–20% (Maniscalco and Edens 2022). Such incidents are more prevalent among less experienced veterinary staff, indicating the need for thorough education in understanding animal body language and proper handling techniques (Voss et al. 2023).

Given this, it is important to develop and implement strategies to mitigate fear and anxiety in pets during their visits to veterinary hospitals (Reimer 2020). Recognizing the signs of fear and anxiety, addressing them early, and implementing techniques and protocols designed to create a more comfortable environment can improve the overall wellbeing of patients and enhance the veterinary experience for both pets and their caregivers (Figure 11.2) (Haywood et al. 2021; Reimer 2020).

Early Recognition of Fear and Anxiety

Recognizing the signs of fear, anxiety, and frustration in pets is the first step in addressing these emotions effectively. Both dogs and cats exhibit a range of behaviors when distressed, including panting, pacing, trembling, vocalizing, hiding, showing aggression, scratching, and biting. Observant caregivers can learn how to identify these signs at home and share their observations with the veterinary team. Early recognition allows for proactive measures to be taken to alleviate fear, anxiety, and frustration before they escalate.

Veterinary Guide to Preventing Behavior Problems in Dogs and Cats, First Edition. Christine D. Calder and Sarah C. Wright.
© 2025 John Wiley & Sons, Inc. Published 2025 by John Wiley & Sons, Inc.

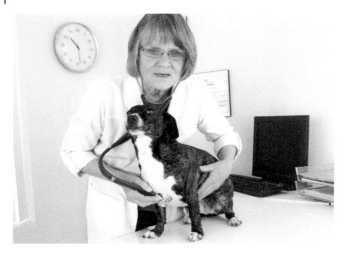

Figure 11.1 This dog is fearful, as is evident from her whale eye (prominent whites of her eyes), ears back, tight mouth, looking away, and stiff body. *Source:* rocketclips/Adobe Stock Photos.

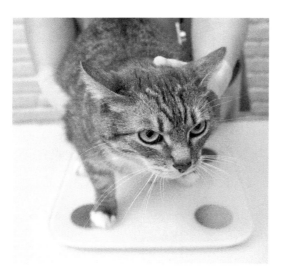

Figure 11.2 This cat is fearful, as evident from the dilated pupils, wide eyes, tight face, and flattened ears. *Source:* Андрей Журавлев/Adobe Stock Photos.

Fear, Anxiety, Frustration, and Stress Start at Home

The stress for pets often begins at home, before they even reach the veterinary hospital. A significant number of pet caregivers notice signs of stress in their animals, particularly cats, before leaving home (Karn-Buehler and Kuhne 2022). Over 50% of cat caregivers report observing stress indicators in their cats while still in their house (Mariti et al. 2016). Factors such as the sight of the carrier, the car journey, and the anticipation of an unknown experience contribute to this stress. Caregivers can help reduce this arousal by implementing training and counterconditioning and desensitization techniques at home (Yin 2009). By lessening the anxiety associated with travel, pets can arrive at the clinic in a more relaxed state, which not only benefits the pets but also makes caregivers less anxious and more likely to return for regular wellness and sick visits (Nibblett et al. 2015; Partners for Healthy Pets 2014).

Carriers

Animals unfamiliar with their carriers or anxious about car travel tend to show increased signs of fear, anxiety, and stress at the clinic (Pratsch et al. 2018; Tateo et al. 2021). Therefore, cats and small dogs should become accustomed to their carriers well in advance of a veterinary visit. The carrier should be seen as a safe space where the pet can willingly enter and remain relaxed, from the moment they enter it, throughout the veterinary appointment, and until they arrive back home.

Selecting a Carrier

There are various styles of carrier available, and veterinary teams can provide guidance to clients on choosing the most suitable one for their pet. The carrier should be appropriately sized, especially for older or arthritic animals who need extra space for comfort. The design should allow for quiet and easy disassembly, enabling veterinary staff to access the pet while they remain comfortable inside (Figures 11.3 and 11.4) (Taylor 2020). For pets that may require sedation injections at the hospital, softer, mesh carriers are advantageous, as they allow for the injections to be administered through the carrier material.

Figure 11.3 A carrier with a shoulder strap can provide stability. *Source:* JackF/Adobe Stock Photos.

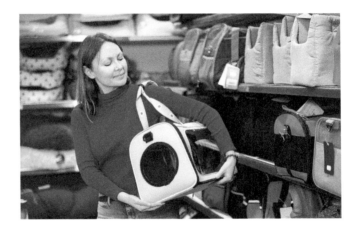

Figure 11.4 Ideally carriers should be able to be easily disassembled for opportunities to conduct examinations where the cat feels safe. *Source:* phoenix021/Adobe Stock Photos.

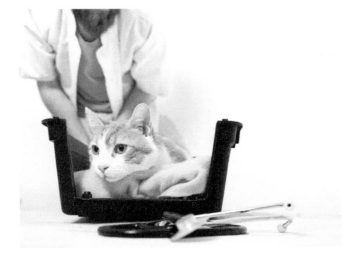

Acclimation to the Carrier

Caregivers can help their pets get comfortable with a carrier by using appealing incentives such as food or toys. Start by placing the pet's meals near the carrier, gradually moving the food bowl further inside to encourage exploration. Scattering treats within the carrier can also entice the pet to explore it at their own pace. For cats, who are naturally curious about enclosed spaces, simply placing the carrier in a common area may prompt them to enter on their own. When they do, rewarding them with food reinforces this behavior. Pets that are more motivated by play than by food might respond well to lure toys or flirt poles, which can be used to engage them in and around the carrier.

Fear of the Carrier

If a pet is initially apprehensive, use a stepwise approach to introduce the carrier. Start with only the bottom half of the carrier, and gradually add the top and door later. Place a soft blanket or towel inside and use calming pheromone sprays such as Feliway® for cats or Adaptil® for dogs (both CEVA Animal Health Ltd, Wooburn Green, UK) (Doonan 2018) to further enhance the carrier's appeal and comfort.

Carrier Training

Studies have shown that carrier training effectively reduces stress in pets during car rides and veterinary visits (Pratsch et al. 2018). The main goal of carrier training is to develop a positive emotional association between the pet and the carrier, sometimes for extended periods (Table 11.1). Such behavior can be encouraged and reinforced through cues like "kennel up" or "crate." Pets should never be forced into carriers; instead, using cues like "kennel up" or "crate" can encourage pets to enter the carrier on their own, reinforcing a positive experience.

Transportation

When transporting pets in their carriers, they need to feel comfortable with the movement involved, such as walking, lifting the carrier, and placing it in the car. Once pets voluntarily enter the carrier and remain relaxed inside with the door closed, caregivers can begin practicing moving the carrier with the animal inside. This process should be gradual to keep the pet's anxiety level low and avoid stress. If the pet shows signs of increased arousal, the caregiver should slow down and return to the previous step where the pet was comfortable. To avoid swaying and bumping, the bottom of the carrier should be supported with both arms for steady and smooth transport, rather than relying on a handle or shoulder strap that allows the carrier to swing (Figure 11.5).

Collars and Harnesses

For animals not being transported in a carrier, they should be properly conditioned to a collar or harness. Avoid using restraint devices that could cause fear, anxiety, stress, or pain such as pinch, prong, choke, or shock collars. Collars or harnesses should be properly fitted for comfort and should not impair movement. Avoid retractable leashes or collars that are too loose, as these could allow pets to escape. A front clip harness with a standard 4–6 ft leash is ideal (Figure 11.6).

Table 11.1 Carrier training steps.

Carrier training for cats: basic training steps	Description and tips
Understanding the basics	Training sessions should be short, lasting only a minute or two, due to cats' quick satiation with treats. The carrier should be a familiar item in the cat's environment before training begins.
Choosing rewards	Use high-value treats, such as cream cheese, tuna, or fish paste. Some cats prefer treats delivered on a spoon to avoid direct touch.
Breaking down the process	Start with the bottom half of a hard carrier if possible. Gradually coax the cat to walk into and stay in the carrier, rewarding each small step of progress.
Step-by-step approach	Begin by rewarding the cat for approaching the carrier. Progressively reward for stepping in with one foot, then both front feet, all feet, and eventually for staying inside.
Adding the carrier top	Once comfortable with the bottom half, add the top (without the door) and repeat the reward process for entering and staying.
Introducing the door	Add the door, keeping it open initially. Reward the cat for being inside with the door moved, then closed, and finally for staying inside with the door closed.
Lifting and moving the carrier	Start by lifting the carrier with the cat inside, then putting it down and treating. Gradually increase time and start walking a few steps while carrying.
Add in car ride	Once the cat is comfortable, it is time to add in a car ride. Take frequent short trips to help the cat feel more comfortable in the carrier and with the movement of the car.
Adapting the method	If using a different type of carrier, adapt the method to reward approach and entry. Use any additional openings for treat delivery. Ensure safety with top-opening carriers.
Duration of training	The amount of time it takes for a cat to feel comfortable varies. Kittens may learn quickly, within days, while adults with negative associations may take months.
Routine training sessions	Two short training sessions per day, about a minute each, are ideal. Incorporate training into daily routines like feeding or playtime.
Long-term benefits	This training eases vet visits and is useful for emergency situations, ensuring quick and safe evacuation if needed.

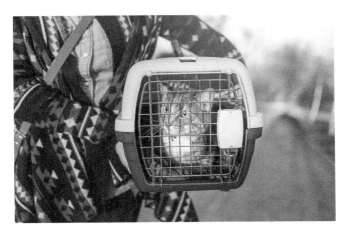

Figure 11.5 Support is needed when carrying a carrier to increase security and stability. *Source:* EdNurg/ Adobe Stock Photos.

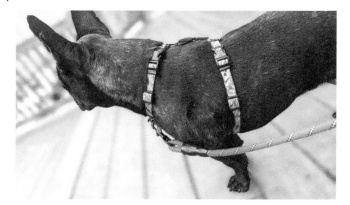

Figure 11.6 A front clip harness is ideal to use for a dog to reduce pulling and provide maximum safety. *Source:* Christine Calder (book author).

Car Rides

Transport can be a source of stress for many animals (Padalino 2015; Van Haaften et al. 2017). Similar to carrier acclimation, helping pets form a positive conditioned emotional response to travel has numerous benefits. Begin the acclimation process below the pet's emotional threshold, breaking the experience down into its simplest components. Start with activities outside the car while the engine is off, gradually encouraging the pet to enter the car on their own. Use ramps or stairs for pets unable to jump. Make the car comfortable with soft bedding, and use pheromone sprays to create a welcoming environment. Food and toy lures can also make the car more inviting.

Practice Car Rides

When riding in the car, pets should be secured in a safe location (Figures 11.7 and 11.8). For cats, the ideal spot is on the floor behind the passenger seat while dogs should be in an impact-resistant crate secured to the floor, not on a seat. Playing music, such as "Through a Dog's Ear" or "Music for Cats," can help create a calm and relaxing environment (https://icalmpet.com).

Once the pet is settled and relaxed in the car with the engine turned off, the caregiver can turn the engine on and offer rewards like food or toys to help the pet adjust to the sounds and vibrations

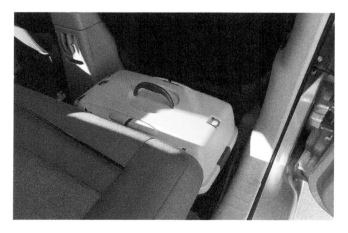

Figure 11.7 The safest location for cats to ride is in a carrier, on the floor behind the passenger seat. *Source:* Bunny Approved LLC / http://bunnyapproved.com/road-trip-transporting-rabbits-in-a-car (accessed February 5, 2024).

Figure 11.8 For dogs the safest location to ride is in the back in an impact-resistant crate. *Source:* lifewithkleekai.com / https://lifewithkleekai.com/impact-collapsible-vs-stationary-dog-crates (accessed February 5, 2024).

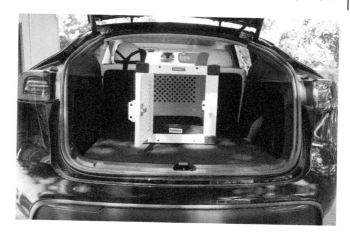

of the engine. Start with short drives, gradually increasing the duration until it matches the time required to reach the clinic. During these rides pets can be given treats in long-lasting toys, such as Kongs® stuffed with frozen, canned food, peanut butter, or cheese. A remote treat dispenser can also used for this purpose.

Motion Sickness and Reactivity

All aspects of an animal's journey during the car ride can affect their behavior and need to be considered. For example, some animals may experience nausea during transport due to the car's movement or the sights and sounds passing by. Administering maropitant citrate at least two hours before travel, along with practicing smooth and safe driving techniques to minimize bumps and rapid turns can help reduce the chance of motion sickness.

Pets may also react to external sights through the car windows, such as other dogs on walks. To address this, accessories like ThunderCaps® or Doggles® can be used to help limit their view, and window clings an be installed to obscure the pet's view from inside the vehicle. For dogs sensitive to the noise of the car, sound-damping ear muffs can be a helpful solution (Figure 11.9).

Figure 11.9 Sound-dampening ear protectors can reduce noise sensitivity when riding in the car. *Source:* Christine Calder (book author).

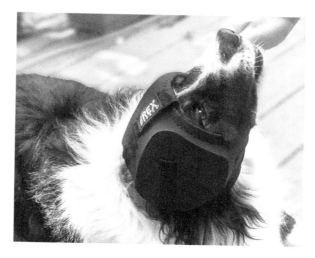

Despite thorough preparation at home and during the car ride to the veterinary hospital, some animals may still experience fear, anxiety, or stress during veterinary visits. Pre-visit pharmaceuticals can help reduce their arousal levels, making the journey and the veterinary experience significantly less stressful.

Preparing the Veterinary Clinic Environment

Entering the veterinary clinic is a significant stressor for many animals. One study indicated that less than 50% of healthy dogs presented to a hospital are able to enter without fear (Doring et al. 2009). Similarly, another study found that only about 25% of cats remain relaxed in the waiting room (Mariti et al. 2016). When animals are fearful, subsequent veterinary visits can exacerbate negative welfare states for both the patient and the client (Reimer 2020; Simpson 1997). Animals learn to associate these negative emotions with the veterinary clinic, leading them to anticipate negative experiences in similar contexts in the future (Overall 2013; Reimer 2020).

To promote positive behavioral and emotional health in patients, veterinary clinics must take proactive steps to create a more welcoming and less intimidating environment. Veterinary professionals need to prioritize preventing negative experiences for both clients and patients (Edwards et al. 2019; Tateo et al. 2021). This approach requires consistent integration and utilization of these methods throughout the veterinary hospital, from the moment the pet enters, continuing for their entire stay.

Design

The entryway and waiting room are among the most stressful areas of the hospital, so creating a low-stress environment should start with the design of these spaces. (Mariti et al. 2015, 2016). Studies indicate that dogs are significantly less stressed when waiting outside rather than inside the waiting room (Lind et al. 2017; Perego et al. 2014). To minimize stress, patients and clients should be directed to go directly to an exam room upon entering the hospital (Engler et al. 2017), bypassing the waiting room whenever possible.

Waiting Rooms

Separate waiting areas for dogs and cats help minimize stress and prevent accidental encounters (Figure 11.10) (Taylor et al. 2022). In the veterinary hospital, dogs should be on a short, nonretractable leash and cat carriers should be placed on elevated surfaces such as a shelf or chair when in the waiting room (Taylor 2020). Covering the carrier with a pheromone-infused towel can block visual stimuli, mute auditory stimuli, and help the cat feel safer and more relaxed (Herron and Shreyer 2014).

Plug-in species-specific pheromone diffusers in the waiting areas can also contribute to a more relaxed atmosphere (Doonan 2018; Engler et al. 2017; Mills et al. 2006). Playing cat and dog-specific music and keeping ambient noise levels to a minimum further reduce stress (Engler et al. 2017; Furgala et al. 2022; Kogan et al. 2012). Efforts should be made to maintain a space free of harsh or unpleasant odors to further reduce stress.

Scales

At the veterinary hospital, the scale often causes significant stress for many patients, sometimes even more than the rest of the waiting room (Hernander 2008). When weighing a patient, they

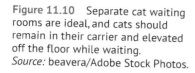

Figure 11.10 Separate cat waiting rooms are ideal, and cats should remain in their carrier and elevated off the floor while waiting.
Source: beavera/Adobe Stock Photos.

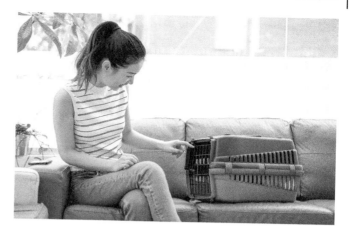

should never be forced onto the scale. Placing a nonslip mat on the scale helps reduce slippage (Doring et al. 2009). Additionally, placing a shelf with food near the scale allows clients to reward their dogs for stepping onto the scale. Teaching dogs to nose target, step up, and station are also effective methods to minimize stress and encourage voluntary cooperation.

Location of the Scale

Placing the scale in an area where animals can walk directly onto and off it without having to enter a confined space or step onto an elevated surface can reduce fear and anxiety associated with the scale. Ideally scales should be recessed into the floor. Use food lures, treat trails, or lickable mats can help encourage an animal to walk onto and stay on the scale until their weight can be accurately measured.

Relaxed Atmosphere

Establishing a relaxed atmosphere within the clinic significantly lowers stress levels in both pets and their caregivers. A calm and welcoming environment encourages clients to routine wellness checks or seek help earlier during an illness, rather than delaying until the pet's condition becomes critical (Volk et al. 2011). Prioritizing the comfort and wellbeing of both pets and their caregivers, can greatly enhance the overall experience at the veterinary hospital.

Reducing Fear in the Exam Room

In addition to the waiting room, the exam room is often a significant source of fear and anxiety for patients. Studies reveal that only about 20% of cats remain relaxed upon entering the exam room, and this number drops to only 15% when they are placed on the exam table (Mariti et al. 2016). Therefore, veterinary professionals must prioritize minimizing patient fear, anxiety, and stress in their patients to promote positive welfare states and conduct accurate physical exam assessments (Bragg et al. 2015; Frank 2014).

Exam Room Strategies

There are numerous strategies that veterinary clinic staff can utilize to make the exam room more comfortable for both clients and patients. Providing a sense of choice, control, and comfort is essential in reducing fear and stress in animals (Mellor 2016). Allowing the patient to explore the exam room during the history-taking and visual exam can help them acclimate and become more at ease. For those in carriers, letting them exit on their own is preferable, and if this is not possible, disassembling the carrier is a better option than forcing them out. If the pet seems to favor a particular area of the exam room such as under the table or near the sink, staff should attempt to examine them in that area if possible. Allowing cats to be "hidden" during the exam is critical to their wellbeing; this can be accomplished by using their carrier, baskets, or loosely wrapped towels (Heath 2020; Taylor 2020).

Patient's Perspective

Consider the exam room from the perspective of the patient's five senses (Taylor et al. 2022). Use species-specific exam rooms and clean thoroughly between each appointment to maintain a welcoming environment. Playing species-specific music can further enhance relaxation and has been shown to reduce stress in both clients and patients during their clinic visits (Engler et al. 2017; Hampton et al. 2020; King et al. 2022). Using pheromones and warmed, pheromone-infused towels can help to make animals feel less anxious and aid in handling (Mills et al. 2006; Pereira et al. 2016). Additionally, nonslip mats should provide secure footing, and offering a variety of treats caters to the patient's preferences for flavor and texture.

The Exam

Research indicates that over 75% of dogs display fear and stress-related behaviors during veterinary exams (Doring et al. 2009; Travain et al. 2015). Similarly, at least 85% of cats exhibit fear-based and stress-related behaviors during exams (Tateo et al. 2021). Therefore, the physical exam in a veterinary clinic should be conducted in a manner that significantly reduces fear, anxiety, and stress for the animal.

Allowing caregivers to stay with their pets during the examination can help minimize stress in patients. They can offer distractions (e.g., food, toys, grooming) to alleviate stress and improve the overall experience (Csoltova et al. 2017). Avoid taking temperatures in healthy animals, and adjust the order of physical examinations from least aversive to most aversive based on the animal's body language. Fecal samples can be collected at home, and caregivers can safely obtain ear swabs and lift lips to assess teeth when needed.

Handling and Restraint

Always use minimal handling, and encourage staff to participate in professional development opportunities that focus on animal welfare (Riemer et al. 2021; Scherk 2022; Taylor 2020). Pursuing handling certifications such as Low Stress Handling® Silver Certification (LSHS-C; www.cattledogpublishing.com), Fear Free™ certification (FFCP; https://fearfreepets.com), and Cat Friendly Practice® certification (CFP; https://catvets.com/cfp/veterinary-professionals) equips veterinary professionals with the skills and knowledge necessary to handle animals in a way that minimizes stress and promotes a positive experience for both the animal and their caregiver (Table 11.2) (Scherk 2022).

the progression of fear, anxiety, and stress in pets. As these emotional states intensify, the response to medication may be slower, and higher doses may be needed to be effective. Such increases in dosage could lead to a higher risk of adverse reactions.

At-Home Oral Medications

Caregivers should administer trial doses at home before the actual veterinary visit, and they should be prepared for the possibility of their pet needing sedation. Medication plans should be tailored to each individual animal, as there is no "one size fits all" approach. Additionally, the use of at-home medications should not be seen as a reason to push an animal beyond their comfort threshold. Body language should be continuously monitored and adjustments made to keep the patient within their comfort zone. This approach requires a collaborative effort between caregivers and veterinary team.

Timing of Medications

Prescribed at-home medications for anxiety can be a valuable tool in preparing a pet for a veterinary appointment. Administering these medications before the visit can significantly reduce the pet's anxiety levels, making the experience at the veterinary hospital more manageable. For optimal effectiveness, these medications are typically given 1–3 hours before the fear-inducing or stressful event such as entering a carrier or car rather than just prior to the appointment time.

Trial Dose

It is advisable for caregivers to test these medications at home before the scheduled appointment day to understand how their pet reacts to the prescribed doses (Table 11.5). However, a pet's response to medication can vary under actual stressful conditions. As a result, multiple visits might be needed to fine-tune the medication plan.

Before starting any medications, baseline lab work, including a complete blood count, serum biochemistry, and urinalysis, should be completed. This helps determine the safety and suitability of the medication for the individual animal, allowing for a more tailored and effective approach to managing their behavior.

Table 11.5 Recordings to be made when trial dosing medications.

Trial dose recording	Description
Time to effectiveness	Record how long it takes for the medication to show its intended effects after administration.
Duration of effectiveness	Note the length of time the medication remains effective in managing or treating the condition.
Observation of side effects	Keep track of any side effects observed after administering the medication, including their nature, severity, and duration.

Gabapentin

Gabapentin influences glutamate, norepinephrine, and substance P (Dooley et al. 2007). Due to its short half-life of less than 12 hours and its excretion through the kidneys, caution is advised when prescribing it to patients with renal disease (Radulovic et al. 1995). Sedation is the most common side effect noted with the use of gabapentin.

For dogs the typical dose range is 10–40 mg/kg bodyweight, and for cats the recommended dose is between 50 and 100 mg per cat (Adrian et al. 2018; Pancratz et al. 2018; Stollar et al. 2022; Van Haaften et al. 2017). It is usually administered about two hours prior to veterinary visits to ensure its effectiveness in reducing anxiety and stress during the appointment. In cats with renal insufficiency, the dose should be reduced by at least 50% (Quimby et al. 2022). Pregabalin, an alternative choice to gabapentin, is specifically labeled to alleviate acute anxiety and fear in cats during transports and veterinary visits (Bonqat® Zoetis).

Trazodone

Trazodone is a serotonin antagonist and reuptake inhibitor (SARI; Stahl 2009). Given its mechanism of action on serotonin, it is important to exercise caution when it is prescribed to patients that are already on other medications influencing serotonin levels, due to the risk of serotonin syndrome (Indrawirawan and McAlees 2014), although at standard dosages the risk of serotonin syndrome is low (Gruen and Sherman 2008).

Trazodone has a short half-life of less than 12 hours (Jay et al. 2013). The most frequently observed side effect in pets taking trazodone is sedation. For dosing, the general guideline for dogs is 3–7 mg/kg bodyweight, and for cats it is between 25 and 50 mg per cat two hours prior to veterinary visits (Erickson et al. 2021; Kim et al. 2022; Orlando et al. 2015; Stevens et al. 2016). Always start with a lower dose and titrate up if needed based on the trial administration.

Dexmedetomidine

Dexmedetomidine, classified as an alpha-2 agonist, is a medication frequently used in veterinary medicine, particularly for dogs (Erickson et al. 2021; Hauser et al. 2020; Hopfensperger et al. 2013). In dogs this medication is typically administered via oral transmucosal (OTM) gel and has a rapid onset of action (approximately 20 minutes). Information regarding the use of OTM dexmedetomidine in cats is limited. However, one study reported that when administered to cats, OTM dexmedetomidine resulted in moderate sedation and all cats vomited (Smith et al. 2020).

Since dexmedetomidine is metabolized by the liver, caution is advised when using it in patients with hepatic disease. The most common side effects observed are sedation and hypersalivation (Zoetis 2015). For dosing, dexmedetomidine oromucosal gel is typically prescribed at a rate of 0.125 mg/m^2. To facilitate ease of administration for caregivers, dosing instructions are often provided in terms of "dots" marked on the dosing syringe (Cohen and Bennett 2015; Dent et al. 2019).

Clonidine

Clonidine, an alpha-2 agonist similar to dexmedetomidine, works by increasing alpha-2 adrenoreceptor activity (Ogata and Dodman 2011). This leads to reduced norepinephrine release from the locus ceruleus, which plays a role in fear-based responses like increased vigilance and arousal (Ogata and Dodman 2011). Such responses can prevent relaxation in stressful situations. Clonidine is often used alongside selective serotonin reuptake inhibitors (SSRIs) such as fluoxetine or tricyclic antidepressants (TCAs) like clomipramine to manage these conditions (Ogata and Dodman 2011).

As an antihypertensive agent in humans, clonidine has a half-life of about 7.7 hours, with diminishing effects over 4–6 hours (Ogata and Dodman 2011). However, specific pharmacokinetic data for dogs are limited. Clonidine is generally administered 1–2 hours before exposure to anticipated stressors and can be used as needed, up to every 8 hours (Ogata and Dodman 2011). It is effective in treating a range of conditions, including noise phobias, separation anxiety, and fear-based aggression (Ogata and Dodman 2011). The dosing range for dogs is 0.01–0.05 mg/kg bodyweight, and the medication is available in tablets of various strengths (Ogata and Dodman 2011). Clonidine is not typically used in cats, so there are no published doses.

Benzodiazepines

Benzodiazepines are a class of drugs that act on the gamma-aminobutyric acid A ($GABA_A$) receptors (Erickson et al. 2021). They bind to specific sites on these receptors, increasing the flow of chloride ions into neurons (Erickson et al. 2021). This action enhances the inhibitory effects of GABAergic neurons, leading to various therapeutic effects (Erickson et al. 2021). Alprazolam, a type of triazolobenzodiazepine, is frequently used in veterinary behavior management due to its rapid onset and effective anxiolytic (anxiety-reducing) and panicolytic (panic-reducing) properties (Chouinard et al. 1982; Erickson et al. 2021).

Benzodiazepines are particularly useful in sedation protocols and for treating animals with profound fears or phobias, as their amnesic properties can help minimize traumatic memories associated with stressful veterinary visits or procedures (Chouinard et al. 1982; Erickson et al. 2021; Overall 2019). Additionally, benzodiazepines induce muscle relaxation independent of sedation, which is beneficial for anxious animals who typically show increased muscle tone (Chouinard et al. 1982; Erickson et al. 2021; Overall 2019). This relaxation aids in reducing overall anxiety and stress levels, thereby making veterinary visits and treatments more manageable for the patient (Erickson et al. 2021; Overall 2019).

For benzodiazepines like alprazolam, the initial dosing range for dogs is typically between 0.02 and 0.04 mg/kg bodyweight, although higher doses up to 0.1 mg/kg bodyweight have been reported (Erickson et al. 2021; Ibañez and Anzola 2009; Reimer 2020). In cats, the documented dose range is 0.0125–0.25 mg/kg bodyweight or 0.125–1 mg per cat (Denenberg and Dubé 2018; Erickson et al. 2021). However, it is important to note that there are no specific dose determination studies for alprazolam in either cats or dogs (Erickson et al. 2021).

The primary adverse effect associated with benzodiazepine use is sedation (Erickson et al. 2021; Overall 2019). Alprazolam tends to be less sedating than diazepam, and most adverse effects, including sedation and ataxia (lack of voluntary coordination of muscle movements), are dose dependent (Erickson et al. 2021; Herron et al. 2018; Overall 2019). Paradoxical excitement and disinhibition of behaviors such as aggression have also been reported in both cats and dogs (Crowell-Davis et al. 2003; Erickson et al. 2021; Overall 2013).

Acepromazine

Acepromazine functions as a dopamine antagonist and is used in veterinary medicine primarily for its tranquilizing effects. However, it is important to note that while it induces tranquilization, acepromazine does not inherently relieve anxiety. Therefore, it is often prescribed in combination with an anxiolytic to ensure both calmness and reduced anxiety in pets.

Compared to the other medications discussed, acepromazine has a slightly longer half-life, approximately 16 hours (Hashem et al. 1992). Among its most common side effects are ataxia (lack of voluntary coordination of muscle movements) and sedation. Additionally, acepromazine can cause hypotension (low blood pressure), necessitating caution in patients with cardiovascular disease (Karas 1999).

When administering acepromazine orally, the recommended dose ranges from 0.5 to 2 mg/kg bodyweight for both dogs and cats. Alternatively, for OTM administration, the dose typically falls within the range of 0.025–0.05 mg/kg bodyweight (Costa et al. 2023). To achieve maximum effectiveness, it is advisable to administer acepromazine approximately 2 hours before the scheduled veterinary visit.

Administering Oral Medications

Administering oral medications to dogs and cats can be challenging due to their natural resistance to taking medications (Table 11.6). Tablet formulations are generally preferred, as they are more readily absorbed and achieve better bioavailability compared to liquid, compounded, or transdermal medications. It is beneficial to start training animals to take medications from a young age, even before they actually need them. This proactive approach can make the process easier when the need for medication arises. However, it is important to note that both dogs and cats are capable of learning to take medications at any age.

Table 11.6   Different strategies to administer oral medications.

Method	Description
Three treat technique	Offer three special treats daily, two to three times at the same time each day. Eventually, conceal the medication in the second treat. Be sure to give treat one, then two, quickly followed by three. You can also count when doing this for added predictability.
Use a lickable mat	Bring out a lickable mat two to three times daily and place three treats on it or use a smearable treat. Gradually, hide a pill in one of the treats on the mat.
Nonsuspicious locations	Administer medications in locations where the pet will not be suspicious, like during a walk or on their cat tree or bed, avoiding typical medication spots like the kitchen or bathroom.
Liquid medication with food	For liquid medications, mix them with canned food or a lickable treat in a syringe. Layer the medication within the food for easier administration.
Medication as rewards	Use treats that conceal the medication as rewards for cued behaviors (e.g., sit or touch) that the dog or cat is already familiar with.

In-Hospital Medications (Injectable)

In some cases injectable sedation may be needed. These medications are customized to each pet's specific needs and should be used alongside other fear-reduction techniques. The sedation should be used before the patient becomes highly aroused for the most effective onset and minimal dosing. Factors to consider when selecting medications and doses include any preadministered medications, the goals of the visit, the patient's pain level, and any potential issues with drug metabolism due to conditions like kidney or liver disease. Combining drugs can provide balanced sedation and analgesia while minimizing the side effects of any individual drug.

Dexmedetomidine

Dexmedetomidine, an alpha-2 agonist, can lead to cardiovascular depression, including bradycardia and reduced cardiac output, particularly when administered as an injectable agent (Erickson et al. 2021). This medication is suitable for both cats and dogs and can be administered either intravenously (IV) or intramuscularly (IM). The level of sedation required determines the dose. Notably, dexmedetomidine's effects can be reversed with an equal volume of atipamezole, providing an additional safety measure in case of adverse reactions or if rapid recovery from sedation is needed (Dent et al. 2019; Ko et al. 2011; Santos et al. 2010; Simon and Steagall 2020).

Acepromazine

Acepromazine is a dopamine antagonist. This medication causes tranquilization but does not have any anxiolytic effect, so it must be used in combination with an anxiolytic. The most common side effects are ataxia and sedation, but it can also cause hypotension, so caution should be used in patients with cardiovascular disease (Karas 1999). Acepromazine is not reversible, so it should be used with caution, particularly at high doses (Mathews et al. 2018; Verstegen et al. 1996).

Opioids

Depending on which opioid is chosen, the drug may have mild to profound analgesic and sedative effects (Moser et al. 2020). These medications can cause significant respiratory depression, so oxygen support and equipment for intubation should be readily accessible if needed. Opioids can be reversed with naloxone, but this is usually only done if significant adverse effects arise (Mathews et al. 2018). Opioids are typically used in combination with alpha-2 agonists and acepromazine, and doses vary depending on which opioid is chosen (Karas 1999; Santos et al. 2010).

Ketamine

Ketamine is a dissociative anesthetic agent. This medication provides excellent sedation and also has anxiolytic properties. Ketamine is typically used when immobilization is needed. Doses vary based on the level of sedation needed (Ko et al. 2011; Mathews et al. 2018; Simon and Steagall 2020).

Benzodiazepines

This class of medications includes diazepam and midazolam. These medications are typically very safe due to their minimal cardiovascular and respiratory effects (Karas 1999). Benzodiazepines are reversible with flumazenil dosed at 0.01–0.02 mg/kg bodyweight IV (Mathews et al. 2018).

Preventing and Treating Fear of the Veterinary Hospital

Prevention and intervention visits play a role in maintaining a positive emotional connection between pets and veterinary hospitals. These visits are distinct from regular medical appointments and serve two primary purposes: to prevent fear in pets who are currently comfortable at the vet, and to intervene in cases where pets are already showing signs of fear, anxiety, and stress (Table 11.7).

Prevention Visits

Prevention visits at veterinary clinics are designed for young animals that do not have a fear of the veterinary hospital, examination, or team members. These visits are strategically scheduled during

Table 11.7   Comparison of prevention and intervention visits.

Aspect	Prevention visits	Intervention visits
Target patients	Young animals without fear of veterinary hospitals, examinations, or team members.	Pets of any age that are already exhibiting signs of stress and fear, especially significant for young animals in critical developmental stages.
Scheduling	During quiet times of the day to minimize stress and ensure no other animals are present.	During quiet times of the day to minimize stress and ensure no other animals are present.
Activities in clinic	Pets can explore the waiting and examination rooms; no physical examination is conducted.	Gradual familiarization with the exam room, exam table, and parts of the physical examination.
Role of caregivers	Encouraged to bring the pet's favorite treats, toys, and comfortable items like mats or beds from home.	Similar role; encouraged to bring comforting items from home to use as part of the familiarization process within the veterinary environment.
Training and preparation	Short visits based on comfort level, interaction encouraged only if initiated by the pet.	Begins at home with specific training like muzzle training for dogs, carrier training for cats, and behavior modification techniques.
Anxiety management	Use of toys, treats, and exploration platforms; specific considerations for kittens, such as encouraging them to emerge from carriers at their own pace.	Addressing fears before the visit; enrichment and relaxation exercises outside the clinic; strategies for specific fears like fear of the scale.
Approach to examination	No physical examination; interaction with veterinary equipment at their own pace.	Incremental approach to examination, focusing on one aspect per visit to avoid overwhelming the pet.
Team member interaction	Interaction based on the pet's choice, with an emphasis on play and positive reinforcement.	Gradual introduction of new staff members, ensuring animal comfort; cooperative care training emphasized.

times of minimal clinic activity. This scheduling approach provides puppies with an opportunity to safely and comfortably explore both the waiting and exam rooms and allows kittens to do the same in the exam room, in a nonthreatening environment. Furthermore, these times are chosen to ensure that no other animals are present, thereby reducing any potential danger or stressors.

During these visits pets are permitted to explore specific areas, such as the scale in the waiting room or features within an exam room. However, a physical exam is not conducted. Caregivers are encouraged to bring their pet's favorite treats and toys to these visits, but it is not necessary or recommended to withhold meals prior to coming.

The duration of these visits should be short and short tailored to the comfort level of the pet. The visit can continue as long as the pet is willing to engage and accept treats. The main goal of these visits is to gradually increase the time spent in the exam room and with the veterinary team members. Interactions should only occur only if the pet initiates them. Initially treats may be tossed rather than offered by hand, and team members are encouraged to engage pets in play using toys (Figures 11.12 and 11.13).

Specific considerations for kittens include placing their carrier on the floor and allowing them ample time to emerge and explore the room at their own pace. Nonslip mats, for both the floor and

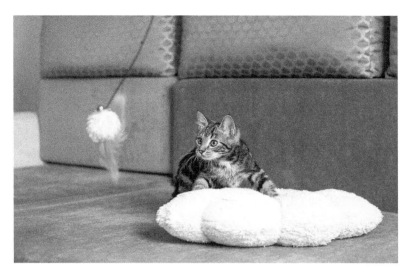

Figure 11.12 Toys can be used in the exam room during prevention visits to encourage play and comfort with the room. Play also helps to build relationships with team members. *Source:* barinovalena/Adobe Stock Photos.

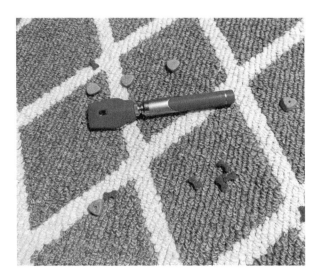

Figure 11.13 Scatter treats around commonly used equipment during veterinary examinations to encourage puppies and kittens to explore and engage. *Source:* Christine Calder (book author).

the examination table improve safety and comfort. A platform in the room encourages exploration and provides an opportunity to reinforce both dogs and cats for choosing to climb on and off the platform at will (Figure 11.14). For dogs, having a variety of toys, including puzzle toys and food-stuffed toys, is suggested. For cats, wand toys are useful for directing kittens onto the scale and facilitating play with team members. Essential items like a water bowl for hydration and a litter box for kittens and cats should be readily available.

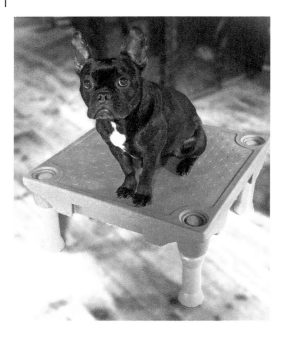

Figure 11.14 Encourage and reinforce dogs and cats for choosing to step up or get onto a platform provided in the room. *Source:* Christine Calder (book author).

While these prevention visits are primarily focused on younger animals, older pets can also benefit from them as well, provided they are not already experiencing fear or anxiety about visiting the veterinary clinic.

Intervention Visits

Intervention visits, different from prevention visits, are designed for patients who already exhibit signs of stress and fear in a veterinary setting. They hold particular importance for young animals at critical developmental stages, such as puppies showing fear at 12 weeks of age and kittens displaying protective emotions at any age. Addressing fearfulness during these early stages is essential, as it can be a reliable indicator of future behavior in adulthood. The main goal of these visits is to alleviate the heightened emotional arousal that animals may experience during various aspects of a veterinary visit. This includes reactions to examinations, injections, restraint, and handling, or even specific areas of the hospital. By focusing on these aspects, intervention visits seek to create a more positive and less stressful experience for both the pet and their caregivers.

Preparation Starts at Home

The preparation for intervention visits usually begins in the pet's home, a familiar and safe space that sets the stage for a more positive experience at the veterinary hospital. In this initial phase, specific training is tailored to the needs of each animal. Dogs, for example, may undergo muzzle training, while both dogs and cats can benefit from carrier training to ease the stress associated with travel to the clinic. Additionally, mat or platform training, coupled with teaching targeting and consent behaviors such as chin, feet, body, and nose touches, is the first step of this process (Jones 2023a). These behaviors help to foster a sense of predictability and prepare the patient for subsequent behavior modification techniques like desensitization and counterconditioning.

Behavior Modification

Behavior modification is the second step in this process and can be highly effective to help change conditioned emotional responses to various aspects of veterinary care, including handling, restraint, and other procedures. First practiced in the home environment, these techniques are later transitioned to the veterinary setting. This process begins without the involvement of the veterinary team but then is progressively adjusted to include them, to give time for the animal to become familiar with their presence in a safe and nonthreatening way.

Fears Beyond the Exam Room

Addressing the fears that pets may experience even before arriving at the veterinary clinic is a critical part of intervention. Managing travel-related anxieties such as car ride anxiety is essential in ensuring the journey to the hospital is as stress free as possible. Distractions and relaxing activities such as playing games in the parking lot or taking leisurely walks around the area can be effective in reducing anxiety levels before the pet enters the hospital. These activities help in creating a positive association with the surroundings of the veterinary clinic.

Specific Strategies

For animals who are nervous about specific aspects of the veterinary visit, like being weighed on a scale, tailored strategies can be used to ease their anxiety (Figure 11.15). Dogs, for instance, may benefit from engaging techniques like following treat trails, participating in specific games, playing with a snuffle mat, or engaging in targeting exercises. These activities are designed to foster engagement and participation. If needed, platform training can be used as the first step in behavior modification to treat scale anxiety.

Cats and Scales

Cats may require a different approach, especially when it comes to being weighed. One method involves covering the scale with a towel to create a less intimidating environment. Another technique is to weigh the carrier separately and then subtract its weight from the total when the

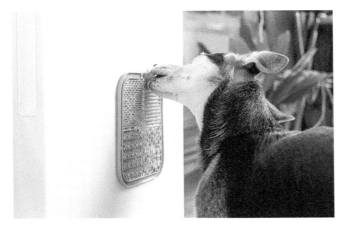

Figure 11.15 Using a lickable mat on the wall near the scale helps to encourage dogs to get on the scale and stand still during weigh-ins. *Source:* dark_blade/Adobe Stock Photos.

cat is inside, thereby avoiding the need to place the cat directly on the scale. These methods are aimed at reducing the stress for cats while still allowing for accurate weight measurements.

Nail Trims

Nail trims are nonurgent procedures and should not be performed if the dog or cat is fearful (Table 11.8). The process of desensitization and counterconditioning, or behavior modification for nail trims, begins by first teaching a start button/signal or consent behaviors (Edwards et al. 2022; Jones 2023a,b; Sydänheimo et al. 2023). These behaviors might include lying on a mat, offering a paw, or engaging in a chin rest behavior. Only after these behaviors are established should the introduction of nail trimmers or a Dremel tool occur, along with handling of the paws.

Nail Board or Scratch Pad

An alternative to regular nail trims is the use of a nail board, which can either be purchased or made at home. These boards come in both rigid and flexible forms (Figure 11.16). Dogs and cats can be taught to file their own nails using these boards.

Hind Feet and Dewclaws

Filing the hind feet of dogs can be effectively managed by harnessing their natural scratching behavior, commonly displayed after elimination. Another method involves using a board placed at an angle against a sturdy, elevated surface like a stool, bench, or platform. The dog is then encouraged to step up to this setup, gradually shaped to scratch their hind feet against the board for nail filing. For dewclaw care, a cut piece of PVC pipe lined with slip-resistant tape on the inside can be used, allowing the dog to safely file their dewclaws.

Table 11.8 Nail trim alternatives for dogs and cats.

Alternatives to nail trims	Description
Nail trim procedures	Nail trims are nonurgent and should not be performed if the pet is fearful. Desensitization and counterconditioning should start with teaching consent behaviors such as lying on a mat, offering a paw, or engaging in chin rest behavior, before introducing nail trimmers or Dremel tools and handling paws.
Nail board or scratch pad	An alternative to traditional nail trims is the use of a nail board. These can be homemade or purchased and are available in rigid and flexible forms. Pets can be trained to file their nails on these boards.
Hind feet and dewclaws (dogs)	Dogs can file their hind nails by harnessing their natural scratching behavior or using a board angled against a raised surface. For dewclaw care, a cut piece of PVC pipe lined with slip-resistant strips can be used.
Cats	Scratch pads can be used for cat nail care. While placing them in litter boxes is an option, placing scratch pads in an additional, empty box is recommended to prevent litter-box aversion, offering cats an alternative space for nail care.

Figure 11.16 Example of a homemade nail board. This is a flexible cutting board with slip-resistant strips attached to the board. *Source:* Christine Calder (book author).

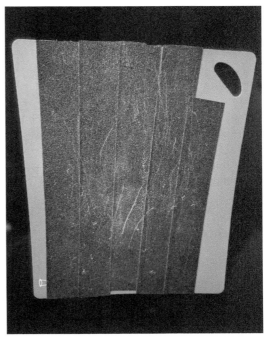

Cats

For cats, introducing scratch pads can assist in grooming needs. These pads can be placed at the bottom of litter boxes. However, it is important to make sure the cat does not find these aversive, as it could lead to house-soiling issues. A more cautious approach would be to place the scratch pads in an additional, empty box. This strategy helps in reducing the likelihood of the cat developing an aversion to the litter box, providing them with an alternative space for their scratching needs.

Expanding to the Examination

Once at the hospital, the main objective of intervention visits is to gradually acclimate the patient to the veterinary environment. This involves familiarizing them with the exam room, the exam table, and various aspects of the physical exam, all done in a step-by-step, not overwhelming manner. For instance, a particular session might be dedicated solely to thoracic auscultation, deliberately avoiding other examination procedures to prevent causing stress to the animal. This incremental approach helps the pet become comfortable with each new aspect of the veterinary experience at their own pace.

Role of the Caregiver and Introduction of Team Members

The role of the pet's caregiver is integral during these visits. They are encouraged to bring items that provide comfort to the pet such as their favorite treats, toys, and a familiar resting area like a mat, bed, or platform. These items can help ease the pet's anxiety and make the veterinary setting feel more like home. Gradual introduction of new team members to the patient is another key element of these sessions. It is important for each animal to be comfortable with each new person, building a sense of trust and safety around them.

Consent and Choice

The guidance of professionals trained in cooperative care is invaluable in these sessions. These experts understand how to give animals a sense of choice and control during their care, which is fundamental to the success of early intervention visits. Emphasizing reinforcement for both engaging and choosing not to engage communicates to the animal that they have options, allowing them to participate in their care at their comfort level. Additionally, providing alternatives for exploration and interaction within the exam room ensures that the animal is consenting to the process (Jones 2024). They should have the freedom to engage in an activity or move to a different one at their discretion. This methodology not only reduces the stress associated with veterinary visits but also fosters a true cooperative relationship between the animal, their caregiver, and the veterinary team.

Returning Home After the Visit

Many animals experience stress and anxiety for hours or even days after returning home from the veterinary clinic (Volk et al. 2011). Veterinary staff can provide clients with recommendations to help ease the transition back into their day-to-day life whether after an annual visit or a hospital stay.

Car Ride Home

Caregivers should be encouraged to use the same techniques for the car ride home as they did for arriving at the clinic. Careful, safe driving can help prevent motion sickness. On arrival at home, pets should be provided with soft bedding with scents from their home environment. This practice aids in eliminating the residual smell of the veterinary clinic. In homes with multiple cats, include bedding with the scent of cats that did not visit the hospital to encourages the natural behavior of allorubbing, which is essential for maintaining healthy relationships among cats in the household (Bradshaw 2016).

Transitioning Home

Once home, clients should provide a safe place for the patient to go. This area should allow the pet to relax independently. Playing calming music, using species-specific pheromones, and providing soft bedding can make this space more welcoming. Caregivers are also advised to place the pet's favorite toys and treats in this area. After a veterinary visit many pets may feel the need to sleep, so ensuring they have a comfortable and quiet space for rest is important. Allowing other cats in the home to smell the carrier and using towels to facilitate allorubbing helps in reintroducing the returning cat's home scent. Generally, with a bit of space and time, pets tend to revert to their normal behavior following a veterinary visit. Caregivers should be advised to contact the veterinary clinic if any abnormal behavior persists or if they have any concerns or questions.

Communicating with Clients

Effective communication between veterinarians and caregivers is essential to provide the best care for patients. Engaging in conversations about a pet's body language can be insightful, as it opens up discussions regarding the pet's behavior at home and enhances the caregiver's understanding of their pet's emotional state. Veterinarians should employ open-ended questions and utilize nonviolent communication strategies to foster a constructive dialogue (Table 11.9) (Rosenberg and Chopra 2015). Avoid using labels and instead ask for specific descriptions of the pet's behavior (Table 11.10).

Table 11.9   The four key components of nonviolent communication.

Nonviolent communication component	Description	Example in veterinary medicine
Observations	Factual descriptions of what is being observed without adding interpretations or judgments	"I noticed that your dog flinched when I touched his ear. He also seems to be tilting his head to one side frequently."
Feelings	Expressing the feelings or emotions that the observation is triggering	"It seems like you might be feeling anxious about your dog's reaction. Are you worried about his comfort or potential pain?"
Needs	Identifying the needs, values, or desires that are connected to the feelings	"It sounds like you need assurance that your dog is not in pain and that we are taking the best possible care of him."
Requests	Making a clear, specific, and actionable request without demanding	"Would you like me to explain the potential causes of your dog's behavior and discuss the treatment options available?"

Table 11.10   Common labels used in veterinary medicine.

Label	More appropriate observation or description
Aggressive	Barking, growling, lunging, snapping, biting are appropriate observations, but there is also a need to know in what context or environment.
Lazy	Prefers to lie down or rest, may not engage in much activity, which could indicate discomfort or physical issues. May also be emotional withdrawal due to being overwhelmed, fearful, or anxious.
Hyper	Exhibits high levels of energy, often active or easily excitable. Often these dogs are anxious or frustrated.
Nervous	Shows signs of anxiety or stress, such as panting, pacing, or hiding, in unfamiliar or challenging situations.
Scared	Displays fearful behavior, like cowering, trembling, or avoidance, in response to certain stimuli or environments.
Dominant	Often used to describe aggressive behavior between humans, other dogs, or in certain environments. Often these animals are anxious and fearful and not confident.
Spoiled	Receives a lot of attention or treats, may show reluctance to comply without rewards or familiar comforts.
Stubborn	Refuses to do certain behaviors when asked. Often this is because there are too many distractions or the behavior was taught with a lure; therefore food in hand is often the cue, and without it the cue is not clear.
Protective	Used to describe a dog that barks, growls, lunges, or displays other aggressive behaviors when around new people and in new environments. Often these dogs are only protecting themselves and are fearful or anxious.

Explaining Procedures

Taking the time to thoroughly explain procedures is an essential aspect of a veterinarian's role. During these conversations, the importance of preventive care and options available for reducing fear in pets should be discussed. Maintaining an open and transparent line of communication ensures that caregivers are well informed and helps them to feel confident about the health-related decisions they make for their pet.

Addressing Concerns

Clear, empathetic, and informative discussions help to ease concerns that caregivers might have and foster a collaborative and trusting relationship between veterinarians and caregivers. Ultimately, effective communication is fundamental to ensuring that pets receive the best possible care, tailored to their individual needs and emotional states.

Conclusion

Reducing fear and anxiety in pets at the veterinary hospital is not only a humane approach but also one that can lead to better medical outcomes and improved compliance with preventative care. By recognizing the signs of fear and anxiety early, preparing the environment, implementing welfare-friendly handling techniques, and considering medications when necessary, veterinarians and caregivers can collaboratively create a veterinary experience that is positive and comfortable for pets. This approach not only benefits clients and pets but also the veterinary team, improving safety, client compliance, and job satisfaction.

References

Adrian, D., Papich, M.G., Baynes, R. et al. (2018). The pharmacokinetics of gabapentin in cats. *Journal of Veterinary Internal Medicine* 32 (6): 1996–2002.

Behnke, A.C., Vitale, K.R., and Udell, M.A.R. (2021). The effect of owner presence and scent on stress resilience in cats. *Applied Animal Behaviour Science* 243: 105444.

Bradshaw, J.W.S. (2016). Sociality in cats: a comparative review. *Journal of Veterinary Behavior* 11: 113–124.

Bragg, R.F., Bennett, J.S., Cummings, A., and Quimby, J.M. (2015). Evaluation of the effects of hospital visit stress on physiologic variables in dogs. *Journal of the American Veterinary Medical Association* 246 (2): 212–215.

Brondani, J.T., Mama, K.R., Luna, S.P.L. et al. (2013). Validation of the English version of the UNESP-Botucatu multidimensional composite pain scale for assessing postoperative pain in cats. *BMC Veterinary Research* 9: 143.

Buckley, L.A. and Arrandale, L. (2017). The use of hides to reduce acute stress in the newly hospitalised domestic cat (*Felis sylvestris catus*). *Veterinary Nursing Journal* 32 (5): 129–132.

Campagna, R.A., Roberts, E., Porco, A., and Fritz, C.L. (2023). Clinical and epidemiologic features of persons accessing emergency departments for dog and cat bite injuries in California (2005–2019). *Journal of the American Veterinary Medical Association* 261 (5): 723–732.

Campbell, W.E. (1985). *Behavior Problems in Dogs*. Schaumburg, IL: American Veterinary Publications.

Chouinard, G., Annable, L., Fontaine, R., and Solyon, L. (1982). Alprazolam in the treatment of general anxiety and panic disorders: a double-blind placebo-controlled study. *Psychopharmacology* 77: 229–233.

Cohen, A.E. and Bennett, S.L. (2015). Oral transmucosal administration of dexmedetomidine for sedation in 4 dogs. *Canadian Veterinary Journal* 56 (11): 1144.

Costa, R.S., Jones, T., Robbins, S. et al. (2023). Gabapentin, melatonin, and acepromazine combination prior to hospital visits decreased stress scores in aggressive and anxious dogs in a prospective clinical trial. *Journal of the American Veterinary Medical Association* 261 (11): 1660–1665.

Crowell-Davis, S.L., Seibert, L.M., Sung, W. et al. (2003). Use of clomipramine, alprazolam, and behavior modification for treatment of storm phobia in dogs. *Journal of the American Veterinary Medical Association* 222: 744–748.

Csoltova, E., Martineau, M., Boissy, A., and Gilbert, C. (2017). Behavioral and physiological reactions in dogs to a veterinary examination: owner-dog interactions improve canine well-being. *Physiology and Behavior* 177: 270–281.

Denenberg, S. and Dubé, M.B. (2018). Tools for managing feline problem behaviors: psychoactive medications. *Journal of Feline Medicine and Surgery* 20: 1034–1045.

Dent, B.T., Aarnes, T.K., Wavreille, V.A. et al. (2019). Pharmacokinetics and pharmacodynamic effects of oral transmucosal and intravenous administration of dexmedetomidine in dogs. *American Journal of Veterinary Research* 80 (10): 969–975.

Dooley, D.J., Taylor, C.P., Donevan, S., and Feltner, D. (2007). Ca^{2+} channel a2d ligands: novel modulators of neurotransmission. *Trends in Pharmacological Sciences* 28 (2): 75–82.

Doonan, C. (2018). The effects of Feliway on the stress of cats during veterinary examination. Honors thesis, Western Michigan University. https://scholarworks.wmich.edu/honors_theses/3100 (accessed March 23, 2024).

Doring, D., Roscher, A., Scheipl, F. et al. (2009). Fear-related behaviour of dogs in veterinary practice. *Veterinary Journal* 182: 38–43.

Edwards, P.T., Smith, B.P., McArthur, M.L., and Hazel, S.J. (2019). Fearful Fido: investigating dog experience in the veterinary context in an effort to reduce distress. *Applied Animal Behaviour Science* 213: 14–25.

Edwards, P.T., Smith, B.P., McArthur, M.L., and Hazel, S.J. (2022). Puppy pedicures: Exploring the experiences of Australian dogs to nail trims. *Applied Animal Behaviour Science* 255: 105730.

Ellis, S.L.H., Rodan, I., Carney, H.C. et al. (2013). AAFP and ISFM feline environmental needs guidelines. *Journal of Feline Medicine and Surgery* 15 (3): 219–230.

Engler, W.J. and Bain, M. (2017). Effect of different types of classical music played at a veterinary hospital on dog behavior and owner satisfaction. *Journal of the American Veterinary Medical Association* 251 (2): 195–200.

Epp, T. and Waldner, C. (2012). Occupational health hazards in veterinary medicine: zoonoses and other biological hazards. *Canadian Veterinary Journal* 53 (2): 144–150.

Erickson, A., Harbin, K., MacPherson, J. et al. (2021). A review of pre-appointment medications to reduce fear and anxiety in dogs and cats at veterinary visits. *Canadian Veterinary Journal* 62 (9): 952–960.

Feyrecilde, M. (2024). *Cooperative Veterinary Care*. Chichester: Wiley.

Frank, D. (2014). Recognizing behavioral signs of pain and disease: a guide for practitioners. *Veterinary Clinics of North America, Small Animal Practice* 44 (3): 507–524.

Fullagar, B., Boysen, S., Toy, M. et al. (2015). Sound pressure levels in 2 veterinary intensive care units. *Journal of Veterinary Internal Medicine* 29 (4): 1013–1021.

Furgala, N.M., Moody, C.M., Flint, H.E. et al. (2022). Veterinary background noise elicits fear responses in cats while freely moving in a confined space and during an examination. *Behavioural Processes* 201: 104712.

Gruen, M.E. and Sherman, B.L. (2008). Use of trazodone as an adjunctive agent in the treatment of canine anxiety disorders: 56 cases (1995–2007). *Journal of the American Veterinary Medical Association* 233 (12): 1902–1907.

Hampton, A., Ford, A., Cox, R.E. et al. (2020). Effects of music on behavior and physiological stress response of domestic cats in a veterinary clinic. *Journal of Feline Medicine and Surgery* 22: 122–128.

Hashem, A., Kietzmann, M., and Scherkl, R. (1992). The pharmacokinetics and bioavailability of acepromazine in the plasma of dogs. *Deutsche Tierarztliche Wochenschrift* 99: 396–398.

Hauser, H., Campbell, S., Korpivaara, M. et al. (2020). In-hospital administration of dexmedetomidine oromucosal gel for stress reduction in dogs during veterinary visits: a randomized, double-blinded, placebo-controlled study. *Journal of Veterinary Behavior* 39: 77–85.

Haywood, C., Ripari, L., Puzzo, J. et al. (2021). Providing humans with practical, best practice handling guidelines during human-cat interactions increases cats' affiliative behaviour and reduces aggression and signs of conflict. *Frontiers in Veterinary Science* 8: 835.

Heath, S. (2020). Environment and feline health: at home and in the clinic. *Veterinary Clinics of North America, Small Animal Practice* 50 (4): 663–693.

Hernander, L. (2008). Factors influencing dogs' stress level in the waiting room at a veterinary clinic. Ethology and Animal Welfare Programme student report, Department of Animal Environment and Health, Swedish University of Agricultural Sciences.

Herron, M.E. and Shreyer, T. (2014). The pet-friendly veterinary practice: a guide for practitioners. *Veterinary Clinics of North America, Small Animal Practice* 44 (3): 451–481.

Herron, M.E., Shofer, F.S., and Reisner, I.R. (2018). Retrospective evaluation of the effects of diazepam in dogs with anxiety-related behavior problems. *Journal of the American Veterinary Medical Association* 233: 1420–1424.

Hopfensperger, M.J., Messenger, K.M., Papich, M.G., and Sherman, B.L. (2013). The use of oral transmucosal detomidine hydrochloride gel to facilitate handling in dogs. *Journal of Veterinary Behavior* 8 (3): 114–123.

Howell, A. and Feyrecilde, M. (2018). *Cooperative Veterinary Care*. Chichester: Wiley.

Ibañez, M. and Anzola, B. (2009). Use of fluoxetine, diazepam, and behavior modification as therapy for treatment of anxiety-related disorders in dogs. *Journal of Veterinary Behavior* 4: 223–229.

Indrawirawan, Y. and McAlees, T. (2014). Tramadol toxicity in a cat: case report and literature review of serotonin syndrome. *Journal of Feline Medicine and Surgery* 16 (7): 572–578.

Jay, A.R., Krotscheck, U., Parsley, E. et al. (2013). Pharmacokinetics, bioavailability, and hemodynamic effects of trazodone after intravenous and oral administration of a single dose to dogs. *American Journal of Veterinary Research* 74 (11): 1450–1456.

Jones, E. (2023a). Cooperative care for companion dogs: Emotional health and wellness. *Companion Animal* 28 (7): 1–6.

Jones, E. (2023b). Preparing fearful dogs for vaccinations with cooperative care. *Animal Behaviour and Welfare Cases* 2023: abwcases20230011.

Jones, E. (2024). *Constructing Canine Consent: Conceptualising and Adopting a Consent-Focused Relationship with Dogs*. Boca Raton, FL: CRC Press.

Karas, A.Z. (1999). Sedation and chemical restraint in the dog and cat. *Clinical Techniques in Small Animal Practice* 14 (1): 15–26.

Karn-Buehler, J. and Kuhne, F. (2022). Perception of stress in cats by German cat owners and influencing factors regarding veterinary care. *Journal of Feline Medicine and Surgery* 24 (8): 700–708.

Kim, S.A., Borchardt, M.R., Lee, K. et al. (2022). Effects of trazodone on behavioral and physiological signs of stress in dogs during veterinary visits: A randomized double-blind placebo-controlled crossover clinical trial. *Journal of the American Veterinary Medical Association* 260 (8): 876–883.

King, T., Flint, H.E., Hunt, A.B. et al. (2022). Effect of music on stress parameters in dogs during a mock veterinary visit. *Animals* 12 (2): 187.

Ko, J.C., Austin, B.R., Bartletta, M. et al. (2011). Evaluation of dexmedetomidine and ketamine in combination with various opioids as injectable anesthetic combinations for cats. *Journal of the American Veterinary Medical Association* 239 (11): 1453–1462.

Kogan, L.R., Schoenfeld-Tacher, R., and Simon, A.A. (2012). Behavioral effects of auditory stimulation on kenneled dogs. *Journal of Veterinary Behavior* 7 (5): 268–275.

Lind, A.K., Hydbring-Sandberg, E., Forkman, B., and Keeling, L.J. (2017). Assessing stress in dogs during a visit to the veterinary clinic: correlations between dog behavior in standardized tests and assessments by veterinary staff and owners. *Journal of Veterinary Behavior* 17: 24–31.

Lloyd, J.K.F. (2017). Minimising stress for patients in the veterinary hospital: why it is important and what can be done about it. *Veterinary Sciences* 4 (2): 22.

Maniscalco, K. and Edens, M.A. (2022). Animal bites. In: *StatPearls*. Treasure Island, FL: StatPearls Publishing https://www.ncbi.nlm.nih.gov/books/NBK430852 (accessed March 23, 2024).

Mariti, C., Raspanti, E., Zilocchi, M. et al. (2015). The assessment of dog welfare in the waiting room of a veterinary clinic. *Animal Welfare* 24: 299–305.

Mariti, C., Bowen, J.E., Campa, S. et al. (2016). Guardians' perceptions of cats' welfare and behavior regarding visiting veterinary clinics. *Journal of Applied Animal Welfare Science* 19 (4): 375–384.

Mariti, C., Pierantoni, L., Sighieri, C., and Gazzano, A. (2017). Guardians' perceptions of dogs' welfare and behaviors related to visiting the veterinary clinic. *Journal of Applied Animal Welfare Science* 20 (1): 24–33.

Mathews, K.A., Sinclair, M., Steele, A.M., and Grubb, T. (2018). *Analgesia and Anesthesia for the Ill or Injured Dog and Cat*. Chichester: Wiley.

McDonald, C. and Zaki, S. (2020). A role for classical music in veterinary practice: does exposure to classical music reduce stress in hospitalized dogs? *Australian Veterinary Journal* 98 (1–2): 31–36.

Mellor, D.J. (2016). Updating animal welfare thinking: moving beyond the "five freedoms" towards "a life worth living". *Animals* 6 (3): 21.

Mills, D., Ramos, D., Estelles, M., and Hargrave, C. (2006). A triple blind placebo-controlled investigation into the assessment of the effect of Dog Appeasing Pheromone (DAP) on anxiety related behaviour of problem dogs in the veterinary clinic. *Applied Animal Behaviour Science* 98: 114–126.

Moser, K.L., Hasiuk, M.M., Armstrong, T. et al. (2020). A randomized clinical trial comparing butorphanol and buprenorphine within a multimodal analgesic protocol in cats undergoing orchiectomy. *Journal of Feline Medicine and Surgery* 22 (8): 760–767.

Nibblett, B.M., Ketzis, J.K., and Grigg, E.K. (2015). Comparison of stress exhibited by cats examined in a clinic versus a home setting. *Applied Animal Behaviour Science* 173: 68–75.

Ogata, N. and Dodman, N.H. (2011). The use of clonidine in the treatment of fear-based behavior problems in dogs: an open trial. *Journal of Veterinary Behavior* 6 (2): 130–137.

Orlando, J.M., Case, B.C., Thomson, A.E. et al. (2015). Use of oral trazodone for sedation in cats: a pilot study. *Journal of Feline Medicine and Surgery* 18 (6): 476–482.

Overall, K. (2013). *Manual of Clinical Behavioral Medicine for Dogs and Cats*. St. Louis, MO: Elsevier.

Overall, K.L. (2019). Fear due to veterinary visits/treatments. In: *Côté's Clinical Veterinary Advisor Dogs and Cats. 4 St* (ed. L.A. Cohen and E. Côté), 324–325. Louis, MO: Elsevier.

Padalino, B. (2015). Effects of the different transport phases on equine health status, behavior and welfare: a review. *Journal of Veterinary Behavior* 10 (3): 272–282.

Pankratz, K.E., Ferris, K.K., Griffith, E.H., and Sherman, B.L. (2018). Use of single-dose oral gabapentin to attenuate fear responses in cage-trap confined community cats: A double-blind, placebo-controlled field trial. *Journal of Feline Medicine and Surgery* 20 (6): 535–543.

Partners for Healthy Pets. (2014). Reversing the decline in veterinary care utilization: Progress made, challenges remain. https://www.scstatehouse.gov/CommitteeInfo/SenateAGSelectSubcommitteeOnAnimalWelfareListeningSessions/October142014Meeting/ReversingTheDeclineInVeterinaryCareUtilization.pdf (accessed March 23, 2024).

Perego, R., Proverbio, D., and Spada, E. (2014). Increases in heart rate and serum cortisol concentrations in healthy dogs are positively correlated with an indoor waiting-room environment. *Veterinary Clinical Pathology* 43 (1): 67–71.

Pereira, J.S., Fragoso, S., Beck, A. et al. (2016). Improving the feline veterinary consultation: the usefulness of Feliway spray in reducing cats' stress. *Journal of Feline Medicine and Surgery* 18: 959–964.

Pratsch, L., Mohr, N., Palme, R. et al. (2018). Carrier training cats reduces stress on transport to a veterinary practice. *Applied Animal Behaviour Science* 206: 64–74.

Quimby, J.M., Lorbach, S.K., Saffire, A. et al. (2022). Serum concentrations of gabapentin in cats with chronic kidney disease. *Journal of Feline Medicine and Surgery* 24 (12): 1260–1266.

Radulovic, L.L., Turck, D., von Hodenberg, A. et al. (1995). Disposition of gabapentin (neurontin) in mice, rats, dogs, and monkeys. *Drug Metabolism and Disposition* 23 (4): 441–448.

Reid, J., Nolan, A.M., Hughes, J.M.L. et al. (2007). Development of the short-form Glasgow composite measure pain scale (CMPS-SF) and derivation of an analgesic intervention score. *Animal Welfare* 16 (S1): 97–104.

Riemer, S., Heritier, C., Windschnurer, I. et al. (2021). A review on mitigating fear and aggression in dogs and cats in a veterinary setting. *Animals* 11 (1): 158.

Rodan, I. and Heath, S. (2016). *Feline Behavioral Health and Welfare*. St. Louis, MO: Elsevier.

Rodan, I., Dowgray, N., Carney, H.C. et al. (2022). 2022 AAFP/ISFM cat friendly veterinary interaction guidelines: Approach and handling techniques. *Journal of Feline Medicine and Surgery* 24 (11): 1093–1132.

Rosenberg, M.B. and Chopra, D. (2015). *Nonviolent Communication: A Language of Life: Life-changing Tools for Healthy Relationships*. Encinitas, CA: Puddle Dancer Press.

Santos, L.C.P., Ludders, J.W., Erb, H.N. et al. (2010). Sedative and cardiorespiratory effects of dexmedetomidine and buprenorphine administered to cats via oral transmucosal or intramuscular routes. *Veterinary Anaesthesia and Analgesia* 37 (5): 417–424.

Scherk, M. (2022). Cats in the clinic. In: *Clinical Handbook of Feline Behavior Medicine* (ed. E. Stelow), 250–273. Chichester: Wiley.

Seksel, K. (2013). The recognition and assessment of pain in cats. In: *Pain Management in Veterinary Practice* (ed. C.M. Egger, L. Love, and T. Doherty), 269–273. Chichester: Wiley.

Simon, B.T. and Steagall, P.V. (2020). Feline procedural sedation and analgesia: when, why and how. *Journal of Feline Medicine and Surgery* 22 (11): 1029–1045.

Simpson, B.S. (1997). Canine communication. *Veterinary Clinics of North America, Small Animal Practice* 27: 445–464.

Siracusa, C., Manteca, X., Cuenca, R. et al. (2010). Effect of a synthetic appeasing pheromone on behavioral, neuroendocrine, immune, and acute-phase perioperative stress responses in dogs. *Journal of the American Veterinary Medical Association* 237 (6): 673–681.

Smith, P., Tolbert, M.K., Gould, E. et al. (2020). Pharmacokinetics, sedation and hemodynamic changes following the administration of oral transmucosal detomidine gel in cats. *Journal of Feline Medicine and Surgery* 22 (12): 1184–1190.

Stahl, S.M. (2009). Mechanism of action of trazodone: a multifunctional drug. *CNS Spectrums* 14 (10): 536–546.

Stella, J., Croney, C., and Buffington, T. (2014). Environmental factors that affect the behavior and welfare of domestic cats (*Felis silvestris catus*) housed in cages. *Applied Animal Behaviour Science* 160: 94–105.

Stellato, A., Jajou, S., Dewey, C.E. et al. (2019). Effect of a standardized four-week desensitization and counter-conditioning training program on pre-existing veterinary fear in companion dogs. *Animals* 9 (10): 767.

Stellato, A.C., Flint, H.E., Dewey, C.E. et al. (2021). Risk-factors associated with veterinary-related fear and aggression in owned domestic dogs. *Applied Animal Behaviour Science* 241: 105374.

Stevens, B.J., Frantz, E.M., Orlando, J.M. et al. (2016). Efficacy of a single dose of trazodone hydrochloride given to cats prior to veterinary visits to reduce signs of transport-and examination-related anxiety. *Journal of the American Veterinary Medical Association* 249 (2): 202–207.

Stollar, O.O., Moore, G.E., Mukhopadhyay, A. et al. (2022). Effects of a single dose of orally administered gabapentin in dogs during a veterinary visit: a double-blinded, placebo-controlled study. *Journal of the American Veterinary Medical Association* 260 (9): 1031–1040.

Stoneburner, R.M., Naughton, B., Sherman, B., and Mathews, K.G. (2021). Evaluation of a stimulus attenuation strategy to reduce stress in hospitalized cats. *Journal of Veterinary Behavior* 41: 33–38.

Sydänheimo, A., Freeman, M., and Hunt, K. (2023). Cooperative care does not scare–use of cooperative care training in routine husbandry in dogs. *Animal Behaviour and Welfare Cases* 2023: abwcases20230010.

Tateo, A., Zappaterra, M., Covella, A., and Padalino, B. (2021). Factors influencing stress and fear-related behaviour of cats during veterinary examinations. *Italian Journal of Animal Science* 20 (1): 46–58.

Taylor, A.F. (2020). Literature review on the handling and restraint of cats in practice and its effect on patient welfare. *Veterinary Nursing Journal* 35 (6): 162–166.

Taylor, S., St. Denis, K., Collins, S. et al. (2022). 2022 ISFM/AAFP Cat Friendly Veterinary Environment Guidelines. *Journal of Feline Medicine and Surgery* 24 (11): 1133–1163.

Travain, T., Colombo, E.S., Heinzl, E. et al. (2015). Hot dogs: thermography in the assessment of stress in dogs (*Canis familiaris*) – a pilot study. *Journal of Veterinary Behavior* 10 (1): 17–23.

Van Haaften, K.A., Forsythe, L.R.E., Stella, E., and Bain, M.J. (2017). Effects of a single preappointment dose of gabapentin on signs of stress in cats during transportation and veterinary examination. *Journal of the American Veterinary Medical Association* 251 (10): 1175–1181.

Verstegen, J., Deleforge, J., Dernblon, D., and Rosillon, D. (1996). Non-linear relationship between bioavailability and dose after oral administration of four single doses of acepromazine in dogs and cats. *Journal of Veterinary Anaesthesia* 23 (2): 47–51.

Volk, J.O., Felsted, K.E., Thomas, J.G., and Siren, C.W. (2011). Executive summary of the Bayer veterinary care usage study. *Journal of the American Veterinary Medical Association* 238 (10): 1275–1282.

Voss, D.S., Boyd, M.V., Evanston, J.F., and Bender, J.B. (2023). An increase in animal-related occupational injuries at a veterinary medical center (2008–2022). *Journal of the American Veterinary Medical Association*.

Yin, S.A. (2009). *Low Stress Handling, Restraint and Behavior Modification of Dogs and Cats: Techniques for Developing Patients Who Love Their Visits*. Davis, CA: CattleDog Publishing.

Zoetis. (2015). SILEO® (dexmedetomidine 0.1 mg/ml oromucosal gel for dogs) [Summary of product characteristics]. https://www.zoetisus.com/products/petcare/sileo (accessed April 8, 2024).

12

Pets and Children

The bond between children and their canine or feline companions is unique and special, yet it comes with its own set of challenges and considerations. This chapter will highlight the important role veterinarians play in helping parents understand and navigate these dynamics. By educating parents about living with both kids and pets, and providing guidance on responsible pet ownership, veterinary team members can significantly enhance the human-animal bond and ensure the safety and well-being of families and their pets.

Potential for Dog and Cat Bites

Educating parents about living with children and pets involves raising awareness of the potential for dog and cat bites. Any dog or cat, regardless of breed or temperament, has the potential to bite under certain circumstances.

Statistics from the United States reveal that approximately 4.5 million people are bitten by dogs annually, with nearly 19% of these incidents requiring medical attention (Table 12.1). Notably, 77% of dog bites occur from pets owned by a family member or friend. Children under the age of 12 are the most at risk (Kerns et al. 2023; Love et al. 2001; Meints et al. 2010; Reisner et al. 2011; Tuckel and Milczarski 2020). These figures emphasize that even pets without previous incidents of aggression can bite if they feel threatened, fearful, or in pain.

The first step in preventing bites is understanding a pet's body language. This knowledge helps parents identify when their pet is uncomfortable, signaling the need for intervention to protect everyone involved, including both the pet and the children. Recognizing these signs allows parents to take proactive measures to prevent bites. Prevention programs educate families about the risks associated with canine interactions, addressing both the obvious and subtle signs of fear, anxiety, and stress in pets. By helping parents recognize these indicators, these programs aim to prevent situations from escalating and keep animals as comfortable as possible, especially in families with young children.

Inquiring About Behavioral Health

During routine visits, veterinarians should assess the behavioral health of their patients, either through direct conversation with the caregiver or by having the client fill out a questionnaire. These assessments should cover the pet's overall behavior, including signs of fear and anxiety

Veterinary Guide to Preventing Behavior Problems in Dogs and Cats, First Edition. Christine D. Calder and Sarah C. Wright.
© 2025 John Wiley & Sons, Inc. Published 2025 by John Wiley & Sons, Inc.

Table 12.1 Overview of the prevalence and nature of dog bites.

Statistic	Value	References
Annual dog bite cases in the United States	Approximately 4.5 million	US Center for Disease Control
Cases requiring medical attention	19%	Reisner (2011); Meints et al. (2010); Tuckel and Milczarski (2020)
Dog bites from a family or friend's pet	77%	Reisner (2011); Meints et al. (2010); Tuckel and Milczarski (2020)
Most likely age group to be bitten	Children under the age of 12	Reisner (2011); Meints et al. (2010); Tuckel and Milczarski (2020)

both at home and in other environments. Understanding how the pet interacts with and responds to both familiar and unfamiliar people, their reactions to various sounds, and any unusual behaviors such as separation-related behaviors or house-soiling helps with early detection and timely intervention to improve safety and quality of life for both the pet and their family.

Dogs that exhibit aggressive reactions when anxious or fearful are more likely to display aggressive behavior toward children. This risk is increased by the unpredictable behavior of young children, such as their high-pitched voices, sudden movements, and potentially inappropriate ways of interacting with dogs (Love et al. 2001). Such actions can provoke defensive or aggressive responses from dogs if they feel threatened or unsafe (Love et al. 2001; Reisner et al. 2007).

Research shows that many dogs that bite children often have other behavioral problems related to anxiety or fear such as separation-related behaviors, storm phobia, and noise sensitivities (Reisner 2003). Conducting an annual behavioral history helps identify any behaviors that need to be addressed. Early intervention and prevention of behavior problems are often more effective than treating them once they have developed. Since living conditions and behavior can change frequently, a pet's behavioral history should be monitored and evaluated at least yearly.

Medical Conditions

Underlying medical conditions, especially those causing pain, can significantly increase the risk of aggression in dogs and cats (Amat et al. 2024). Diseases and discomfort related to pain can make pets more irritable and affect their behavior. Therefore, a comprehensive evaluation is necessary for all dogs and cats presented with behavioral concerns, regardless of their biting history. This evaluation should include a thorough physical examination to assess the pet's overall health, an orthopedic examination to identify any musculoskeletal issues contributing to defensive behaviors, and a neurologic examination to rule out or identify any neurologic disorders that could influence the pet's behavior.

Baseline bloodwork and other diagnostic tests provide additional insights into the pet's overall health and can reveal underlying medical conditions that might not be detected during a physical examination. Including these tests allows veterinarians to gain a more comprehensive understanding of the root causes of behavior changes, develop effective management plans, and provide tailored treatment plans based on the individual needs of each patient.

Understanding Body Language

Recognizing and understanding the signs of stress in a pet's body language can help avoid potentially dangerous situations. Clients need to be aware of indications that a pet is anxious or uncomfortable, as behaviors often labeled as unprovoked aggression in animals are typically preceded by numerous warning signs. This interpretation can be particularly challenging for children, who may not accurately read subtle cues and may not respond appropriately in risky situations (Kerns et al. 2023). Misinterpretations, such as assuming a dog's rigid, wagging tail or a cat's arched back signifies happiness, can lead to unintended consequences like bites or scratches.

Canine behavior, often perceived as unpredictable and complex, is primarily communicated through body language. This can lead to misunderstandings by humans, who might misinterpret dog behaviors based on human social norms (Mariti et al. 2012). For example, a dog placing its paws on a human's shoulders is often wrongly seen as a hug. However, in canine behavior this action could indicate anxiety, frustration, or uncertainty. Many dogs are uncomfortable with typical human social behaviors such as hugs and kisses, which can feel invasive (Figure 12.1).

This is a particularly challenging concept for children, who may naturally express affection toward dogs in these familiar ways, not realizing that their actions might cause the dog stress or discomfort (Aldridge and Rose 2019). Therefore, educating children about respecting a dog's personal space and understanding their body language is key to ensuring safe and harmonious interactions.

Feline behavior, like that of canines, can often be misinterpreted due to the differences in communication styles between cats and humans. Cats are generally nonconfrontational and express themselves through less obvious body language signals, including tail flicking, ear positioning, and different vocalizations. These signals can represent a spectrum of emotions, ranging from relaxation to fear (Figure 12.2). For instance, while a cat's purring is commonly associated with happiness, it can also indicate pain or distress.

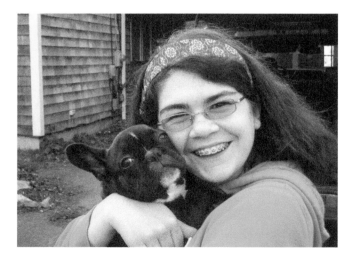

Figure 12.1   Many dogs will tolerate hugs but not necessarily enjoy them. In this picture the dog is avoiding eye contact, his ears are back and slightly down, his facial expression is tight, and there is evidence of a whale eye. *Source:* Christine Calder (book author).

Figure 12.2 This cat's body language could be indicative of pain. The body is tucked, tail curled around the cat, ears slightly to the side, eyes closed, whiskers down, and mild piloerection around the spine and back. *Source:* Petra Richli/Adobe Stock.

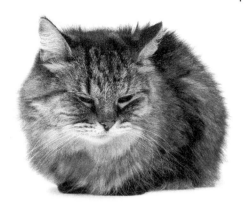

Respecting a cat's personal space is just as important as it is with dogs. Intruding into their space can stress or threaten a cat. Additionally, cats typically prefer to be petted around their cheeks and temples rather than stroked down their back. Understanding and adhering to these preferences can help prevent discomfort and foster a more comfortable and trusting relationship between humans and cats.

Visual Aids and Educational Resources

Resources such as diagrams, body language posters, videos, and books help clients visualize and understand the behavior of their dogs and cats more effectively (Table 12.2). By enhancing their comprehension of their pets' emotional states, caregivers are more likely to respond appropriately and prevent situations that might lead to distress and bites.

Table 12.2 Educational websites for parents.

Website	Focus of education
www.familypaws.com	Education about coexisting with pets and children
www.thefamilydog.com	Guidance for families on integrating dogs into their homes
www.petsandpeopleinharmony.com	Strategies for harmonious living between pets and people
www.yourdogsbestfriend.org	Resources for building strong relationships between dogs and their human families
www.livingwithkidsanddogs.com	Advice for managing a household with both children and dogs
www.doggonesafe.com	Information on dog bite prevention and safe interactions between dogs and people
www.thebluedog.org	Educational resources focusing on preventing dog bites in children and promoting safe interactions
www.doggonecrazy.ca	Interactive tools and resources for understanding canine body language and behavior

Educating Parents on Responsible Pet Ownership

When parents are well informed they are better equipped to make decisions that significantly reduce the risk of bites and foster a positive relationship between children and their pets. This education not only improves family safety but also enhances the overall quality of life for both the family and their pets.

Choosing the Right Pet

Assisting parents in selecting the appropriate pet for their family offers numerous benefits. When selecting a pet, and especially when considering a dog, various factors need to be taken into account to ensure compatibility with the family's lifestyle. These factors include the breed, size, temperament, and energy level of the pet, as well as the ages of the children in the family (Levine 2023).
Key questions to ask include:

- Why does the family want a dog?
- Are they seeking an active pet that can join in family activities such as hiking or sports?
- What is the family's living environment? On a farm, in a city, a house with a yard, or an apartment that would necessitate regular walks?

For families considering a cat, consider the cat's age, the presence of other pets at home, the family's ability to meet the cat's basic needs, and whether they can provide enough space for the cat (Levine 2023).

Age and Behavior

When selecting a new pet for a home with children, consider the ages of both the pet and the children (Table 12.3). Puppies, in their early stages, explore their environment and experiment with behaviors, including object play using their teeth and paws. Without proper redirection to

Table 12.3 Developmental stages of children and how they affect interactions with pets.

Developmental stage	Description
Newborn to 6 months	Infants introduce new smells and sounds, might grab pet's fur or ears, increasing risk of pet-related injuries. Dogs may bite; cats may hiss, swat, or bite.
6–24 months	Rapid development in gross motor skills; toddlers' interactions with pets can lead to accidental provocation or rough handling. Pets may react with growling, hissing, or snapping.
2–5 years	Improved gross motor coordination; increased curiosity and onset of empathy. Children include pets in play, which can be stressful for pets. Pets may react defensively to unfamiliar stimuli during play dates.
5–9 years	More independence and testing limits; difficulty understanding outcomes of actions. Children may engage in rough play or teasing, leading to pet frustration and potential aggressive reactions.
9–12 years	Gaining skills in organizing facts, problem-solving, and empathizing. Capable of more responsibility in pet care, but may engage in rough play or teasing, testing a pet's limits.

Source: Adapted from Love et al. (2001).

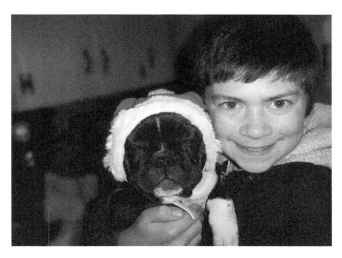

Figure 12.3 Dressing pets up in clothing can be aversive. This dog is uncomfortable, as evident from his closed eyes, lack of eye contact, and tight mouth *Source:* Christine Calder (book author).

appropriate toys, mouthy behaviors in puppies can persist into adulthood and potentially cause injuries to children. Puppies may be attracted to children's movements, food, and clothing, and children might find it challenging to effectively redirect these behaviors, which could escalate to aggressive responses from the puppy (Figure 12.3) (Love et al. 2001).

As dogs approach sexual maturity, typically between 6 and 9 months of age, they may exhibit behaviors such as increased attention to smells, marking, roaming, fighting, and mounting. These changes can be confusing for children, who might unintentionally encourage them or respond too harshly. This stage requires more adult supervision to guide both the dog and the child, particularly in areas like housetraining (Love et al. 2001).

Upon reaching social maturity, around 18–24 months of age, dogs refine their social skills and may display different or unexpected behaviors. Interactions that were harmless during the puppy phase can become problematic. The dog may react defensively to actions like pushing, taking objects from them, or chasing, which previously resulted in avoidance or escape. Caregivers need to recognize these changes and adjust the approach to dog–child interactions, fostering a safe and respectful relationships as the dog matures (Figure 12.4) (Love et al. 2001).

Older dogs, possibly affected by medical conditions like arthritis or sensory decline, may have decreased tolerance for physical play. Children might not understand these changes and continue to engage in ways that are uncomfortable for the dog, potentially leading to irritable or defensive reactions. In some cases older dogs may respond aggressively due to pain or fear. Understanding these stages of canine development and adjusting interactions accordingly ensure safe and positive experiences for both children and dogs (Love et al. 2001).

Cats' behavior, similar to that of dogs, is also influenced by developmental stages. Kittens actively explore their environment and learn about human interaction through play, often using claws and teeth. If not redirected to appropriate activities, these behaviors may continue into adulthood, leading to play aggression and potential scratches or bites. Kittens are also drawn to the movements and items associated with children, posing challenges in guiding their behaviors.

As cats reach sexual maturity, usually between 6 and 9 months of age, they may display increased territorial behavior, including marking and agonistic interactions. Older cats, like older dogs,

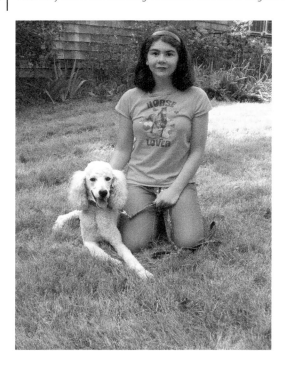

Figure 12.4 By age 12, children are capable of taking on more responsibility in regard to pet care, including feeding, grooming, and training. *Source:* Christine Calder (book author).

may not openly show signs of pain but experience age-related changes such as reduced mobility and diminished senses, leading to decreased tolerance for activities like active play and cuddling. These changes can be difficult for children to understand, increasing the risk of defensive behaviors and injury. Caregivers should help children recognize and adapt to these changes in cat behavior to maintain safe and positive interactions.

How to Approach

When approaching a dog or cat, personal space needs to be respected, and they should be given the choice to interact on their own terms. Extending a hand for them to sniff, a common human gesture like a handshake, can be startling and even threatening to animals, potentially leading to fearful or defensive behavior (Figure 12.5). Direct eye contact, which is seen as polite among humans, can be perceived as a threat by both dogs and cats. In contrast, some consider slow blinking a reassuring signal for cats (Beaver 2003). A soft gaze and relaxed facial expression are more appropriate when greeting pets. Items that obscure the face such as hats, sunglasses, or facial hair, along with wheelchairs, canes, or objects carried in the hands, may also be intimidating to animals.

Observe Body Language

Avoid approaching a dog or cat from overhead or directly from behind, as most pets do not appreciate being loomed over. It is better to gently pet a dog on the chest or shoulder area first, and for cats start with petting around the temple area, steering clear of back stroking initially. Observing body language is a must! A relaxed dog typically displays soft, almond-shaped eyes, relaxed ears, and a

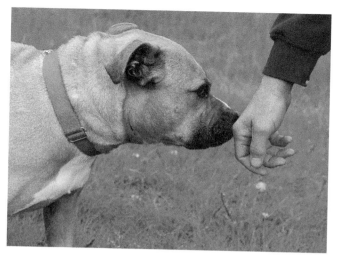

Figure 12.5 Extending a hand in greeting can be perceived as threatening to a dog. *Source:* Alex/Adobe Stock.

loosely wagging tail, whereas a comfortable cat will have upright ears, a relaxed face and whiskers, and possibly a tail curved into a question mark.

Teaching Children Respect and Boundaries

Teach children not to pull on ears, tails, or fur. Instead, under adult supervision, children can use the "touch" cue with dogs or engage pets with appropriate toys such as a wand or feather toy for cats and a ball or other favorite toy for dogs (Figure 12.6). Another option is to gently toss treats behind the pet, allowing them the choice to return for more. By attentively monitoring a pet's body language, caregivers can determine if the pet is enjoying the interaction or not, making sure the experience is positive for both the child and the pet (Table 12.4).

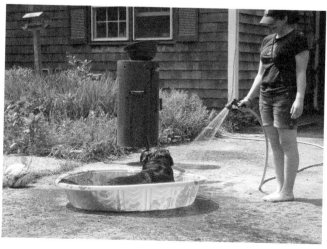

Figure 12.6 Engaging in activities that the pet enjoys helps to build a stronger bond between children and pets. *Source:* Christine Calder (book author).

Table 12.4 The Dial Method: Pat, Pet, Pause by Justine Schuurmans.

Step	Action	Description	Responses from the dog
Pat	Pat your leg	Invite the dog over. If the dog does not come, respect their choice and leave them be.	More please: if the dog snuggles up for more, pet for another three seconds, then pause and check again.
Pet	Pet the dog for 3 seconds	Pet the dog slowly and gently with one hand on the body to allow an exit strategy for the dog.	"All done" or "Okay, bye": if the dog freezes or walks away, it means "I am all done, thank you," and you should stop the interaction.
Pause	Pause and observe	Check if the dog is still enjoying the interaction. Give them the option to leave if they are not.	

Source: Adapted from Justine Schuurmans' The Dial Method (www.thefamilydog.com).

Be a Tree

Dogs and cats are hardwired to notice movement and noise. Children tend to run, jump, scream, and be loud, which can be overly stimulating and overwhelming for pets. This can result in dogs chasing, grabbing, nipping, and jumping, or cats running, hissing, and swatting. To prevent bites and reduce arousal, one of the most valuable skills children can learn is to stand still and "be a tree" if a strange dog approaches or jumps on, nips, or chases them (www.doggonesafe.com). This advice applies to encounters with any dog, including their own.

Be a Tree involves:

- Stop and be quiet.
- Fold in your branches (hands folded in front).
- Watch your roots grow (look at your feet).
- Count your breaths in your head until help comes or the dog goes away.
- "Trees" are boring to dogs, and they will usually just sniff and then go away. No matter what the dog does, just stand still, avoid eye contact (by looking at your feet), and stay quiet.

Children should practice this technique when dogs are not around so they become proficient and prepared to apply it in real-life situations if they feel threatened by a dog in any way.

Preparing Pets for Children

When preparing pets for the arrival of a baby or toddler, start by making necessary changes to the home well in advance (Bergman and Gaskins 2008; Levine 2023). Relocate resources such as litter boxes and feeding areas to places accessible to the pet but out of reach of children, like a home office or bathroom. These areas can be secured from child access using a baby gate or a door propped open just enough for a cat to pass through (Figure 12.7). Additionally, make changes to sleeping arrangements and dog-walking schedules in advance of the child's arrival.

Implementing these changes well before the baby arrives gives pets time to adapt to the new household dynamics without the added pressure of a new child. Taking a proactive approach allows caregivers to observe how well the pet is adjusting and, if needed, provide extra support or further modify routines to facilitate a smooth integration of the pet with the new family member.

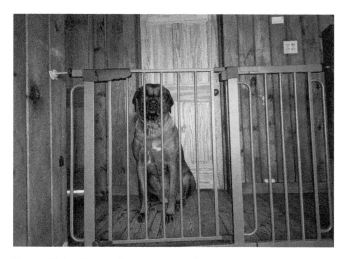

Figure 12.7 The confinement area should be secure (e.g., behind a gate), and the pet should feel comfortable in this area before it is used. *Source:* Christine Calder (book author).

Before the Baby Arrives

Introducing pets, particularly dogs and cats, to the various items and sounds associated with infants is the first step in preparing them for the arrival of a baby (Bergman and Gaskins 2008; Levine 2023). This preparation should include setting up the baby's room (Table 12.5). Place a gate in the doorway to keep the pet out of the baby's room when unsupervised, while still providing an opportunity for the pet to see and smell the new items in the room (lotions, powders, diapers, etc.). Supervised trips into the room, allow the pet time to explore and familiarize themselves with the items at their own pace.

Table 12.5 Steps to prepare pets for the arrival of a baby.

Action	Description
Change pet's environment gradually	Introduce new furniture or create a nursery in small stages. Pets need time to adjust to changes in their environment. Once an area is ready, playing with the pet in the area can help to create positive associations.
Create barriers to areas of the home	Install gates or close doors to manage pet access, especially when caring for an infant alone. Gradually practicing keeping pets in a separate area or level of the home can accustom them to this arrangement.
Prepare pet for baby sounds	Use prerecorded videos/sounds of baby noises to habituate pets. Start at a low volume during feeding or playtime, gradually increasing the volume to make pets more comfortable with these sounds.
Prepare pet for baby smells	Associate the smell of baby detergent, lotions, and powders with high-value treats to create positive connections with baby-related scents for the pet.
Start training now	For both dogs and cats, start training well before the baby is due. Practice basic social skills and foundational behaviors (relaxation on a mat) while simulating common baby-related tasks, like walking around with a doll or blanket in the hand. Toss treats to help the pet associate these items and actions with positive associations.

Sounds and Baby Items

Before the baby's arrival, pets should be gradually exposed to the sounds they will hear, such as baby's cry, and the high-pitched music and noises from baby toys and devices. Desensitization and counterconditioning should begin in a controlled environment without the baby present. This strategy allows for careful observation of the pet's reactions. Once these noises no longer elicit signs of fear or anxiety, the pet should be exposed to real-life sounds of crying and laughing infants. This can be done in person, but a physical barrier is needed for safety. High-quality audio recordings can serve as an intermediate step if needed.

During these sessions, pair the noise with food distractions or tasty treats, such as a frozen puzzle toy, a snuffle mat, or a lickable mat, to create a positive conditioned emotional response to these sounds. If a pet shows signs of fear or becomes overly aroused by these sounds, indicated by behaviors like barking, hair standing on end (piloerection), hypervigilance, or appearing overly alert, seek professional intervention from a board-certified veterinary behaviorist or other qualified animal behavior professional for guidance. This should be done well before the baby's arrival to give ample time to effectively address any concerning behaviors before arrival.

Babies and Dogs

In households with infants and dogs, caregivers must never leave dogs unattended with a young child or infant. Designate safe spaces for spending time with the baby, both during the day and at night, making sure there is a way to physically separate the dog from the child. Sometimes using a crib or playpen for the baby is more practical than confining the dog. However, if the dog can reach or knock over a playpen, other arrangements are necessary. Dogs should not be allowed near a baby in a swing due to similar risks.

For families practicing co-sleeping, careful consideration is required regarding where the dog will sleep, especially if they are accustomed to sleeping in the same bed. Nighttime confinement of the dog may be necessary to prevent access to the family bed. Baby toys and supplies such as bottles, pacifiers, and teething rings can be attractive to dogs due to their similarity to dog toys and possible residues of saliva or food (Bergman and Gaskins 2008). Avoid leaving these items within the dog's reach, as training dogs to ignore them can be challenging. Dirty diapers are also appealing to many dogs, so using a secure diaper pail helps manage this behavior (Bergman and Gaskins 2008).

Babies and Cats

Although it is less essential to separate immobile babies from cats than from dogs, some cats still need to learn how to be comfortable with confinement in a separate room or in a cat crate or condo, especially if they are fearful or anxious. While it is a myth that cats can suffocate babies by "snatching their breath", there have been cases of infants suffocated by cats seeking warm places to sleep (Bergman and Gaskins 2008). Cats should be prevented from sleeping in cribs or strollers before the baby's arrival. Installing a screen door on the nursery can keep a cat out of the room while still allowing for airflow and sound to pass through (Bergman and Gaskins 2008). Confining cats at night and providing them with alternative sleeping or hiding spots, should be set up before the child arrives.

Introducing Pets to the New Baby

Introducing a pet to a baby starts with acclimating the pet to the baby's scent. New parents should bring items carrying the baby's scent, such as clothing or blankets, and allow the pet to sniff them, offering high-value rewards for positive interactions. Initial meetings between the pet and parents should occur without the baby present to reduce overexcitement and minimize anxious or fearful reactions.

The first meeting between the pet and the baby should take place when the baby is quiet. The dog should be leashed or safely behind a gate, and the interaction should be supervised by an adult. How the introduction proceeds depends on the dog's history with children and their behavior in new situations. Most dogs can be leashed and rewarded with treats for remaining calm and engaged with their caregiver. Pets should never be forced to interact with the baby; they should be allowed to explore at their own pace. If the dog becomes too excited or fearful, redirect their attention onto another activity. In case of fear, anxiety, or aggressive behavior, calmly remove the dog without punishment.

After the initial introduction, continue to build a positive relationship between the pet and the baby by offering treats and attention when the baby is nearby. Treats and attention should still be provided even when the baby is not present.

Understanding Pets' Needs

Parents should be made aware of the physical and emotional needs of their pets, including a safe space, adequate resources, positive human interactions, mental enrichment, and appropriate (not excessive) physical exercise.

Safe Spaces

Pets should always have access to a comfortable resting area where they can retreat when desired. Caregivers must be able to physically separate pets from people or other animals when necessary (Figure 12.8). This chosen area may also serve as a confinement space if needed. Addressing any preexisting behaviors like confinement anxiety, noise phobias, fear-related aggression, or general anxiety is essential before using the area for separation purposes. Medications may be needed if the pet is struggling with confinement.

For cats, a comfortable resting place should include access to valuable resources such as individual resting areas, hiding spots, litter boxes, toys, food, and water dishes. This setup allows cats to access what they need while avoiding discomfort, reducing the risk of protective or defensive behaviors.

Pets unaccustomed to confinement and separation may display signs of distress such as vocalizing or destructive behavior when isolated. Therefore, gradual acclimatization to a designated space should occur before the baby arrives. This can be achieved by providing puzzle toys and food dispensers and creating a positive association with the area through soft music, lighting, comfortable bedding, and pheromone diffusers. Start by offering the food-dispensing or puzzle toy while in the room, gradually exiting the room and shutting the gate or door for short periods of time. The space should be secure and inviting, especially for cats, and spacious enough to accommodate a litter box and a comfortable resting area.

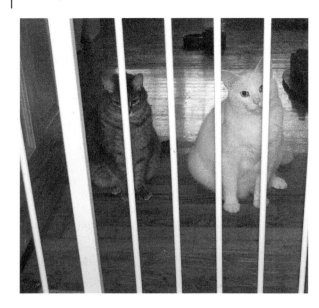

Figure 12.8 A gate can also be used to designate a safe space for cats. *Source:* Christine Calder (book author).

Sleeping in the Bed

Unless pets exhibit aggression in bed or become disturbed while sleeping, there is no need to prevent them from sharing a bed with their humans (Bergman and Gaskins 2008). However, dogs and cats should be comfortable sleeping apart from their humans, regardless of the arrival of a new family member. This helps reduce distress if there is a change in routine or the pet cannot access their caregiver's for whatever reason.

Alternative sleeping arrangements include providing access to a dog bed, a crate in the bedroom, or designating a separate room for sleeping. If a pet has never spent a night away from the caregiver, be prepared for a few sleepless nights during the initial separation period. Follow the same protocol as safe space training described earlier to ease the transition.

Feeding

In households with children, meal feeding is preferred over free-choice feeding (Bergman and Gaskins 2008). This allows for portion control and minimizes competition for food. Meal feeding also provides an opportunity to monitor appetites and food consumption. For pets prone to resource guarding, it is best to feed them in a safe space, separate from children and other pets, and behind a gate or closed door. Food bowls should be promptly removed after meals.

Feeding pets out of food-dispensing or puzzle toys helps reduce overeating and encourages problem-solving (Figure 12.9). Resource guarding, a common issue in pets, can lead to children being bitten and may be more pronounced during periods of stress or environmental changes (Bergman and Gaskins 2008). To reduce such incidents, keep children's food away from pets. Stationing a pet to a mat or platform, or confining them behind a gate during meal preparation and eating time, can effectively manage and prevent potential issues (Figure 12.10). A remote treat dispenser is an excellent tool to teach and reinforce this behavior from a safe distance.

Figure 12.9 The use of a snuffle mat helps with portion control and to monitor food intake. It also provides enrichment and more natural feeding opportunities (foraging and sniffing). *Source:* Christine Calder (book author).

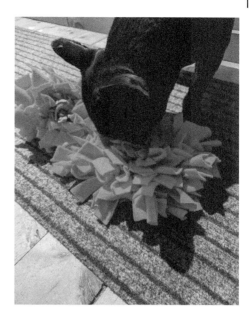

Figure 12.10 Teaching a pet to station to a mat or platform is one effective strategy to manage a dog (or cat) around food. *Source:* Christine Calder (book author).

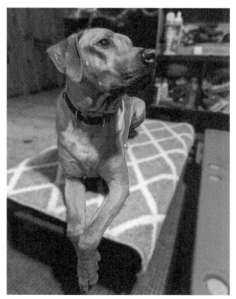

Handling

Helping pets feel more comfortable with handling, especially in households with children, begins with brief handling sessions paired with food distractions. If a pet shows signs of fear or discomfort when touched in certain areas, such as pulling away, looking away, yawning, or licking lips, seek assistance from a qualified professional.

Behavior modification for handling involves introducing touch at a level that does not cause fear, anxiety, or frustration, while simultaneously offering food to keep the pet engaged and comfortable. Gradually increase the intensity of touch to simulate real-life handling situations. For example, if a cat is uneasy about having their paws touched, start by gently stroking the cat's legs, watching for any signs of discomfort such as ear flicking or tail twitching before touching the paw. Offering a favorite treat (e.g., a lickable treat, cream cheese, squeeze cheese) can help during this process. Over time, as the cat becomes more comfortable, extend the stroking down to the paws and eventually progress to holding the paws, all while continuing to pair the handling with treats.

Caregivers should routinely handle their pets gently over their entire bodies. As pets become more accustomed to gentle handling, gradually introduce clumsier handling that resembles that of a toddler. This should be done cautiously to avoid scaring or harming the pet, and food should be paired with the handling. If at any point the pet displays signs of aggression or other concerning behaviors, stop the exercises immediately and arrange for a full behavioral consultation, especially if the pet has a history of aggression during handling.

Socialization and Training in Preventing Dog and Cat Bites

Socialization and training play an important role in preventing dog and cat bites. Socialization provides pets, especially dogs, the chance to engage in a variety of experiences and interactions with various people, animals, and environments during their early developmental stages. Training, on the other hand, focuses on teaching pets desirable and safe behaviors. Both socialization and training are key aspects of responsible pet ownership and contribute significantly to learning important social skills and improving communication, providing a safe living environment for pets and children.

Socialization

Early and continuous socialization helps pets, particularly dogs, feel more comfortable in different situations and around various individuals, including children. Socialized pets are less prone to responding with protective emotions when faced with new people, animals, or environments. Providing opportunities for pets to have consistent and positive interactions allows them to make choices and have control over these interactions (Figure 12.11). Using food helps with this process.

Training

Appropriate training is a fundamental aspect of responsible pet ownership. Training involves teaching pets new behaviors that are desirable and safe for both the pet and the family. Positive reinforcement training is a highly effective and humane approach that uses rewards such as treats and toys to motivate animals. This method strengthens the bond between pets and humans while promoting desirable behavior. Positive reinforcement training encourages a positive and cooperative relationship between pets and children, improving communication and reducing the risk of defensive behaviors. It also helps pets understand boundaries and expectations within the household.

The use of negative reinforcement and positive punishment for behavior modification and training is not appropriate. Negative reinforcement involves using aversive stimuli or actions to encourage a pet to increase the frequency of a behavior by removing or reducing the unpleasant stimulus when the behavior is exhibited. In contrast, positive punishment involves adding an aversive stimulus or

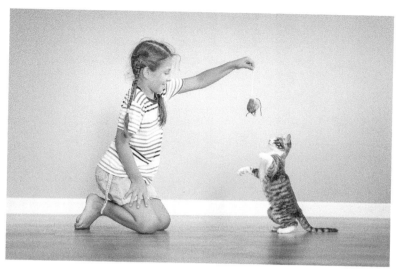

Figure 12.11 Appropriate play is a great way for kids to form relationships and to interact with pets. *Source:* candy1812/Adobe Stock.

action to decrease an unwanted behavior. These methods can lead to fear, anxiety, frustration, and aggressive responses in pets. Caregivers should be educated about the potential harm and negative consequences of using these techniques, emphasizing the long-lasting benefits of positive reinforcement training in creating a safe and enjoyable environment for pets and children in the household.

Children and Training

Children, even at a young age, can participate in training both dogs and cats. They tend to easily grasp the concepts of clicker training, which involves using a clicker to mark and reinforce desired behaviors. Supervision by an adult particularly for younger children is needed. The adult can manage the clicker while the child offers the reward such as a treat. Simple training behaviors that kids can learn to teach pets include targeting (guiding the pet to touch their nose to the child's hand or an object) or teaching the pet to station and relax on a mat. These activities not only aid in training the pet but also help in developing a bond between the child and the animal (Figure 12.12).

Understanding Triggers

Common reasons why dogs and cats bite include fear, pain, illness, and feeling threatened or unsafe. All of these emotions can be triggered by real or perceived threats. Educating parents to identify and recognize specific triggers that cause distress or discomfort in their pets helps them take proactive measures to reduce the risk of exposure and keep their pets feeling safe. Identifying specific triggers can also guide decisions about whether medications might be beneficial and which ones will improve learning and coping skills.

For dogs and cats experiencing fear or anxiety, behavior modification strategies can be highly effective. These strategies include managing the environment to reduce exposure to triggers and prevent escalation of the behavior, reinforcing alternative behaviors to change a pet's response to a

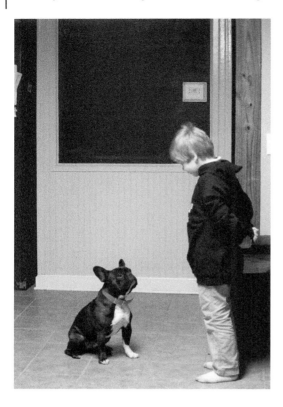

Figure 12.12 Even younger children can be active participants in training dogs and cats in the home. *Source:* Christine Calder (book author).

trigger, desensitization, and counterconditioning. Implementing these techniques can help pets become more comfortable with the triggers that cause them distress.

Conclusion

Veterinarians play an important role in educating parents about living with children and pets, including dogs and cats. By highlighting the potential for dog and cat bites and emphasizing the importance of responsible pet ownership, we can help create a safer and more enjoyable environment for both children and their pets. Educating parents about triggers for bites, the role of socialization and training, and the selection of the right pet can contribute to a harmonious relationship between families and their four-legged members. Together, veterinarians and parents can work toward fostering a bond built on trust, respect, and understanding, ensuring the wellbeing of all family members, both human and animal.

References

Aldridge, G.L. and Rose, S.E. (2019). Young children's interpretation of dogs' emotions and their intentions to approach happy, angry, and frightened dogs. *Antrozoos* 32: 361–374.

Amat, M., Le Brech, S., and Manteca, X. (2024). The relationship between aggression and physical disease in dogs. *Veterinary Clinics of North America, Small Animal Practice* 54 (1): 43–53.

Beaver, B.V. (2003). *Feline Behavior*. Philadelphia, PA: Elsevier Health Sciences.

Bergman, L. and Gaskins, L. (2008). Expanding families: preparing for and introducing dogs and cats to infants, children, and new pets. *Veterinary Clinics of North America, Small Animal Practice* 38 (5): 1043–1063.

Kerns, K.A., Dulmen, M.H., Kochendorfer, L.B. et al. (2023). Assessing children's relationships with pet dogs: a multi-method approach. *Social Development* 32 (1): 98–116.

Levine, E.D. (2023). Pets and the family dynamic. In: *Behavior Problems of the Dog and Cat* (ed. L. Ackerman and G. Landsberg), 49. St. Louis, MO: Elsevier Health Sciences.

Love, M. and Overall, K.L. (2001). How anticipating relationships between dogs and children can help prevent disasters. *Journal of the American Veterinary Medical Association* 219 (4): 446–453.

Mariti, C., Gazzano, A., Moore, J.L. et al. (2012). Perception of dogs' stress by their owners. *Journal of Veterinary Behavior* 7: 213–219.

Meints, K., Syrnyk, C., and De Keuster, T. (2010). Why do children get bitten in the face? *Injury Prevention* 16 (Suppl. 1): A172–A173.

Reisner, I.R. (2003). Differential diagnosis and management of human-directed aggression in dogs. *Veterinary Clinics of North America, Small Animal Practice* 33 (2): 303–320.

Reisner, I.R., Nance, M.L., Zeller, J.S. et al. (2011). Behavioural characteristics associated with dog bites to children presenting to an urban trauma centre. *Injury Prevention* 17 (5): 348–353.

Reisner, I.R., Shofer, F.S., and Nance, M.L. (2007). Behavioral assessment of child-directed canine aggression. *Injury Prevention* 13 (5): 348.

Tuckel, P.S. and Milczarski, W. (2020). The changing epidemiology of dog bite injuries in the United States, 2005–2018. *Injury Epidemiology* 7 (1): 57.

Index

Note: *Italic* page numbers refer to *figure* and **Bold** page numbers reference to **tables**.